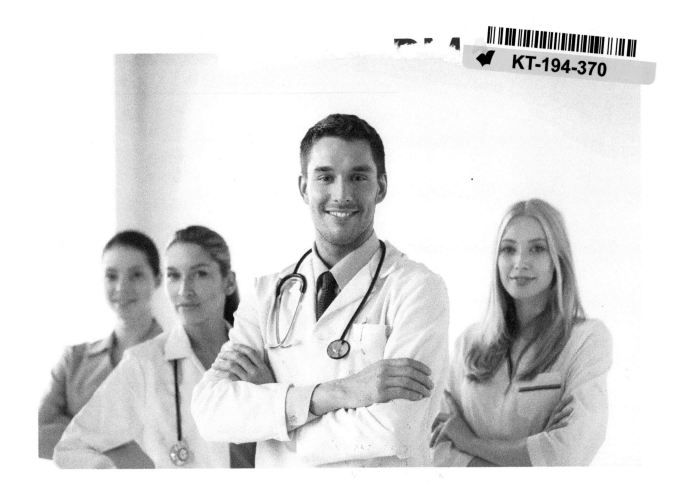

BMJ Clinical Review:

General Practice

Edited by
Babita Jyoti & Ahmed Hamad

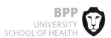

First edition August 2015

ISBN 9781 4727 3931 5
eISBN 9781 4727 4406 7
eISBN 9781 4727 4414 2

British Library Cataloguing-in-Publication Data
A catalogue record for this book is available
from the British Library

Published by
BPP Learning Media Ltd
BPP House, Aldine Place
London W12 8AA

www.bpp.com/health

Printed in the United Kingdom by
Ashford Colour Press Ltd

Unit 600, Fareham Reach,
Fareham Road,
Gosport, Hampshire,
PO13 0FW

Your learning materials, published by BPP Learning
Media Ltd, are printed on paper sourced from
sustainable, managed forests.

The content of this publication contains articles from The
BMJ which have been selected, collated and published
by BPP Learning Media under a licence.

The contents of this book are intended as a guide
and not professional advice. Although every effort
has been made to ensure that the contents of this
book are correct at the time of going to press, BPP
Learning Media, the Editor and the Author make no
warranty that the information in this book is accurate
or complete and accept no liability for any loss or
damage suffered by any person acting or refraining
from acting as a result of the material in this book.

Every effort has been made to contact the copyright
holders of any material reproduced within this
publication. If any have been inadvertently overlooked,
BPP Learning Media will be pleased to make the
appropriate credits in any subsequent reprints or
editions.

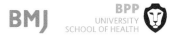

About the publisher

BPP Learning Media is dedicated to supporting aspiring professionals with top quality learning material. BPP Learning Media's commitment to success is shown by our record of quality, innovation and market leadership in paper-based and e-learning materials. BPP Learning Media's study materials are written by professionally-qualified specialists who know from personal experience the importance of top quality materials for success.

About The BMJ

The BMJ (formerly the British Medical Journal) in print has a long history and has been published without interruption since 1840. The BMJ's vision is to be the world's most influential and widely read medical journal. Our mission is to lead the debate on health and to engage, inform, and stimulate doctors, researchers, and other health professionals in ways that will improve outcomes for patients. We aim to help doctors to make better decisions. BMJ, the company, advances healthcare worldwide by sharing knowledge and expertise to improve experiences, outcomes and value.

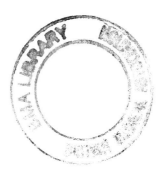

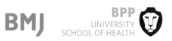

Contents

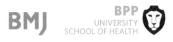

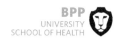

About the editors

Dr Babita Jyoti is a Radiation Oncologist with a special interest in Paediatric Proton Therapy. She graduated in Medicine in India followed by training in UK and obtained MRCP (UK) & FRCR (UK). She trained as a Clinical Oncologist at Clatterbridge Cancer Centre. She is currently working at the University of Florida Health Proton Therapy Institute in Paediatric Proton Therapy. She has been a PBL tutor and an OSCE examiner at Manchester Medical School.

Mr. Ahmed Hamad is a Registrar in General Surgery with special interest in Breast Surgery at Mid Cheshire Hospitals NHS Trust. He graduated in 1992 from Cairo University School of Medicine in Egypt. Initially trained in Surgical Oncology, he received a Masters Degree in Surgery in 1997 from Cairo University. After completing his training in General Surgery, he worked as a Specialist in Surgery in different hospitals in Egypt, Saudi Arabia and Kuwait. He has become a Member of the Royal College of Surgeons of England in 2009 and in 2010, he joined the NHS, initially in General Surgery and is currently developing more experience in Breast Surgery.

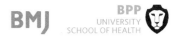

Introduction to General Practice

"Transforming Primary Care is the next step towards safe, personalised, proactive out-of-hospital care for all."

– Jeremy Hunt, Secretary of State, Department of Health, April 2014

As the bedrock of healthcare, General Practice is coming increasingly under focus by various concerned bodies. The maintenance of up-to-date knowledge in this challenging environment remains the key to provision of world-class medical care.

As primary care physicians spearhead the twenty first century's NHS, this book is an attempt to support General Practitioners and Family Physicians in the provision of this service.

Furthermore, doctors in other specialties are also invited to refresh and update their knowledge in topics related to general practice since collaboration with their general practice counterparts is indispensable.

Although systematic reviews and meta-analyses provide more comprehensive details, evidence and statistical analysis of certain topics, clinical reviews are of no less importance as they tend to be more applicable to the local situation than a systematic review, as it may take into account local shortages of equipment or personnel*.

In addition to relevance to day-to-day practice, we believe the fascinating diversity in this book is an advantage.

This compilation in a simple format, with summarised tips and advice can be of great value, especially with the increasing workload and pressure experienced by healthcare professionals.

*Dr Norman Vetter, University of Wales College of Medicine, Cardiff, Wales, UK

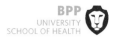

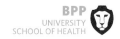

Managing patients with multimorbidity in primary care

Emma Wallace, general practice lecturer[1], Chris Salisbury, professor in primary health care[2], Bruce Guthrie, professor of primary care medicine[3], Cliona Lewis, general practice lecturer[1], Tom Fahey, professor of general practice[1], Susan M Smith, associate professor of general practice[1]

[1]HRB Centre for Primary Care Research, Royal College of Surgeons in Ireland Medical School, Dublin 2, Ireland

[2]Centre for Academic Primary Care, University of Bristol, Bristol, UK

[3]Quality, Safety and Informatics Research Group, University of Dundee, Dundee, UK

Correspondence to: E Wallace emmawallace@rcsi.ie

Cite this as: *BMJ* 2015;350:h176

DOI: 10.1136/bmj.h176

http://www.bmj.com/content/350/bmj.h176

Multimorbidity, commonly defined as the presence of two or more chronic medical conditions in an individual,[1] is associated with decreased quality of life, functional decline, and increased healthcare utilisation, including emergency admissions, particularly with higher numbers of coexisting conditions.[2 3 4 5 6] The management of multimorbidity with drugs is often complex, resulting in polypharmacy with its attendant risks.[7 8 9] Patients with multimorbidity have a high treatment burden in terms of understanding and self managing the conditions, attending multiple appointments, and managing complex drug regimens.[10] Qualitative research highlights the "endless struggle" patients experience in trying to manage their conditions well.[11] Psychological distress is common: in an Australian survey of 7620 patients in primary care, 23% of those with one chronic condition reported depression compared with 40% of those with five or more conditions.[12]

Multimorbidity presents many challenges, which may at times seem overwhelming. This review provides evidence based practice points that are feasible to implement in general practice and offers guidance for general practitioners in organising care delivery.

How common is it?
Recent estimates suggest that one in six patients in the United Kingdom has more than one of the conditions outlined in the Quality and Outcomes Framework, and these patients account for approximately one third of all consultations in general practice.[13] A recent, large scale Scottish study reported that approximately 65% of those aged more than 65 years and almost 82% of those aged 85 years or more had two or more chronic conditions.[14] Although prevalence increases substantially with age, in absolute terms multimorbidity is more prevalent in those aged 65 years or less and is much more common in socioeconomically deprived areas.[14] A recent systematic review included 11 studies relating to patterns of multimorbidity. The most common pair of conditions across studies was osteoarthritis and a cardiometabolic condition, such as hypertension, diabetes, obesity, or ischaemic heart disease.[15] This review also attempted to identify meaningful groups of conditions. In four studies that used factor analysis to identify common factors across combinations of conditions, three were consistent across studies; a cardiometabolic condition factor, a mental health condition factor (most commonly depression or anxiety), and a painful condition factor.[15]

What is the impact of multimorbidity?
Box 1 summarises some commonly encountered problems for patients with multimorbidity. In a recent systematic review, general practitioners identified four areas where they experience difficulties in caring for patients with multimorbidity: disorganisation and fragmentation of care, inadequacy of current disease specific guidelines, challenges in delivering patient centred care, and barriers to shared decision making (box 2).[16] General practitioners also highlighted the sense of professional isolation they experience in managing these patients.

What are the challenges of chronic disease management in multimorbidity?
Inadequacy of single disease clinical guidelines
Managing several chronic conditions with the current single disease focus of clinical guidelines and research is a challenge general practitioners face daily. Guidelines rarely deal with comorbidity, in part because they are designed to be based on evidence from randomised controlled trials and because trials routinely exclude older people and people with multiple chronic conditions.[23 24 25] This leads to a situation where every individual recommendation made by a guideline may be rational and evidence based, but the sum of all recommendations in an individual is not. Consider the application of five UK clinical guidelines for a hypothetical 78 year old woman with previous myocardial infarction, type 2 diabetes, osteoarthritis, chronic obstructive pulmonary disease, and depression.[26] She would be prescribed a minimum of 11 drugs, with potentially up to 10 others recommended depending on symptoms and progression of disease, and she would be advised to engage in at least nine lifestyle modifications. In addition to any unplanned appointments, she would be expected to annually attend 8-10 routine primary care appointments for her physical conditions and 8-30 psychosocial intervention appointments for depression and advised to attend multiple appointments for smoking cessation support and pulmonary rehabilitation.[26]

SOURCES AND SELECTION CRITERIA

We based this article on the authors' experience and information from published literature. We carried out searches of PubMed and the Cochrane library using the search terms "co-morbidity" or "comorbidity" or "multimorbid" or "multimorbidity" or "multi-morbidity". No MeSH term exists for multimorbidity. The searches were supplemented by a review of authors' personal archives as well as relevant articles from the International Research Community on Multimorbidity archive at the University of Sherbrooke, Quebec, Canada (http://crmcspl-blog.recherche.usherbrooke.ca/?page_id=248).

THE BOTTOM LINE

- Multimorbidity is commonly defined as the presence of two or more chronic medical conditions in an individual and it can present several challenges in care particularly with higher numbers of coexisting conditions and related polypharmacy
- Practices should actively identify patients with complex multimorbidity and adopt a policy of continuity of care for these patients by assigning them a named doctor
- The adoption of a policy for routine extended consultations should be considered for particularly complex patients or the introduction of occasional "specific extended consultations," allowing protected time to deal with problems encountered in the management of chronic diseases

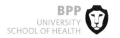

One potential solution is for future developers of guidelines to consider addressing more common clusters of chronic conditions.[27] Although this is an important step, guidelines to cover all combinations of conditions are unlikely and so the value of clinical judgment should be recognised and supported.[28] At times clinical judgment may mean an acceptance that in certain circumstances pursuing stringent disease specific targets is unlikely to be beneficial and may in fact be harmful. Alternatively it may mean prioritising the treatment of depression, which has been shown to impact the ability of patients to manage their other chronic conditions.[29] Policy makers who base performance related payments on disease specific targets need to be aware that such trade-offs based on clinical judgment may represent better patient centred care. Other performance measures that truly capture quality of care for this patient group should be considered.

BOX 1: PROBLEMS COMMONLY EXPERIENCED BY PATIENTS WITH MULTIMORBIDITY

Fragmentation and poor coordination of care
- Results from seeing multiple health professionals in primary and secondary care.[16] [17]

Polypharmacy
- Attendant risk of adverse drug events, potentially inappropriate prescribing, and problems with drug concordance[7] [18]

Treatment burden
- Results from the necessity of learning about and adhering to management plans and lifestyle changes suggested for different conditions and engaging with multiple healthcare professionals[19]

Mental health difficulties
- Anxiety and depression are more common in patients with multimorbidity and can impact on patients' ability to manage other long term conditions[2] [12]
- Patients living in deprived areas are particularly vulnerable to multimorbidity that includes mental health conditions [20]
- Those with cognitive impairment are also particularly vulnerable and may have added difficulties in managing their conditions[21]

Functional difficulties
- Functional difficulties increase with increasing number of conditions and in people aged more than 75 years[5] [6]

Reduced quality of life
- Associated with the number of chronic medical conditions[6]

Increased healthcare utilisation
- Includes an increased risk of emergency admission to hospital[4] [22]

BOX 2: PRACTICE POINTS FOR DEALING WITH CHALLENGES IN CARING FOR PATIENTS WITH MULTIMORBIDITY

Disorganisation and fragmentation of care
- Identify patients as having complex multimorbidity and adopt a practice policy of continuity of care by assigning them a named doctor

Chronic disease management
- Some evidence supports focusing on functional optimisation of patients with multimorbidity and on shared risk factors for several conditions, such as blood pressure and smoking cessation
- In the absence of meaningful clinical guidelines, clinical judgment is especially important in the decision making process

Medicines management
- Plan regular reviews (at least annually) of drugs (explicit prescribing tools for potentially inappropriate prescribing may be useful in reviewing polypharmacy)

Promoting patient centred care
- *Shared decision making*—asking patients at the outset of a consultation "What is bothering you most?" or "What would you like to focus on today?" can help prioritise management to those aspects of care that will have the most impact on patients
- *Self management of multimorbidity*—research to date is mixed about the benefit of self management, but it may be an option for patients expressing an interest in group based support

Short consultation times
- Consider adopting a practice policy of routine extended consultations for particularly complex patients or introducing occasional "specific extended consultations," allowing protected time to deal with problems encountered in the management of chronic diseases
- Ensure practice systems are in place to maximise the value of the general practice consultation for both patient and doctor in reaching management decisions—for example, by seeing the practice nurse ahead of an appointment with the doctor
- Arrange multidisciplinary team involvement, where appropriate

Targeting function not disease
The Cochrane systematic review of community based interventions to improve outcomes for patients with multimorbidity identified only 10 randomised controlled trials.[30] Of these, six involved changes to the organisation of care delivery, usually through case management, and the remaining four interventions were predominantly patient oriented, including support for self management. Although results were mixed, interventions directed towards particular risk factors shared across comorbid conditions or generic functional difficulties experienced by patients seem promising. One randomised controlled trial delivered by occupational therapists and physiotherapists targeted functional difficulties of 319 patients aged 70 years or older with multimorbidity and improved health outcomes including a statistically significant reduction in mortality two years post-intervention. This highlights the potential importance of a multidisciplinary approach in management and a focus on generic outcomes relevant across conditions.[31]

Medicines management
A recent study of 180 815 adults in primary care reported that approximately 20% of patients with two conditions were prescribed four to nine drugs and 1% were prescribed 10 or more drugs.[32] For patients with at least six conditions, these values increased to 48% and 42%, respectively. Polypharmacy is associated with drug related morbidity such as adverse drug events, potentially inappropriate prescribing, and reduced drug adherence.[8] The prevalence of polypharmacy is increasing, owing largely to changes in population demographics and increasing multimorbidity.

A major difficulty for general practitioners is that many prescriptions are initiated by specialists but repeat prescribing occurs in primary care.[8] Without clear communication it can be difficult to judge the rationale of drug treatment. Optimising drug regimens is an important component of care, and to achieve this regular drug reviews are required for patients with multimorbidity.[8] The evidence for pharmacist led drug reviews for complex polypharmacy in the community is mixed.[33] [34] [35] Close collaboration between pharmacists and doctors seems the most sensible approach for this patient group.

Drug reviews should encompass "deprescribing," which involves stopping drugs that are not indicated, have inadequate prognostic benefit, or are causing side effects.[36] Explicit prescribing criteria, such as the Screening Tool of Older Persons' potentially inappropriate Prescriptions (STOPP) and the Screening Tool to Alert doctors to Right Treatment (START), can be useful in maximising the effectiveness of drugs.[37] STOPP consists of 65 indicators of potentially inappropriate prescribing in older populations (aged ≥65 years), which have been validated in both

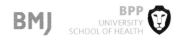

hospital and community settings and have been found to be associated with adverse drug events.[38] [39] START comprises 22 evidence based prescriptions for long term conditions relevant to older people.[40] For younger patients, the Prescribing Optimally in Middle Aged People's Treatments (PROMPT) prescribing criteria have recently been developed. Although yet to be validated, these criteria are important steps in recognising and dealing with treatment burden in those aged less than 65 years.[41]

How can organisation and continuity of care be improved?

Patients with complex multimorbidity often see many different healthcare providers working across multiple sites. Communication between providers is frequently suboptimal, which can impact negatively on patient outcomes.[16] Changes in the delivery of general practice service have reduced the provision of continuity of care.[42] [43] Patients value continuity, with over 80% of older patients (aged ≥75 years) in a recent UK survey reporting a preference for seeing a particular doctor in their general practice.[44] Continuity of care is also associated with improved outcomes, such as the delivery of preventive care and reduced preventable admissions.[45] [46] In a recent US study, higher levels of continuity were associated with lower rates of hospital and emergency department visits, lower complication rates, and less healthcare expenditure.[47] General practitioners are uniquely positioned to provide the necessary relational, informational, and managerial continuity of care, and the importance of this function should not be underestimated.[28] [48] A great strength of primary care is the access it affords patients, and regular planned reviews may be helpful in "ordering the chaos" for this group.[49] Another key aspect for general practitioners is rationalising specialist referrals and considering the components of secondary care that will have most impact on patients' wellbeing.

Clinicians are encouraged to identify patients as having complex multimorbidity and adopt a practice policy of continuity of care for these patients by assigning them a named doctor. Identification is not straightforward: the most common research definition of multimorbidity (the presence of ≥2 conditions) will identify large numbers of patients, many of whom will not have particularly complex needs. Evidence is lacking to guide practice in this area, but groups with multimorbidity and demonstrably higher care needs include patients with "complex" multimorbidity, defined as three or more chronic conditions affecting three or more body systems[50]; patients with comorbid physical conditions and depression[51]; patients prescribed 10 drugs or more[8] [52]; and patients who are housebound or resident in nursing homes. Practices could also consider running specific multimorbidity clinics that address common clusters of conditions, as there is evidence that targeting risk factors common to comorbid conditions such as diabetes, heart disease, and depression is effective,[30] and this would also reduce treatment burden for patients as they would need less frequent visits.[19] Currently it may not be easy for practices to identify such patients and this is a priority for general practice software systems.

What measures can be used to promote patient centred care?

Shared decision making

Shared decision making has been defined as "an approach where clinicians and patients share the best available evidence when faced with the task of making decisions, and where patients are supported to consider options, to achieve informed preferences."[53] Research shows that shared decision making improves patients' knowledge about their condition and treatment options, increases patient satisfaction with care, and improves patient self confidence and self care skills.[54] In the context of multimorbidity it is first important to elicit what matters most to the patient. Asking this at the outset of the consultation allows the rest of the consultation to be utilised most effectively.

A recent model has been proposed to support clinicians in implementing shared clinical decision making in clinical practice.[55] This concerns three key steps: firstly, "choice talk," which refers to the step of making sure that patients know that reasonable options are available, "option talk," which refers to providing more detailed information about options, and "decision talk," which relates to supporting the work of considering preferences and deciding what is best. A range of online shared decision making tools is also available to support this process.[56]

Another tool named the "Adriadne principles" has recently been developed to support decision making specifically during general practice consultations involving multimorbidity.[57] This model places the setting of realistic treatment goals at the centre of the multimorbidity consultation and this is achieved by a thorough interaction assessment of the patient's conditions, treatments, consultation, and context; the prioritisation of health problems that take into account the patient's preferences; and individualised management to determine the best options of care to achieve these goals.

In practice, asking a patient at the outset of a consultation "What is bothering you most?" or "What would you like to focus on today?" can help prioritise the management of aspects of care that will have the most impact for patients. Once patient priorities are identified, using available shared decision making tools may help support the process.

Self management in patients with multimorbidity

Some evidence supports lay led self management education programmes for single chronic diseases in improving certain outcomes, such as self efficacy and self rated health.[58] The evidence for such an approach with multimorbidity is, however, mixed.[30] Patient preference should guide the utilisation of lay led self management groups.

The evaluation of the UK expert patient programme showed improved self efficacy and energy levels at six month follow-up but no reduction in healthcare utilisation.[59] In a recent randomised controlled trial in the United Kingdom general practice staff were trained about available resources, including an assessment tool for the support needs of patients, guidebooks on self management, and a web based directory of local resources. At 12 month follow-up there were no reported improvements in shared decision making, self efficacy, or generic health related quality of life.[60]

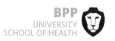

QUESTIONS FOR FUTURE RESEARCH

- What is the role of complex interventions to improve function in multimorbidity?
- The UK National Institute for Health Research is examining a complex intervention for multimorbidity patients in general practice (http://public.ukcrn.org.uk/search/StudyDetail.aspx?StudyID=16067). The intervention is a coordinated three dimensional review of multimorbidity and includes the assessment of quality of life, patients' priorities and disease measures, the identification and treatment of depression, and measures relating to simplification of drug regimens and adherence
- What is the role of integrated chronic disease prevention and management in patients with multimorbidity?
- In Canada, the Patient-Centred Innovations for Persons with Multimorbidity (PACE) team is developing and testing interventions of integrated chronic disease prevention and management for patients with multimorbidity in primary care (http://crmcspl-blog.recherche.usherbrooke.ca/?p=716)
- Will extended general practice consultation times improve outcomes for people with multimorbidity?
- The ongoing Scottish CARE PLUS randomised controlled trial, which is examining a general practice system-wide approach, including extended general practitioner consultation time, to improve outcomes for people with multimorbidity living in deprived areas will add to the limited evidence base in this area

ADDITIONAL EDUCATIONAL RESOURCES

Resources for healthcare professionals

- Medicines optimisation: helping patients to make the most of medicines. Good practice guidance for healthcare professionals in England (www.rpharms.com/promoting-pharmacy-pdfs/helping-patients-make-the-most-of-their-medicines.pdf)—This guide, developed as a collaboration between patients and practitioners, describes four principles of medicines optimisation
- American Geriatrics Society Expert Panel on the Care of Older Adults with Multimorbidity. Guiding principles for the care of older adults with multimorbidity: an approach for clinicians. *J Am Geriatr Soc* 2012;60:E1-25 (www.guideline.gov/content.aspx?id=39322)—This guide summarises the evidence for clinicians in managing older patients with multimorbidity across five domains; patient preferences, interpreting the evidence, prognosis, clinical feasibility, and optimising therapies and care plans

Resources for patients

- US Department of Health & Human Services. Agency for Healthcare Research and Quality. Questions to ask your doctor (www.ahrq.gov/patients-consumers/patient-involvement/ask-your-doctor/index.html)—Tips for patients to get the most out of their doctor appointments
- Ottawa Health Research Institute. Ottawa personal decision guide (http://decisionaid.ohri.ca/decguide.html)—A resource to support patients in making decisions about their health

What can be achieved in a 10 minute consultation?

Internationally, general practitioners have highlighted lack of time as a barrier to providing care for patients with multimorbidity.[61 62] Some evidence suggests that longer consultations result in more preventive health advice, less prescribing, and increased patient satisfaction rates.[63] However this review was limited by the inclusion of only five older studies with short term follow-up. In deprived areas, increased consultation times have been shown to increase patient enablement and reduce general practitioners' stress.[64]

With demand for general practitioner services increasing, it is difficult to schedule extra consultation time for patients with multimorbidity. Practices may decide to flag certain patients with complex needs to allocate longer routine consultation times, or arrange "specific extended consultations" to allow protected time on occasion to review chronic disease management and drugs. Having robust practice systems in place to ensure appropriate monitoring with the practice nurse before the appointment with a general practitioner would facilitate the most efficient and effective use of both patients' and doctors' time. Practice nurses or other multidisciplinary team members can contribute in specific ways, including undertaking target assessment of chronic disease and psychological or functional capacity assessments that can support doctor and patient shared decision making. Multidisciplinary input is an essential component of care for these patients, and referrals to relevant disciplines should be arranged when indicated and available.

Contributors: All authors contributed to the development, content, and practice points presented in this article, and all agreed on the final version. EW wrote the manuscript. SS is the guarantor.

Funding: EW is funded by the Health Research Board (HRB) of Ireland under the research training fellowship for healthcare professionals award (HPF/2012/20). This review was conducted as part of the HRB PhD scholars programme in health services research (PHD/2007/16) at the HRB Centre for Primary Care Research (HRC/2007/1).

Competing interests: We have read and understood the BMJ policy on declaration of interests and declare that: BG is the chair of the National Institute of Health and Care Excellence Guideline Development Group for "Multimorbidity: clinical assessment and management." The views and opinions expressed are those of the authors, and do not represent NICE. CS has received fees as an external speaker on the topic of multimorbidity for the Ministry of Health in Singapore and has a role in the Royal College of General Practitioners in the United Kingdom, which includes consideration of care for multimorbidity.

Provenance and peer review: Not commissioned; externally peer reviewed.

1 Fortin M, Bravo G, Hudon C, Vanasse A, Lapointe L. Prevalence of multimorbidity among adults seen in family practice. *Ann Fam Med* 2005;3:223-8.
2 Fortin M, Bravo G, Hudon C, Lapointe L, Dubois MF, Almirall J. Psychological distress and multimorbidity in primary care. *Ann Fam Med* 2006;4:417-22.
3 Fortin M, Lapointe L, Hudon C, Vanasse A, Ntetu AL, Maltais D. Multimorbidity and quality of life in primary care: a systematic review. *Health Qual Life Outcomes* 2004;2:51.
4 Condelius A, Edberg AK, Jakobsson U, Hallberg IR. Hospital admissions among people 65+ related to multimorbidity, municipal and outpatient care. *Arch Gerontol Geriatr* 2008;46:41-55.
5 Bayliss EA, Bayliss MS, Ware JE Jr, Steiner JF. Predicting declines in physical function in persons with multiple chronic medical conditions: what we can learn from the medical problem list. *Health Qual Life Outcomes* 2004;2:47.
6 Marengoni A, Angleman S, Melis R, Mangialasche F, Karp A, Garmen A, et al. Aging with multimorbidity: a systematic review of the literature. *Ageing Res Rev* 2011;10:430-9.
7 Gandhi TK, Weingart SN, Borus J, Seger AC, Peterson J, Burdick E, et al. Adverse drug events in ambulatory care. *N Engl J Med* 2003;348:1556-64.
8 Duerden M, Avery T, Payne R. Polypharmacy and medicines optimisation. King's Fund, 2013.
9 Guthrie B, McCowan C, Davey P, Simpson CR, Dreischulte T, Barnett K. High risk prescribing in primary care patients particularly vulnerable to adverse drug events: cross sectional population database analysis in Scottish general practice. *BMJ* 2011;342:d3514.
10 Gallacher K, May CR, Montori VM, Mair FS. Understanding patients' experiences of treatment burden in chronic heart failure using normalization process theory. *Ann Fam Med* 2011;9:235-43.
11 O'Brien R, Wyke S, Guthrie B, Watt G, Mercer S. An 'endless struggle': a qualitative study of general practitioners' and practice nurses' experiences of managing multimorbidity in socio-economically deprived areas of Scotland. *Chronic Illn* 2011;7:45-59.

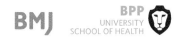

12 Gunn JM, Ayton DR, Densley K, Pallant JF, Chondros P, Herrman HE, et al. The association between chronic illness, multimorbidity and depressive symptoms in an Australian primary care cohort. *Soc Psychiatry Psychiatr Epidemiol* 2012;47:175-84.

13 Salisbury C, Johnson L, Purdy S, Valderas JM, Montgomery AA. Epidemiology and impact of multimorbidity in primary care: a retrospective cohort study. *Br J Gen Pract* 2011;61:e12-21.

14 Barnett K, Mercer S, Norbury M, Watt G, Wyke S, Guthrie B. The epidemiology of multimorbidity in a large cross-sectional dataset: implications for health care, research and medical education. *Lancet* 2012;380:37-43.

15 Violan C, Foguet-Boreu Q, Flores-Mateo G, Salisbury C, Blom J, Freitag M, et al. Prevalence, determinants and patterns of multimorbidity in primary care: a systematic review of observational studies. *PLoS One* 2014, 9:e102149.

16 Sinnott C, Mc Hugh S, Browne J, Bradley C. GPs' perspectives on the management of patients with multimorbidity: systematic review and synthesis of qualitative research. *BMJ Open* 2013;3:e003610.

17 Bodenheimer T. Coordinating care—a perilous journey through the health care system. *N Engl J Med* 2008;358:1064-71.

18 Tinetti ME, Bogardus ST Jr, Agostini JV. Potential pitfalls of disease-specific guidelines for patients with multiple conditions. *N Engl J Med* 2004;351:2870-4.

19 May C, Montori VM, Mair FS. We need minimally disruptive medicine. *BMJ* 2009;339.

20 Mercer SW, Watt GC. The inverse care law: clinical primary care encounters in deprived and affluent areas of Scotland. *Ann Fam Med* 2007;5:503-10.

21 Drewes YM, den Elzen WP, Mooijaart SP, de Craen AJ, Assendelft WJ, Gussekloo J. The effect of cognitive impairment on the predictive value of multimorbidity for the increase in disability in the oldest old: the Leiden 85-plus Study. *Age Ageing* 2011;40:352-7.

22 Glynn LG, Valderas JM, Healy P, Burke E, Newell J, Gillespie P, et al. The prevalence of multimorbidity in primary care and its effect on health care utilization and cost. *Fam Pract* 2011;28:516-23.

23 Wyatt KD, Stuart LM, Brito JP, Carranza Leon B, Domecq JP, Prutsky GJ, et al. Out of context: clinical practice guidelines and patients with multiple chronic conditions: a systematic review. *Med Care* 2014;52(Suppl 3):S92-S100.

24 Zulman DM, Sussman JB, Chen X, Cigolle CT, Blaum CS, Hayward RA. Examining the evidence: a systematic review of the inclusion and analysis of older adults in randomized controlled trials. *J Gen Intern Med* 2011;26:783-90.

25 Fortin M, Dionne J, Pinho G, Gignac J, Almirall J, Lapointe L. Randomized controlled trials: do they have external validity for patients with multiple comorbidities? *Ann Fam Med* 2006;4:104-8.

26 Hughes LD, McMurdo ME, Guthrie B. Guidelines for people not for diseases: the challenges of applying UK clinical guidelines to people with multimorbidity. *Age Ageing* 2013;42:62-9.

27 National Institute for Health and Care Excellence. Depression in adults with a chronic physical health problem: treatment and management. (Clinical guideline 91.) 2009. www.nice.org.uk/guidance/cg91.

28 Roland M, Paddison C. Better management of patients with multimorbidity. *BMJ* 2013;346:f2510.

29 Lin EH, Katon W, Von Korff M, Tang L, Williams JW Jr, Kroenke K, et al. Effect of improving depression care on pain and functional outcomes among older adults with arthritis: a randomized controlled trial. *JAMA* 2003;290:2428-9.

30 Smith S, Soubhi H, Fortin M, Hudon C, O'Dowd T. Interventions for improving outcomes in patients with multimorbidity in primary care and community settings. *Cochrane Database Syst Rev* 2012;4:CD006560.

31 Gitlin LN, Hauck WW, Dennis MP, Winter L, Hodgson N, Schinfeld S. Long-term effect on mortality of a home intervention that reduces functional difficulties in older adults: results from a randomized trial. *J Am Geriatr Soc* 2009;57:476-81.

32 Payne RA, Avery AJ, Duerden M, Saunders CL, Simpson CR, Abel GA. Prevalence of polypharmacy in a Scottish primary care population. *Eur J Clin Pharmacol* 2014;70:575-81.

33 Avery AJ, Rodgers S, Cantrill JA, Armstrong S, Cresswell K, Eden M, et al. A pharmacist-led information technology intervention for medication errors (PINCER): a multicentre, cluster randomised, controlled trial and cost-effectiveness analysis. *Lancet* 2012;379:1310-9.

34 Holland R, Desborough J, Goodyer L, Hall S, Wright D, Loke YK. Does pharmacist-led medication review help to reduce hospital admissions and deaths in older people? A systematic review and meta-analysis. *Br J Clin Pharmacol* 2008;65:303-16.

35 Holland R, Lenaghan E, Harvey I, Smith R, Shepstone L, Lipp A, et al. Does home based medication review keep older people out of hospital? The HOMER randomised controlled trial. *BMJ* 2005;330:293.

36 Steinman MA, Hanlon JT. Managing medications in clinically complex elders: "there's got to be a happy medium". *JAMA* 2010;304:1592-601.

37 Gallagher P, Baeyens J-P, Topinkova E, Madlova P, Cherubini A, Gasperini B, et al. Inter-rater reliability of STOPP (Screening Tool of Older Persons' Prescriptions) and START (Screening Tool to Alert doctors to Right Treatment) criteria amongst physicians in six European countries. *Age Ageing* 2009;38:603-6.

38 Hamilton H, Gallagher P, Ryan C, Byrne S, O'Mahony D. Potentially inappropriate medications defined by STOPP criteria and the risk of adverse drug events in older hospitalized patients. *Arch Intern Med* 2011;171:1013-9.

39 Cahir C, Bennett K, Teljeur C, Fahey T. Potentially inappropriate prescribing and adverse health outcomes in community dwelling older patients. *Br J Clin Pharmacol* 2013;77:201-10.

40 Gallagher P, Ryan C, Byrne S, Kennedy J, O'Mahony D. STOPP (Screening Tool of Older Person's Prescriptions) and START (Screening Tool to Alert doctors to Right Treatment). Consensus validation. *Int J Clin Pharmacol Ther* 2008;46:72-83.

41 Cooper JA, Ryan C, Smith SM, Wallace E, Bennett K, Cahir C, et al. The development of the PROMPT (PRescribing Optimally in Middle-aged People's Treatments) criteria. *BMC Health Serv Res* 2014;14:484.

42 Campbell SM, Kontopantelis E, Reeves D, Valderas JM, Gaehl E, Small N, et al. Changes in patient experiences of primary care during health service reforms in England between 2003 and 2007. *Ann Fam Med* 2010;8:499-506.

43 Sharma G, Fletcher KE, Zhang D, Kuo YF, Freeman JL, Goodwin JS. Continuity of outpatient and inpatient care by primary care physicians for hospitalized older adults. *JAMA* 2009;301:1671-80.

44 Aboulghate A, Abel G, Elliott MN, Parker RA, Campbell J, Lyratzopoulos G, et al. Do English patients want continuity of care, and do they receive it? *Br J Gen Pract* 2012;62:e567-75.

45 Saultz JW, Lochner J. Interpersonal continuity of care and care outcomes: a critical review. *Ann Fam Med* 2005;3:159-66.

46 Nyweide DJ, Anthony DL, Bynum JP, Strawderman RL, Weeks WB, Casalino LP, et al. Continuity of care and the risk of preventable hospitalization in older adults. *JAMA Intern Med* 2013;173:1879-85.

47 Hussey PS, Schneider EC, Rudin RS, Fox DS, Lai J, Pollack CE. Continuity and the costs of care for chronic disease. *JAMA Intern Med* 2014;174:742-8.

48 Guthrie B, Saultz JW, Freeman GK, Haggerty JL. Continuity of care matters. *BMJ* 2008;337:a867.

49 Haggerty JL. Ordering the chaos for patients with multimorbidity. *BMJ* 2012;345.

50 Harrison C, Britt H, Miller G, Henderson J. Examining different measures of multimorbidity, using a large prospective cross-sectional study in Australian general practice. *BMJ Open* 2014;4:e004694.

51 Multimorbidity clinical assessment and management. NICE in development [GID-CGWAVE0704]. www.nice.org.uk/guidance/indevelopment/gid-cgwave0704/documents.

52 Brilleman SL, Salisbury C. Comparing measures of multimorbidity to predict outcomes in primary care: a cross sectional study. *Fam Pract* 2013;30:172-8.

53 Elwyn G, Laitner S, Coulter A, Walker E, Watson P, Thomson R. Implementing shared decision making in the NHS. *BMJ* 2010;341:c5146.

54 Da Silva D. Helping people share decision making. Health Foundation, 2012.

55 Elwyn G, Frosch D, Thomson R, Joseph-Williams N, Lloyd A, Kinnersley P, et al. Shared decision making: a model for clinical practice. *J Gen Intern Med* 2012;27:1361-7.

56 Tools for shared decision making. NHS England. 2014. www.england.nhs.uk/ourwork/pe/sdm/tools-sdm/.

57 Muth C, van den Akker M, Blom JW, Mallen CD, Rochon J, Schellevis FG, et al. The Ariadne principles: how to handle multimorbidity in primary care consultations. *BMC Med* 2014;12:223.

58 Foster G, Taylor SJ, Eldridge SE, Ramsay J, Griffiths CJ. Self-management education programmes by lay leaders for people with chronic conditions. *Cochrane Database Syst Rev* 2007;4:CD005108.

59 Kennedy A, Reeves D, Bower P, Lee V, Middleton E, Richardson G, et al. The effectiveness and cost effectiveness of a national lay-led self care support programme for patients with long-term conditions: a pragmatic randomised controlled trial. *J Epidemiol Community Health* 2007;61:254-61.

60 Kennedy A, Bower P, Reeves D, Blakeman T, Bowen R, Chew-Graham C, et al. Implementation of self management support for long term conditions in routine primary care settings: cluster randomised controlled trial. *BMJ* 2013;346:f2882.

61 Smith SM, O'Kelly S, O'Dowd T. GPs' and pharmacists' experiences of managing multimorbidity: a 'Pandora's box'. *Br J Gen Pract* 2010;60:285-94.

62 Fiscella K, Epstein RM. So much to do, so little time: care for the socially disadvantaged and the 15-minute visit. *Arch Intern Med* 2008;168:1843-52.

63 Wilson AD, Childs S. Effects of interventions aimed at changing the length of primary care physicians' consultation. *Cochrane Database Syst Rev* 2006;1:CD003540.

64 Mercer SW, Fitzpatrick B, Gourlay G, Vojt G, McConnachie A, Watt GCM. More time for complex consultations in a high-deprivation practice is associated with increased patient enablement. *Brit J Gen Pract* 2007;57:960-6.

Related links

bmj.com/archive

- The prevention and management of rabies (*BMJ* 2015;350:g7827)
- Heparin induced thrombocytopenia (*BMJ* 2014;349:g7566)
- The management of chronic breathlessness in patients with advanced and terminal illness (*BMJ* 2015;350:g7617)
- Ebola virus disease (*BMJ* 2014;349:g7348)
- Managing perineal trauma after childbirth (*BMJ* 2014;349:g6829)

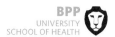

Telehealthcare for long term conditions

Susannah McLean, clinical research fellow[1], Denis Protti, professor of health informatics[2], Aziz Sheikh, professor of primary care research and development[1]

[1]eHealth Research Group, Centre for Population Health Sciences, University of Edinburgh, Edinburgh EH8 9AG, UK

[2]University of Victoria, Victoria, BC, Canada

Correspondence to: A Sheikh
aziz.sheikh@ed.ac.uk

Cite this as: *BMJ* 2011;342:d120

DOI: 10.1136/bmj.d120

http://www.bmj.com/content/342/bmj.d120

Telehealthcare is the provision of personalised healthcare over a distance.[1] It has the three following essential components[2w1]:

- The patient provides data such as a voice recording, video, electrocardiography, or oxygen saturation that gives information about the illness.
- Information is transferred electronically to a healthcare professional at a second location.
- The healthcare professional uses clinical skills and judgment to provide personalised feedback tailored to the individual.

Telehealthcare can be delivered by both synchronous and asynchronous (such as store and forward) technologies (fig 1). For example, telephone and video conferencing enable consultations in real time. An example of asynchronous communication would be storing two weeks' of spirometry results in a batch and forwarding these on to a healthcare provider, who responds by email or telephone.

Telehealthcare is related to, but distinct from telemedicine, where technology is used to share information over a distance between healthcare providers.[2]

Why is interest in telehealthcare increasing?

Healthcare systems globally are facing major challenges such as ageing populations, increasing numbers of people living with long term conditions, patients in remote areas or with limited mobility, and increasing expectations for patient centred healthcare.[w2w3] Telehealthcare offers potential solutions to these challenges (see box 1),[3] but the acceptability and effectiveness, and the safety considerations associated with its adoption need careful consideration.

SOURCES AND SELECTION CRITERIA

We identified systematic reviews and original research studies on telehealthcare and long term conditions. We used searches from our ongoing Cochrane systematic reviews to find randomised controlled trials for telehealthcare interventions for asthma and chronic obstructive pulmonary disease. Search terms were telehealth, tele-health, telemedicine, tele-medicine, internet, computer, web, interactive, telecommunication, telephone, phone, SMS, tele-monitor, telemonitor, telemanagement, tele-management, teleconsultation, tele-consultation, telecare, tele-care, telematic, telepharmacy, and tele-pharmacy. We searched PubMed (1948 to March 2010) using search terms telehealthcare, telehealth, telecare, telemedicine, systematic review or randomised controlled trial, and selected relevant studies from these.

We searched the internet for so called grey literature, including legal and strategic documents, and official government healthcare websites. We also used our private libraries of research papers and completed and ongoing work on telehealthcare.

SUMMARY POINTS

- Telehealthcare is personalised healthcare delivered over a distance; data are transferred from the patient to the professional, who then provides feedback
- In patients with severe long term conditions, such as problematic asthma and diabetes, telehealthcare can reduce hospital admissions without increasing mortality
- Potential pitfalls include user interface problems, technical problems, and safety concerns such as data loss and confidentiality
- Telehealthcare can alter the doctor-patient relationship so try to humanise the interaction
- Consider workflows, to minimise unintended disruptions to normal routines
- Careful assessment of effectiveness, cost effectiveness, and safety considerations is needed before introduction

---

Acceptability to professionals and patients

Professionals

Telehealthcare can greatly alter the healthcare encounter. In the United States there was some resistance to adopting telehealthcare until state insurers (such as Medicare) recognised it as a reimbursable medical act. A similar reimbursement related barrier has been seen in parts of the European Union.[w4] In fact, in countries with insurance based health systems, collocation of patient and practitioner was sometimes a requirement for reimbursement.[w4] However, the European Commission now regards telehealthcare as a legitimate medical act, drawing attention to the points listed in box 2.[w5]

Patients

Patients' attitudes to telehealthcare have been extensively studied. A 2007 systematic review of patients with a range of long term conditions found that most patients saw telehealthcare as a positive development.[3] Telehealthcare improves access to care, which increases patients' understanding of their condition and can lead to a greater sense of empowerment and willingness to engage with self care.[3 4]

Telehealthcare is not just suited to the technologically literate. A 1998 study of people with little experience of technology using a new asthma telehealthcare system daily for three weeks found that 88% of them felt safer while being monitored by the system; 94% were interested in using the same system in the future.[5]

Descriptive studies provide only limited data on patients' and carers' perspectives on these new models of care. A 2000 systematic review found that despite a large body of literature on patients' satisfaction with telehealthcare, the research lacked depth. The authors urged caution when interpreting the largely positive findings reported in many studies.[6]

Qualitative approaches can generate a more rounded, nuanced appreciation of patients' experiences and expectations. A 2009 study convened a so called citizens' panel to help understand patients' perspectives on telehealthcare.[7] The panel discussions generated important insights. Although the policy discourse on telehealthcare is full of positive references to a shift in the patient's role from passive to active—becoming "informed," "expert," and "self managing"—the panel thought that existing power relationships were often reinforced, with passive patients being monitored by a now distant medical professional. They also concluded that telehealthcare could not take the place of face to face interaction and that a combination of face to face and telehealthcare consultations was optimal. The panel emphasised the need for increased discourse with the public regarding the boundaries for these technologies, because of a concern that telehealthcare could take attention away from personal care needs. However, the panel recognised that such interventions could potentially make a valuable contribution to modern healthcare provision so long as the patient still had the option of face to face care, if required.

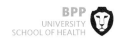

BMJ   BPP
UNIVERSITY
SCHOOL OF HEALTH

BOX 1 HOW MIGHT TELEHEALTHCARE SYSTEMS BENEFIT PATIENTS?[3]

- Allows patients to be cared for in their preferred location, typically at home
- Provides patient education and support for preventive care in, for example, those trying to lose weight
- Videophone or web based clinical consultations, such as those for asthma or chronic obstructive pulmonary disease, or diabetes annual reviews, can replace routine visits such as face to face annual reviews
- Improves adherence to drugs and other treatments
- Proactive education and support, such as via web forums, may facilitate self management and help with coping (for example, in people with chronic back pain) or prevent exacerbations of conditions such as asthma
- Use of monitoring techniques can enable earlier detection of disease exacerbations, thereby facilitating timely management and support
- Allows greater opportunities for continuity of care with the same clinician and more frequent assessments
- Reduces costs to patients by obviating the need for time off school or work and for travel

BOX 2 SUMMARY OF THE EUROPEAN ECONOMIC AND SOCIAL COMMITTEE'S OPINION ON TELEHEALTHCARE[W5]

- Telehealthcare cannot and should not replace conventional medicine. It is a complementary technique, limited by the absence of clinical examinations.
- The status of the health practitioner should be clearly indicated
- The patient must benefit from the latest medical knowledge
- The patient must be able to give his or her free consent
- Medical confidentiality must be ensured
- Resulting documents must be secure and recorded in the medical file
- Continuity of care must be ensured
- The medical act must be of at least equivalent quality to a traditional act

BOX 3 AN EXAMPLE OF A SUCCESSFUL TELEHEALTHCARE INTERVENTION IN TYPE 2 DIABETES[13] [14]

The IDEATel trial (http://clinicaltrials.gov/ct2/show/NCT00271739) found that when people monitored their blood glucose and blood pressure with telehealthcare input from specialist nurses and endocrinologists, their glycated haemoglobin decreased, as did their blood pressure, and low density lipoprotein-cholesterol. All cause mortality was similar in the intervention and control arms of the trial. The study was not powered to find differences in mortality from cardiovascular disease. Further analysis showed that improvement in self efficacy in older ethnically diverse patients with diabetes resulted in an improvement in glycaemic control. The telehealthcare intervention had a direct effect and an indirect effect—mediated by a change in self-efficacy—on glycaemic control. Blood pressure and low density lipoprotein-cholesterol improved, but this effect was not mediated by a change in self efficacy.

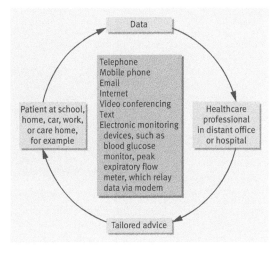

Fig 1 Key elements of telehealthcare

telehealthcare and described being "looked after" at home. They also experienced "freedom" in contrast to being "under surveillance" while in hospital.

Age and cognitive function are relevant when considering the acceptability of telehealthcare to different populations. Incipient dementia or mental health problems can affect patients' ability to use the technology. As vision, hearing, and dexterity change with age, even mentally competent older people may struggle with the technology. Further, setting up systems that increase the social isolation of this group of vulnerable people is a concern. Each individual's suitability for telehealthcare interventions needs to be carefully considered.[w7w8]

Effectiveness and cost effectiveness

Effectiveness

The effectiveness of telehealthcare is often assumed by industry and policymakers.[8] However, effectiveness depends on the context of the introduction of a specific system. The aim of introducing telehealthcare must be clear from the start.[9] Such aims might be to widen access, improve clinical end points, aid the early detection of disease exacerbations, reduce the risk of hospital admissions, reduce mortality, or reduce the degree of dependency in old age. Agreement on why telehealthcare has been introduced, followed by focused implementation and evaluation to see if the specific need has been dealt with, helps determine when and if aims have been realised.

Several examples of clinically successful telehealthcare projects exist (see box 3 for an example in patients with diabetes). In chronic obstructive pulmonary disease, interventions with a dedicated chronic obstructive pulmonary disease case manager have reduced the numbers of exacerbations and related admissions to hospital.[10] [11] [12] For example, in one trial, case managers provided an enhanced service during working hours, monitoring patients with increased frequency using media including video conferencing (see fig 2). In a 2003 trial of patients with chronic obstructive pulmonary disease related respiratory failure requiring long term oxygen therapy or mechanical ventilation, or both, case managers alternated physical visits to the patient's home with virtual home visits via telehealthcare to conduct reviews and reduce the need for admission.[10]

Our systematic review identified several telehealthcare trials in asthma with similar findings.[15] It found little evidence of improvements in measures of disease specific

Other qualitative studies have identified similar concerns. The subjects in a 2008 study registered some annoyance with their partner or informal carer for being "too concerned" during a period of telehealthcare in the home. Interviews with the partners showed that they felt "forced to take responsibility," despite feeling insecure and worried because they lacked confidence in the technology.[w6] More positively, patients also described feeling secure with

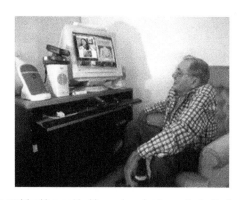

Fig 2 Telehealthcare with video conferencing for a patient with chronic obstructive pulmonary disease

quality of life in most patients with mild or moderate disease, but hospital admissions were reduced in carefully selected patients who had severe asthma or had recently been admitted to hospital (or both) and are consequently at high risk of readmission.[15]

A 2009 systematic review found that telehealthcare for people with diabetes can help improve glycaemic control.[16] The number of admissions to hospital and the length of stay associated with admission were reduced. People with more severe problems benefitted most from the regular tailored feedback.[6] The data suggested that outcomes were more likely to improve if these contacts helped establish and maintain the continuity of a close therapeutic relationship. Patients were likely to become better at self management and increase their self efficacy so that, over time, they depended less on feedback.[13 16] Conversely, patients with high baseline self efficacy may be less likely to benefit from a management regimen that involves frequent testing and reporting.

Overall, the evidence shows that telehealthcare based initiatives may be particularly helpful for people with accessibility problems, or where a need for careful monitoring and regular feedback has been identified, or both. These newer models of care seem to be less effective in people with relatively mild disease and those in whom control is already considered optimal.[13 15 16 17]

Cost effectiveness

Evidence suggests that only some classes of low cost telehealthcare interventions in certain contexts (such as telephone follow-up to improve attendance or text messaging reminders for monitoring) are likely both to improve outcomes and reduce costs.[18] Overall, the evidence for cost effectiveness is limited. Where studies have been conducted, they were often short term or did not consider the full range of perspectives (those of the patient, healthcare provider, and society). There are only a limited number of more detailed analyses, such as cost-utility analysis or estimations of opportunity costs.[14 w9w10w11]

Safe implementation
Protocols and procedures

Professionals and their respective bodies have been hesitant to introduce telehealthcare partly because of safety concerns. The worry is that specialist emergency care might be precluded for an ill patient managed outside of the hospital environment—as in the case of a patient experiencing an exacerbation of chronic obstructive pulmonary disease, for example—should an unpredictable acute deterioration occur. However, in most cases acute deterioration can be anticipated, and the death rates of

patients managed in the community are, so far as has been demonstrated in trials, not higher than those managed in hospital.[19 20] This concern helps to explain the increased intensity of monitoring when telehealthcare systems are introduced into people's homes. Frequency of contact is often necessary to gain the confidence of both patients and healthcare professionals using the technologies. However, to tackle these concerns more research with full reporting of adverse events is needed.

Access to healthcare professionals via telephone, email, and the internet or other networked interventions may lead to breaches of confidentiality or loss of electronic data (or both), as has been illustrated by several recent high profile cases.[w12w13] Appropriate encryption software should be used and secure data transfer built into systems. Doctors should follow the advice from national professional regulatory bodies on telephone and email consulting, such as the General Medical Council's advice for UK practitioners (box 4).[w14]

More fundamentally, doctors need to consider whether a remote consultation is appropriate in the first place. Most defence unions emphasise that no email, text message, or telephone consultation is a substitute for a standard face to face consultation and examination.[21w15w16] In the UK, general practices are contractually obliged to offer patients a physical examination if considered appropriate.

Workflow changes

The potential for disruption to existing workflow patterns should not be underestimated and is a major factor in the failure of many IT based service redesigns.[22 23] Healthcare professionals need to have protected time and resources to respond to the work generated by telehealthcare. More broadly, a theoretical framework such as normalisation process theory can help identify the barriers to change in this type of situation.[w17]

For example, consider the implications of a trial of a telehealthcare intervention in patients with chronic heart failure in which patients monitored their own weight and blood pressure and recorded their own electrocardiogram to transmit to a hospital based specialist nurse. The nurse, in consultation with a cardiologist, provided tailored advice to the patient over the telephone on managing the illness.[w18]

Several important workflow points were highlighted:
- The role and responsibility of the nurse has changed; nurses are increasingly involved in decision making, which requires further training.
- The general practitioner is somewhat marginalised, because patients with increasingly complex management regimens default to a trusted specialist relationship.
- There is a need to maintain accountability; this can be achieved by protocols and guidelines for case managers, describing how much they can undertake themselves and when to involve a senior medical practitioner, though such protocols and guidelines may prove burdensome.

Training of staff and patients

The integration of telehealthcare into health service workflows often means adding to the roles and responsibilities of healthcare professionals. This was the case in the Columba telehealthcare initiative,[w19] where extensive protected training opportunities had to be provided for staff. During these sessions, staff learnt how to use the technologies and in turn contributed ideas for the adaptation and integration of the technologies into existing workflow patterns.

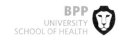

Patients may also need training. Ideally, to help establish trust and confidence, the first interaction of a telehealthcare system should be face to face. Training should be tailored to patients' baseline familiarity with technology. Once confident with using the technology, patients can continue to operate it independently (see fig 3).

Looking ahead, future research should seek to understand how best to humanise the remote relationship and find ways of maintaining and, if possible, enhancing the all important therapeutic relationship.[w5]

Conclusions

Telehealthcare based interventions are proliferating rapidly and are underpinned by variable quality of evidence. To implement telehealthcare effectively and safely, the aims of introducing telehealthcare to a care process must be clear. Such aims might be to improve access, increase satisfaction, avoid emergency admissions, or reduce costs. Less complex interventions, such as those based on the telephone, have a more robust evidence base, but even with such established technologies healthcare providers must remain vigilant to the dangers of compromising safety in the absence of a face to face consultation.[24] Contextual factors such as type of illness, type of technology, age, and ability of the patients to interface with technology must be considered. Robust cost-benefit evaluations must be performed before making these technologies mainstream, to avoid increased cost and widespread disappointments.[25w20]

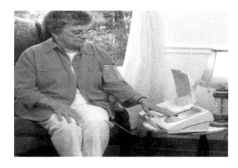

Fig 3 Once confident with using the technology, patients can continue to operate it independently

Contributors: AS conceived the idea for this paper. SMcL drafted the paper, which was commented on by DP and revised by AS. SMcL and AS are guarantors.

Competing interests: All authors have completed the Unified Competing Interest form at www.icmje.org/coi_disclosure.pdf (available on request from the corresponding author) and declare that this work was supported by grants from NHS Connecting for Health Evaluation Programme (NHS CFHEP 001) and an Academic Fellowship for General Practice funded by NHS Education for Scotland; support was also received from the Chief Scientist's Office of the Scottish Government; the authors have no financial relationships with any organisations that might have an interest in the submitted work in the previous three years; no other relationships or activities that could appear to have influenced the submitted work.

Provenance and peer review: Commissioned; externally peer reviewed.

1 McLean S, Sheikh A. Does telehealthcare offer a patient-centred way forward for the community-based management of long-term respiratory disease? *Prim Care Resp J* 2009;18:125-6.
2 Sood S, Mbarika V, Jugoo S, Dookhy R, Doarn CR, Prakash N, et al. What is telemedicine? A collection of 104 peer-reviewed perspectives and theoretical underpinnings. *Telemed J E Health* 2007;13:573-90.
3 Finkelstein J, Friedman RH. Potential role of telecommunication technologies in the management of chronic health conditions. *Dis Manage Health Outcome* 2000;8:57-63.
4 Pare G, Jaana M, Sicotte C. Systematic review of home telemonitoring for chronic diseases: the evidence base. *J Am Med Inform Assoc* 2007;14:269-77.
5 Finkelstein J, Hripcsak G, Cabrera MR. Patients' acceptance of Internet-based home asthma telemonitoring. *Proc AMIA Symp* 1998:336-40.
6 Mair F, Whitten P. Systematic review of studies of patient satisfaction with telemedicine. *BMJ* 2000;320:1517-20.
7 Mort M, Finch T, May C. Making and unmaking telepatients: identity and governance in new health technologies. *Sci Technol Hum Val* 2009;34:9-33.
8 McKinstry B, Pinnock H, Sheikh A. Telemedicine for management of patients with COPD? *Lancet* 2009;374:672-3.
9 Catwell L, Sheikh A. Evaluating eHealth interventions: the need for continuous systemic evaluation. *PLoS Med* 2009;6:e1000126.
10 Bourbeau J, Julien M, Maltais F, Rouleau M, Beaupre A, Begin R, et al. Reduction of hospital utilization in patients with chronic obstructive pulmonary disease: a disease-specific self-management intervention. *Arch Intern Med* 2003;163:585-91.
11 De Toledo P, Jimenez S, del Pozo F, Roca J, Alonso A, Hernandez C. Telemedicine experience for chronic care in COPD. *IEEE Trans Inf Technol Biomed* 2006;10:567-73.
12 Vitacca M, Bianchi L, Guerra A, Fracchia C, Spanevello A, Balbi B, et al. Tele-assistance in chronic respiratory failure patients: a randomised clinical trial. *Eur Respir J* 2009;33:411-8.
13 Trief P, Teresi JA, Eimicke JP, Shea S, Weinstock RS. Improvement in diabetes self-efficacy and glycaemic control using telemedicine in a sample of older ethnically diverse individuals who have diabetes: the IDEATel project. *Age Ageing* 2009;38:219-25.
14 Moreno L, Dale SB, Chen AY, Magee CA. Costs to Medicare of the Informatics for Diabetes Education and Telemedicine (IDEATel) home telemedicine demonstration: findings from an independent evaluation. *Diabetes Care* 2009;32:1202-4.
15 McLean S, Chandler D, Nurmatov U, Liu J, Pagliari C, Car J, et al. Telehealthcare for asthma. *Cochrane Database Syst Rev* 2010;10:CD007717.
16 Polisena J, Tran K, Cimon K, Hutton B, McGill S, Palmer K. Home telehealth for diabetes management: a systematic review and meta-analysis. *Diabetes Obes Metab* 2009;11:913-30.
17 Polisena J, Tran K, Cimon K, Hutton B, McGill S, Palmer K, et al. Home telemonitoring for congestive heart failure a systematic review and meta-analysis. *J Telemed Telecare* 2010;16:68-76.

BOX 4 REMOTE PRESCRIBING GUIDANCE FROM THE UK GENERAL MEDICAL COUNCIL[w14]

In all circumstances, ensure that you have an appropriate dialogue with the patient to:

- Establish the patient's history and current medical conditions and current or recent use of drugs, including non-prescription ones
- Carry out an adequate assessment of the patient's condition
- Identify the likely cause of the patient's condition
- Ensure that there is sufficient justification to prescribe the drugs or treatment proposed. Where appropriate discuss other treatment options with the patient
- Ensure that the treatment or drug(s) are not contraindicated for the patient
- Make a clear, accurate, and legible record of all drugs prescribed

---

ADDITIONAL EDUCATIONAL RESOURCES

- McLean S, Chandler D, Nurmatov U, Liu J, Pagliari C, Car J, et al. Telehealthcare for asthma. *Cochrane Database Syst Rev* 2010;10:CD007717.
- Bunn F, Byrne G, Kendall S. Telephone consultation and triage: effects on health care use and patient satisfaction. *Cochrane Database Syst Rev* 2004;4:CD004180.
- Currell R, Urquhart C, Wainwright P, Lewis R. Telemedicine versus face to face patient care: effects on professional practice and health care outcomes. *Cochrane Database Syst Rev* 2000;2:CD002098.
- Inglis SC, Clark RA, McAlister FA, Ball J, Lewinter C, Cullington D, et al. Structured telephone support or telemonitoring programmes for patients with chronic heart failure. *Cochrane Database Syst Rev* 2010;8:CD007228.
- Martin S, Kelly G, Kernohan WG, McCreight B, Nugent C. Smart home technologies for health and social care support. *Cochrane Database Syst Rev* 2008;4:CD006412.
- Mistiaen P, Poot E. Telephone follow-up, initiated by a hospital-based health professional, for postdischarge problems in patients discharged from hospital to home. *Cochrane Database Syst Rev* 2006;4:CD004510.
- Murray E, Burns J, See TS, Lai R, Nazareth I. Interactive Health Communication Applications for people with chronic disease. *Cochrane Database Syst Rev* 2005;4:CD004274.
- Eysenbach G, Powell J, Englesakis M, Rizo C, Stern A. Health related virtual communities and electronic support groups: systematic review of the effects of online peer to peer interactions. *BMJ* 2004;328:1166.

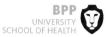

18 Pinnock H, Adlem L, Gaskin S, Harris J, Snellgrove C, Sheikh A. Accessibility, clinical effectiveness, and practice costs of providing a telephone option for routine asthma reviews: phase IV controlled implementation study. *Br J Gen Pract* 2007;57:714-22.

19 Casas A, Troosters T, Garcia-Aymerich J, Roca J, Hernandez C, Alonso A, et al. Integrated care prevents hospitalisations for exacerbations in COPD patients. *Eur Respir J* 2006;28:123-30.

20 Gruffydd-Jones K, Hollinghurst S, Ward S, Taylor G. Targeted routine asthma care in general practice using telephone triage. *Br J Gen Prac* 2005;55:918-23.

21 Car J, Sheikh A. Telephone consultations. *BMJ* 2003;326:966-9.

22 Cresswell K, Sheikh A. The NHS Care Record Service (NHS CRS): recommendations from the literature on successful implementation and adoption. *Inform Prim Care* 2009;17:153-60.

23 Pinnock H, Hanley J, Lewis S, MacNee W, Pagliari C, Van der Pol M, et al. The impact of a telemetric chronic obstructive pulmonary disease monitoring service: randomised controlled trial with economic evaluation and nested qualitative study. *Prim Care Respir J* 2009;18:233-5.

24 McKinstry B, Hammersley V, Burton C, Pinnock H, Elton R, Dowell J, et al. The quality, safety and content of telephone and face-to-face consultations: a comparative study. *Qual Saf Health Care* 2010;19:298-303.

25 Boddy D, King G, Clark JS, Heaney D, Mair F. The influence of context and process when implementing e-health. *BMC Med Inform Decis Mak* 2009;9:9.

Related links

bmj.com/archive

- The assessment and management of rectal prolapse, rectal intussusceptoin, rectocoele, and enterocoele in adults (2011;342:c7099)
- Preventing exacerbations in chronic obstructive pulmonary disease (2011;342:c7207)
- Islet transplantation in type 1 diabetes (2011;342:d217)
- Diagnosis and management of hereditary haemochromatosis (2011;342:c7251)
- Diagnosis and management of soft tissue sarcoma (2010;341:c7170)

bmj.com/podcasts

- Podcast: Aziz Sheikh discuss telehealthcare for long term conditions

doc2doc

- Discuss telemedicine on doc2doc, BMJ Group's global clinical community

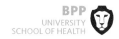

Management of medication overuse headache

Drug and Therapeutics Bulletin

[1]Drug and Therapeutics Bulletin Editorial Office, London WC1H 9JR

dtb@bmjgroup.com

Cite this as: *BMJ* 2010;340:c1305

DOI: 10.1136/bmj.c1305

http://www.bmj.com/content/340/bmj.c1305

Headache is one of the most frequent reasons for medical consultation in both general practice and specialist neurology clinics.[1] Prescribed and over-the-counter medications are taken to alleviate headaches, but may be used incorrectly.[2] In particular, use of some drugs both frequently and regularly can have a paradoxical effect, causing headaches rather than relieving them, and leading to medication overuse headache (MOH).[3] Such overuse is a common cause of frequent headache. Here we review MOH and its management.

About MOH

The *International Classification of Headache Disorders*, 2nd edition states that for a diagnosis of MOH, all of the following criteria must be present:

- headache occurring on 15 or more days per month;
- regular overuse for more than 3 months of one or more acute/symptomatic treatment drugs (ergotamine, triptans, opioids or combined analgesic medications [typically simple analgesics plus opioids or caffeine] on 10 or more days per month; or simple analgesics alone or any combination of ergotamine, triptans and analgesic opioids on 15 or more days per month); and
- development or marked worsening of headache during medication overuse.[4]

The preceding headache problem

Headaches may be primary (eg, migraine, tension-type headache, cluster headache) or secondary (eg, associated with trauma, subarachnoid haemorrhage, intracranial neoplasm, infection or the use or withdrawal of substances such as alcohol or drugs).[3][5] MOH occurs only in patients with a history of primary headache.[6][7] It is most likely to affect patients with migraine and/or tension-type headache,[7][8] but can also arise in association with cluster headache, particularly if there is a personal or family history of migraine or regular headache.[9]

Epidemiology

Studies from various countries suggest that the prevalence of MOH is around 1% of adults and 0.5% of adolescents (aged 13–18 years) in the general population;[10] around 25–64% in those attending tertiary care headache centres;[7][11] and 90% in patients experiencing chronic daily headache.[12] MOH is most prevalent in those aged around 40–50 years and affects about three times more women than men.[8][13]

Which drugs cause MOH and how?

Overuse of any acute or symptomatic headache treatment can cause MOH.[14][15] The mechanism by which overuse of NSAIDs (including aspirin), paracetamol, codeine or dihydrocodeine can cause the condition probably involves changes in neural pain pathways.[1] Combination analgesics containing caffeine and codeine may encourage development of MOH as a consequence of their addictive properties.[16] Ergot is very slowly eliminated from the body and readily accumulates if taken more than twice a week; it is thought that this may lead to chronic activation of central

5-hydroxytryptamine (5-HT) receptors, leading to their downregulation, reducing the activity of central serotonergic pain-reducing systems and thereby increasing headache.[1][17] Triptans do not accumulate but chronic use probably results in a similar downregulation of 5-HT receptors.[1][17]

Many patients with MOH use very large quantities of medication (eg, 35 doses per week; six different drugs); however, much lower quantities can induce MOH (eg, ergot or triptans taken on 10 or more days per month).[1] It is the frequency of doses rather than the absolute quantity of drug consumed that is important; lower daily doses carry a greater risk of causing MOH than larger weekly doses.[1]

A study of 96 patients with MOH found that the delay between frequent intake of the medication and onset of daily headache was shortest for triptans (around 1.7 years), longer for ergots (around 2.7 years), and longest for simple analgesics (around 4.8 years).[13]

Similarly, the number of doses associated with development of MOH was lowest for triptans (18 single doses per month), higher for ergots (37 single doses per month) and highest for analgesics (114 single doses per month).[13]

Clinical features of MOH

The type of headache that develops in MOH varies; for example, patients with underlying migraine who overuse triptans report a migraine-like daily headache (unilateral pulsating headache with autonomic disturbances) or marked increase in frequency of migraine attacks.[13] Those with tension-type headache who overuse combination analgesics generally develop a constant, pressing, diffuse (ie, tension-type) daily headache.[13] Those with cluster headache generally develop a migraine-like daily headache. MOH is often present and at its worst on waking in the morning.[1] Patients with MOH develop tolerance (reduced efficacy of medication and need for higher doses to achieve analgesic effect) and withdrawal symptoms (rebound headache), which are similar to signs of dependence on drugs traditionally classified as addictive.[18]

In a study of 200 patients fulfilling the criteria for MOH, 79% had additional symptoms, including "asthenia" (weakness), nausea, restlessness, irritability, depression, concentration difficulties and memory problems.[19] Patients with MOH who have had pre-existing tension-type headache are more likely to have co-morbid psychiatric or mood disorders than those with chronic tension-type headache without medication overuse.[20]

Diagnosis of MOH

The diagnosis of MOH is made from the patient's history and clinical presentation. Among the pointers to check for are use of analgesics, including for reasons other than headache; use of over-the-counter as well as prescription drugs; acute medications becoming less effective; and escalation to using more drugs. Investigations are generally not required to diagnose MOH.[21] Assessment should also search for possible complications of regular drug intake (eg, recurrent gastric ulcers, anaemia).[13]

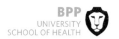

Prevention of MOH

Patients with primary headaches should be informed about the risk of medication overuse, and be encouraged to keep a diary to monitor headache frequency and drug use.[22] Prescriptions for acute migraine should be monitored closely to prevent overuse.[22] Medication for acute headache should be restricted in frequency: use of triptans to below 10 treatment days per month and analgesics to below 15 days per month; migraine drugs containing caffeine, opioids, or tranquillisers should be avoided.[23] Early migraine prophylaxis, with medical or behavioural treatment or acupuncture, aims to reduce the use of acute medication and may therefore help to prevent MOH.[23] [24] A Cochrane systematic review, including data from two randomised controlled trials, involving a total of 241 patients, found that acupuncture and prophylactic drug treatment of migraine produced a similar reduction in analgesic use.[24]

Aims of management for MOH

The objectives in managing patients with MOH are to reduce the frequency and/or severity of headache; to reduce consumption of acute medication (and possibly dietary caffeine); to improve responsiveness to acute and preventive medication; and to alleviate disability and improve quality of life.[22] These are addressed by the following means:

- stopping the overused medication;
- managing withdrawal symptoms;
- reviewing and reassessing the underlying primary headache disorder; and
- preventing relapse.[1]

Stopping the overused medication

General principles of withdrawal

Guidelines from the British Association for the Study of Headache state that patients with MOH fare better if they are motivated and understand that their 'treatment' is likely to be causing their frequent headache.[1] They should be forewarned that withdrawal initially aggravates symptoms (eg, withdrawal headache, which may be accompanied by nausea, vomiting, tachycardia, sleep disturbances, restlessness, anxiety, and nervousness).[1] [13] Withdrawal should be planned in advance to avoid unnecessary lifestyle disruption, and done under the supervision of a doctor or headache specialist nurse.[1] It may be necessary to arrange absence from work for 1–2 weeks.[1] The guidelines also recommend a diary to record symptoms and medication use during withdrawal, and that good hydration should be maintained.[1]

Most drugs causing MOH can be stopped abruptly; the Scottish Intercollegiate Guideline Network suggests that opioids and benzodiazepines should be withdrawn gradually.[14] As with other drugs that produce a withdrawal syndrome, gradual reduction in caffeine intake may be preferable to abrupt withdrawal.[22] [25]

How drug type affects outcome

The duration of withdrawal headache and associated autonomic symptoms varies depending on the types of medication that have been overused. For example, in a study involving 98 patients with MOH undergoing withdrawal as inpatients, the mean duration of withdrawal headache was 4.1 days for triptans; 6.7 days for ergots; and 9.5 days for analgesics.[17] Similarly, the number of days with associated symptoms (eg, nausea, vomiting, sleep disturbance) was lower for triptans than for either ergots or analgesics (1 day vs. 2.5 or 2.2 days,

respectively). Overall improvement occurs within 7–10 days when the causative drug is a triptan; after 2–3 weeks when it is a simple analgesic; and after 2–4 weeks when it is an opioid.[1]

How headache type affects outcome

The initial type of headache appears to affect outcome. Evidence for this comes from a retrospective cohort study based on headache diaries from 337 patients with probable MOH, treated by withdrawal of the drug responsible without any other headache treatment for 2 months.[8] In the study, the response in patients with a previous diagnosis of migraine was better than in those with both migraine and tension-type headache (median reduction in headache frequency 67% vs. 37%) or tension-type headache alone or other type of headache (no reduction).

When withdrawal fails

The mean success rate for withdrawal therapy (defined as at least a 50% reduction in headache days) over 1–6 months is around 72% (based on data from 17 studies, involving a total of 1 101 patients).[21] Factors that affect the likelihood of successful withdrawal include:

- the duration of regular drug intake (a longer duration is associated with a worse prognosis);
- the specific drug overused (eg, withdrawal from triptans has a better prognosis than other drugs);
- the underlying headache type (eg, tension-type headache plus combined tension-type and migraine have a higher relapse risk than other headache types);
- low self-reported sleep quality (associated with a worse prognosis); and
- high self-reported bodily pain (associated with a worse prognosis).[23] [26]

Any lack of commitment from the patient to the withdrawal process should be addressed by greater efforts to inform and support him/her; evidence of psychological dependence may require referral for cognitive behavioural therapy (CBT).[1] In either of these scenarios, there is a potential role for counselling, but this has not been formally assessed in MOH.[1]

Sometimes, withdrawal of overused medication does not lead to recovery, with chronic daily headache persisting more or less unabated. This requires a review of the diagnosis and is an indication for specialist referral.[1]

Managing withdrawal symptoms

Treatment of vomiting

Patients with vomiting during withdrawal can be treated with an antiemetic (eg, metoclopramide, domperidone).[13]

Use of NSAIDs

Withdrawal headache can be managed by offering the patient naproxen (250 mg three times daily or 500 mg twice daily), to be taken regularly or as symptoms require.[1] [27] Some specialists recommend that naproxen is prescribed for a course of 3–4 weeks, and not repeated, or taken for a 6 week course (three times daily for 2 weeks, twice daily for 2 weeks, once daily for 2 weeks) and then stopped.[1] There are no published studies to support or refute these strategies, and manufacturers of NSAIDs have pointed out that this is an unlicensed indication.

Use of corticosteroids

Studies on the management of withdrawal headache using prednisolone have produced mixed results.[28] [29]

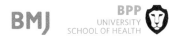

A randomised placebo-controlled trial, involving 100 patients with probable MOH undergoing drug withdrawal (with the first 3 days in hospital), assessed prednisolone with an initial dose 60 mg daily, tapered down over 6 days.[28] There was no difference between the prednisolone and placebo groups on a combined measure of the intensity and number of days with headache in the first 6 days after withdrawal.

A much smaller randomised placebo-controlled trial, involving 20 patients undergoing inpatient withdrawal for MOH, showed that withdrawal headache was reduced in the group taking prednisolone 100 mg daily for 5 days (number of hours with severe or moderate headache in the first 72 hours of withdrawal, the primary outcome measure: 18.1 vs. 36.7 on placebo, p=0.031).[29]

Use of triptans

In a non-blinded trial, 150 patients with MOH, who were abruptly withdrawing symptomatic medication as outpatients, were randomised to one of three strategies (in addition to receiving "orientation" and education before withdrawal): naratriptan 2.5 mg twice daily for 6 days; prednisolone 60 mg daily tapered over 6 days; or no regular medication.[30] There was no significant difference between the groups in the proportion of patients having severe, moderate, mild or no headache over the first 6 days. Fewer patients on naratriptan or prednisolone reported withdrawal symptoms over the first 6 days (68.6% and 81.8%, respectively, vs. 97.5% on no treatment, p=0.003 for difference between the three groups). Compared with the no-treatment group, fewer patients on naratriptan or prednisolone required symptomatic medication (17.2% with naratriptan vs. 46.4%, p=0.007, or 20.5% with prednisolone, p=0.011).

Addressing the primary headache

The patient should be reviewed after 2–3 weeks to ensure withdrawal has been achieved.[1] Recovery continues slowly for weeks to months and follow-up is necessary.[1] Most patients revert to their original headache type within 2 months.[1]

Symptomatic relief

Overused medications (if needed) may be reintroduced for symptomatic relief after 2 months, with explicit restrictions to ensure that the frequency of use does not usually exceed 2 days per week on a regular basis.[1]

Prophylaxis for primary headache

In patients whose headache stops responding to prophylactic treatment while overusing symptomatic medications, the prophylactic efficacy may return after successful withdrawal of the overused medication.[14]

Recent studies suggest that topiramate offers a modest benefit in reducing headache frequency, even in the absence of drug withdrawal.[15][31][32] The rationale for the use of this drug is based on the fact that patients with chronic headache and medication overuse have upregulation of cerebral cortex activity; the effect of topiramate is to inhibit neuronal activity.[32] However, topiramate also has potential unwanted effects (eg, cognitive impairment, depression) which may limit its use.

Preventing relapse

Definition of relapse into medication overuse

Relapse is defined as frequent use of any acute headache medication on more than 15 days per month for at least 3 months after recovery from previous MOH.[33]

What are the risks for relapse?

Most relapses occur within the first year after withdrawal.[34] For example, a prospective 4-year follow-up study of 96 patients with MOH treated with drug withdrawal found that 31% of participants relapsed within the first 6 months after withdrawal; 41% had relapsed by 1 year and 45% by 4 years after withdrawal.[34] Reported risk factors for relapse include tension-type headache or a combination of migraine plus tension-type headache, rather than migraine alone; longer duration of migraine with more than 8 headache days per month; lower improvement after drug withdrawal; greater number of previous preventive treatments tried; male gender; and intake of combined analgesic drugs (eg, combination of one or more NSAIDs with caffeine or codeine).[34][35][36]

How can relapse be prevented?

Patients with risk factors for relapse should be informed about these and monitored regularly, and combination drugs should be avoided; many patients require extended support to prevent relapse.

The primary headache must be treated using a different approach rather than medication.[22] Massage, acupuncture and behavioural therapies (eg, CBT, stress reduction, biofeedback training) may help.[22] Amitriptyline can also help to alleviate associated symptoms of MOH, particularly mood and sleep disorders; however, evidence on this is limited[37] and the drug may have troublesome unwanted effects.

Prophylactic treatment can be introduced and is more likely to be effective in the absence of MOH; it should follow the standard recommendations of titration to an effective tolerated dose and continuation for 3-6 months.[1][38]

Comparison of management strategies

A non-blinded randomised controlled trial comparing strategies to manage medication withdrawal involved 120 patients with migraine, probable MOH and low medical needs (ie, not requiring specific additional medical interventions, with exclusion criteria such as no overuse of opioids, barbiturates or benzodiazepines; no significant physical or psychiatric co-morbidity; no previous experience of detoxification).[39] Participants were allocated to one of three strategies: advice to withdraw the overused medication; outpatient detoxification with advice, prednisolone (tapered down from 60 mg daily over 8 days) and personalised prophylaxis; or inpatient detoxification with advice, prednisolone (as above), prophylaxis, parenteral fluid replacement and antiemetics (intravenous metoclopramide 10 mg twice daily). Treatment was considered successful if, 2 months after starting withdrawal, the patient had no headache or reverted to episodic headache and to an intake of symptomatic medication on fewer than 10 days per month. There was no difference in outcome between the three treatment groups, with around 75% of patients in each being treated successfully.

In a non-blinded study, 56 patients with MOH were randomised to one of three treatment strategies for 5 months: outpatient detoxification without prophylaxis; prophylactic treatment without detoxification; or neither new preventive medication nor direct advice to stop medication (the control group; after 5 months, these patients were offered a choice of withdrawal or prophylactic treatment).[40] The reduction in headache days per month at month 3 (the major primary outcome measure) did not differ significantly between groups (a reduction of 4.1 days in the detoxification group, 7.2 days in the prophylactic treatment group and 1.6 days in the control group).

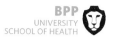

When to refer

UK guidelines suggest that patients with MOH should be referred to a neurologist if attempted withdrawal in primary care fails.[14] [41] Patients who also have psychiatric co-morbidity or dependence behaviour should have these conditions treated additionally; referral to a psychiatrist or clinical psychologist may be necessary.[14]

Conclusion

Medication overuse headache (MOH) is common, and should be suspected in a patient with increasing headache frequency, taking triptans, ergots, combined analgesics or opioids on 10 or more days a month, or analgesics or NSAIDs on 15 or more days a month, over a number of months. The type of headache may be tension-type daily headache and/or migraine-like attacks. Associated symptoms can include nausea and gastrointestinal symptoms, irritability, anxiety, depression, concentration difficulties and memory problems.

Measures to prevent the development of MOH include restricting consumption of the medications commonly responsible, and avoiding dietary caffeine and drugs containing caffeine or codeine. Early prophylaxis, either medical or behavioural, may be appropriate in patients with frequent headaches.

Once MOH has developed, management involves education of the patient on the cause, as well as drug withdrawal. Amitriptyline or topiramate may help reduce withdrawal symptoms, but there are few data to support these interventions and their unwanted effects should be borne in mind. Patients should be reviewed following drug withdrawal and, if frequent headaches persist, specialist referral should be considered. Patients with frequent headache not taking prophylaxis may find previously ineffective prophylactic drugs become effective once MOH has been diagnosed and the patient treated; acupuncture is an alternative. Patients should be followed up regularly to prevent relapse, which is most likely in the first year after withdrawal.

- This article was originally published in *Drug and Therapeutics Bulletin* (*DTB* 2010;48:2-6).
- *DTB* is a highly regarded source of unbiased, evidence based information and practical advice for healthcare professionals. It is independent of the pharmaceutical industry, government, and regulatory authorities, and is free of advertising.
- *DTB* is available online at http://dtb.bmj.com.

---

1   Steiner TJ et al, 2007. Guidelines for all healthcare professionals in the diagnosis and management of migraine, tension-type, cluster and medication-overuse headache. 3rd edition. http://216.25.88.43/upload/NS_BASH/BASH_guidelines_2007.pdf.

2   Watson DP. Easing the pain: challenges and opportunities in headache management. *Br J Gen Pract* 2008;58:77–8.

3   Headache Classification Subcommittee of the International Headache Society (IHS). The International Classification of Headache Disorders 2nd edition 1st revision (May, 2005). *Cephalalgia* 2005;25:460–5.

4   Olesen J et al. New appendix criteria open for a broader concept of chronic migraine. *Cephalalgia* 2006;26:742–6.

5   Headache Classification Subcommittee of the International Headache Society (IHS). The International Classification of Headache Disorders (2nd edition). *Cephalalgia* 2004;24(suppl 1):1–160.

6   Bahra A et al. Does chronic daily headache arise de novo in association with regular use of analgesics? *Headache* 2003;43:179–90.

7   Wilkinson SM et al. Opiate use to control bowel motility may induce chronic daily headache in patients with migraine. *Headache* 2001;41:303–9.

8   Zeeberg P et al. Probable medication-overuse headache: the effect of a 2-month drug-free period. *Neurology* 2006;66:1894–8.

9   Paemeleire K et al. Medication-overuse headache in patients with cluster headache. *Neurology* 2006;67:109–13.

10 Stovner LJ et al. The global burden of headache: a documentation of headache prevalence and disability worldwide. *Cephalalgia* 2007;27:193–210.

11 Meskunas CA et al. Medications associated with probable MOH reported in a tertiary care headache center over a 15-year period. *Headache* 2006;46:766–72.

12 D'Amico D et al. Application of revised criteria for chronic migraine and MOH in a tertiary headache centre. *Neurol Sci* 2008;29:S158–60.

13 Diener H-C, Katasarva Z. Analgesic/abortive overuse and misuse in chronic daily headache. *Curr Pain Headache Rep* 2001;5:545–50.

14 Scottish Intercollegiate Guidelines Network, 2008. 107: Diagnosis and management of headache in adults. A national clinical guideline. www.sign.ac.uk/pdf/sign107.pdf.

15 Joint Formulary Committee. British National Formulary. Edition 58. London: BMJ Group and RPS Publishing, September 2009.

16 Bigal ME et al. Acute migraine medications and evolution from episodic to chronic migraine: a longitudinal population-based study. *Headache* 2008;48:1157–68.

17 Katsarava Z et al. Clinical features of withdrawal headache following overuse of triptans and other headache drugs. *Neurology* 2001;57:1694–8.

18 Grande RB et al. The Severity of Dependence Scale detects people with medication overuse. The Akershus study of chronic headache. *J Neurol Neurosurg Psychiatr* 2009;80:784–9.

19 Mathew NT et al. Drug induced refractory headache—clinical features and management. *Headache* 1990;30:634–8.

20 Atasoy HT et al. Psychiatric comorbidity in MOH patients with pre-existing headache type of episodic tension-type headache. *Eur J Pain* 2005;9:285–91.

21 Diener H-C, Limmroth V. Medication-overuse headache: a worldwide problem. *Lancet Neurol* 2004;3:475–83.

22 Rapoport AM. MOH: awareness, detection and treatment. *CNS Drugs* 2008;22:995–1004.

23 Katsarava Z et al. MOH. *Curr Neurol Neurosci Rep* 2009;9:115–9.

24 Linde K et al. Acupuncture for migraine prophylaxis. *Cochrane Database Syst Rev* 2009, Issue 1. Art No.: CD001218.

25 Silverman K et al. Withdrawal syndrome after the double-blind cessation of caffeine consumption. *N Engl J Med* 1992;327:1109–14.

26 Bøe MG et al. Chronic daily headache with medication overuse: predictors of outcome 1 year after withdrawal therapy. *Eur J Neurol* 2009;16:705–12.

27 Mathew NT. Amelioration of ergotamine withdrawal symptoms with naproxen. *Headache* 1987;27:130–3.

28 Bøe MG et al. Prednisolone does not reduce withdrawal headache: a randomized, double-blind study. *Neurology* 2007;69:26–31.

29 Pageler L et al. Prednisone vs. placebo in withdrawal therapy following MOH. *Cephalalgia* 2008;28:152–6.

30 Krymchantowski AV, Moreira PF. Out-patient detoxification in chronic migraine: comparison of strategies. *Cephalalgia* 2003;23:982–93.

31 Diener H-C et al. Topiramate reduces headache days in chronic migraine: a randomized, double-blind, placebo-controlled study. *Cephalalgi a* 2007;27:814–23.

32 Mei D et al. Topiramate and triptans revert chronic migraine with medication overuse to episodic migraine. *Clin Neuropharmacol* 2006;29:269–75.

33 Katsarava Z et al. Rates and predictors for relapse in MOH: a 1-year prospective study. *Neurology* 2003;60:1682–3.

34 Katsarava Z et al. MOH: rates and predictors for relapse in a 4-year prospective study. *Cephalalgia* 2005;25:12–5.

35 Suhr B et al. Drug-induced headache: long-term results of stationary versus ambulatory withdrawal therapy. *Cephalalgia* 1999; 19: 44–9.

36 Rossi P et al. MOH: predictors and rates of relapse in migraine patients with low medical needs. A 1-year prospective study. *Cephalalgia* 2008;28:1196–200.

37 Descombes S et al. Amitriptyline treatment in chronic drug-induced headache: a double-blind comparative pilot study. *Headache* 2001;41:178–82.

38 Zeeberg P et al. Discontinuation of medication overuse in headache patients: recovery of therapeutic responsiveness. *Cephalalgia* 2006;26:1192–8.

39 Rossi P et al. Advice alone vs. structured detoxification programmes for MOH: a prospective, randomized, open-label trial in transformed migraine patients with low medical needs. *Cephalalgia* 2006;26:1097–105.

40 Hagen K et al. Management of MOH: 1-year randomized multicentre open-label trial. *Cephalalgia* 2009;29:221–32.

41 Clinical Knowledge Summaries. Headache—medication overuse. August 2009. www.cks.nhs.uk/headache_medication_overuse#-393230.

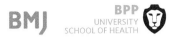
Clinical management of stuttering in children and adults

Susan O'Brian, senior research fellow[1], Mark Onslow, director[1]

[1]Australian Stuttering Research Centre, University of Sydney, Lidcombe, NSW 2060, Australia

Correspondence to: M Onslow mark. onslow@sydney.edu.au

Cite this as: BMJ 2011;342:d3742

DOI: 10.1136/bmj.d3742

http://www.bmj.com/content/342/bmj.d3742

Stuttering, also known as stammering, is a common speech disorder of neural speech processing that typically begins during the first years of life. An Australian cohort study (n=1619) of children recruited at 8 months of age found that 8.5% had begun to stutter a 36 months of age, and 12.2% by 48 months.[1] A review of 44 studies shows a prevalence of around 1% for schoolchildren worldwide (range 0.03-5.2%).[w1] Stuttering is essentially a movement disorder of speech, with observable effects on the jaw and mouth, but also facial muscles and sometimes upper limbs. Those who stutter are at risk of developing social anxiety or mental health problems.

Evidence from randomised trials has shown that treatment before 6 years of age reduces the chance of stuttering becoming intractable. Children can recover without formal intervention, but it is not possible to predict who will recover spontaneously. It is therefore best to take advantage of the window of opportunity within which children may be treated with best effect, which is within one year of onset. For adults with long term stuttering, early randomised trials of behavioural and cognitive interventions show promise.

What causes stuttering?

Stuttering usually begins during the early years of life, and it affects all races and cultures. The cause of stuttering is not known, but the findings of research using brain imaging point towards a deficit of the neural processing that underpins spoken language.[w2] A small case-control study found increased odds of structural and functional anomalies in areas of the brain responsible for spoken language in adult patients with persistent developmental stuttering.[2] Similar findings have been reported for children.[3] About two thirds of patients who stutter report a family history. Studies show greater concordance between monozygotic twins than dizygotic twins and suggest that 70% of cases can be accounted for genetically.[4] A recent study that combined genetic linkage data and brain imaging data has generated what seems to be a tenable hypothesis—that the onset of stuttering is linked to abnormal myelogenesis of speech related fibre tracts.[5]

SOURCES AND SELECTION CRITERIA

We consulted our own archive and searched the Institute of Scientific Information Web of Science and PubMed databases of peer reviewed journals using the search terms "stutter*" and "stammer*".

SUMMARY POINTS

- Stuttering is a common speech disorder of neural speech processing that usually begins during the first three or four years of life and may affect as many as 10% of children
- Educational, occupational, and social problems are common if chronic stuttering is not treated early
- Mental health problems, in particular social anxiety, are likely to develop with chronic stuttering
- Early intervention is recommended, preferably within one year of onset of stuttering
- Randomised controlled trials have shown an early parent implemented behavioural intervention to be efficacious for stuttering control in preschool children
- Speech restructuring can rehabilitate speech in people with chronic stuttering

How is a diagnosis made?

The diagnosis is usually straightforward because affected adults and adolescents almost always describe their condition accurately.

What is not stuttering?

Stuttering is occasionally comorbid with a rare fluency disrupting speech disorder known as cluttering.[w3] Cluttering is usually distinguishable from stuttering in that the speech pattern is typically rapid and irregular, and affected patients usually lack awareness of the problem. Disturbed fluency can occasionally be the result of an acute neurological insult, in which case the clinical presentation will be clearly different from that seen with stuttering.[w4] Stuttering tends to occur on the first word of utterances and the first syllables of words, but "neurogenic stuttering" is distributed evenly across utterances, and extraneous non-verbal behaviours, commonly found with stuttering, do not occur. In rare cases, neurogenic stuttering can be psychogenic in origin.[w5]

How do patients or parents usually present?

Young children

Parents will usually present saying that their child has begun to stutter. The onset of stuttering can be particularly distressing for parents, for three reasons. Firstly, stuttering usually begins unexpectedly after a period of normal and uneventful language development, often when children start to put words together into short utterances. The onset of stuttering has not been associated with child temperament, social, or environmental variables. Secondly, the onset of stuttering may be sudden. Observational evidence suggests that half of cases develop over the course of a week and a third of cases over a single day.[1] [6] Parents may report that their child went to bed speaking normally but was stuttering at breakfast the next morning. Thirdly, the disfiguring features of the disorder described below do not develop insidiously but can be present soon after onset.[7] Parents may report that their preschool child is distressed by the onset of stuttering.[6]

Older children and adults

The speech problems of stuttering can mean a lifelong struggle to speak. Patients openly complain of stuttering and often mention associated anxiety. Repeated movements of the jaw and mouth occur for sounds, syllables, words, or phrases. Normal speech involves continuous movements of the mouth and jaw, but stuttering can be associated with periods when movement stops, giving the impression that the speaker is "blocked." Tic-like movements and extraneous vocalisations often occur and cause disfigurement during speech. With severe stuttering fixed postures can last for more than 30 seconds. These "blocks" can be accompanied by extraneous non-verbal behaviours such as grimacing, twitching, and other body movements. Stuttering may cause the patient to speak slowly and effortfully, with reduced speech output. People who stutter speak, on average, at three quarters of the rate of controls, but in severe cases the rate of speech may be

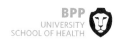

less than a quarter of normal. The severity of stuttering ranges greatly, from people who are mildly affected (just a few stutters each day), who often never seek help, to those who are very severely affected and essentially cannot communicate. Patients who stutter may fail to fulfil their educational and occupational potential. A survey of more than 200 adults who stutter found that about 70% thought that their stuttering had stood in the way of a promotion, whereas 20% had turned down a promotion because of it.[8] In addition, a seminal survey of employers' attitudes found that many employers agreed that stuttering reduces employability and promotion prospects.[9]

Patients with long term stuttering may have mental health problems, and these may begin early in childhood after the onset of stuttering.[10] [11] A recent observational study in adults who stutter found that stuttering affects quality of life as adversely as life threatening conditions such as neurotrauma and coronary heart disease,[12] but in contrast to those diseases it is present for a lifetime. People who stutter may be affected by social anxiety, and an observational study estimated that people with chronic stuttering have a 34-fold increased risk of having a formal diagnosis of social phobia compared with matched controls.[13] Case reports of social phobia and stuttering are common,[14] and comorbid stuttering has been reported in 40-60% of clinical cohorts of people with social phobia.[13] [15] [16] Anxiety disorders, mood disorders, substance misuse, and personality disorders are also highly prevalent in people who stutter,[17] [18] and the presence of mental health problems reduces the likelihood that speech rehabilitation will be successful.[19] We suggest that healthcare personnel fully explore anxiety experiences of patients with stuttering because of their potential clinical relevance.

Why not let stuttering resolve naturally?

Although natural recovery from stuttering does occur and published estimates have been generally similar to the 74% reported from a prospective cohort,[20] much "natural recovery" may be attributable to treatment. In the absence of control for such interventions, and without studies of children before the onset of stuttering, we think that the correct natural recovery rate is much lower. In our opinion, the important question is how many children recover naturally during the known window of clinical opportunity. Findings from the above prospective cohort suggested that less than 5% of children recover within a year of the onset of stuttering, although many more recover later. It is not possible to predict which children will recover naturally, so intervention shortly after onset is best practice.

In addition, negative conditioning experiences during the school years may be implicated in the development of mental health problems in those who stutter. An observational study showed that in children who stutter, negative attitudes to speech and communication measured in 6 and 7 year olds worsened progressively during later school years (7-12 year olds), whereas attitudes to communication in control children become healthier.[21] Schoolchildren who stutter are more susceptible to bullying than those who do not.[22] Non-stuttering peers perceive stuttering school age children negatively,[23] and schoolchildren who stutter find it more difficult to establish peer relationships than controls.[24] Adults often report that their stuttering had catastrophic effects on their school life. In a survey of 276 adult members of a national association of stutterers,[25] most (96%) reported immediate negative emotional effects of childhood bullying and 46% reported some long term effects on social and emotional functioning.[26]

How is stuttering treated?

Children

A meta-analysis of clinical cohorts established a guideline that early intervention should begin within a year of onset.[27] Although delaying the start of the intervention for one year after onset within the preschool years did not seem to jeopardise responsiveness to subsequent intervention, the possibility of intractability during the school age years (presumably because of decreasing plasticity within the speech motor system as neural networks for speech become established) leads us to advise early referral for intervention. A monitoring period of up to one year after onset may be appropriate in some cases, particularly when natural recovery clearly is occurring. Referrals can be made in the first instance to speech-language therapists (United Kingdom), speech-language pathologists (North America), or speech pathologists (Australia).

A simple intervention known as the Lidcombe Programme, developed in Australia, has been evaluated in randomised trials. This programme is a behavioural treatment, which is administered by parents under the direction of a clinician. The child and parent visit the speech clinic for an hour each week, during which time the clinician teaches the parent how to control the child's stuttering. This is done with a method that relies on laboratory findings that early stuttering is one of the many problem behaviours with operant properties, meaning that "stimulus control" can be attained with environmental contingencies for those problem behaviours. With the Lidcombe programme, the contingencies for stuttering are verbal; parents are taught to indicate to the child occasionally during the day when they hear a stutter, and occasionally to ask the child to self correct a stuttered utterance. Children can normally make such a self correction. Most importantly, parents are taught to praise their children during the day when stuttering does not occur. To confirm that the treatment is proceeding satisfactorily, parents measure the child's stuttering severity each day, using a scale where "1" equals "no stuttering" and "10" equals "extremely severe stuttering." This scale is also useful if the clinician decides to delay treatment to determine whether natural recovery is occurring. The treatment ends when stuttering is absent or at a very low level. The manual for the Lidcombe programme is publicly available at the website of the Australian Stuttering Research Centre.

There is much low level evidence from phase I and phase II clinical trials for this early stuttering intervention.[28] Two independent phase III randomised controlled trials (total n=100) have been published—one with New Zealand preschool children and one with German preschool children.[29] [30] The studies show that the treatment can control stuttering and resulted in normal speech in these children, and that the programme reduces stuttering more quickly than allowing natural recovery to occur. A meta-analysis of all sources of randomised controlled evidence for the treatment—including brief exposure experiments not considered here to be clinical trials—indicated an odds ratio of 7.7.[28] This result means that preschool children who received the Lidcombe programme in clinical trials were 7.7 times more likely to recover than children who did not receive the treatment. A randomised phase II trial showed that the treatment can be adapted to telehealth delivery.[31]

Although treatment might simply speed up the natural process, at the very least it shortens the exposure of these children to the negative effects of early stuttering.

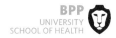

However, the Lidcombe programme may control stuttering with mechanisms that are independent of natural recovery. Studies showing that this treatment reduces stuttering in school age children who are unlikely to recover naturally support this possibility.[w6 w7]

Two other treatments are currently being evaluated in phase I and phase II clinical trials—two phase I trials of parent-child interaction therapy,[w8 w9] and phase I and II trials of the Westmead programme.[w10-w12] Parent-child interaction therapy is a family based treatment designed to modify the parental style of everyday interaction with the child. In the Westmead programme, children are taught to control stuttering with a syllable-timed speech pattern, similar to talking in time to a metronome. However, until randomised controlled trials are published, the efficacy of these treatments is not clear.

Adolescents and adults

Speech rehabilitation for adults and adolescents requires a different approach. Nearly all recently published clinical trials investigating treatment for chronic stuttering have incorporated variants of a technique called "speech restructuring."[w13] Patients are trained to use a new speech pattern to reduce or eliminate stuttering while sounding as natural as possible. During speech restructuring, patients learn to speak initially with a slow drawling speech pattern that is stutter free. The speech pattern is then shaped toward stutter-free speech that is reasonably natural sounding. The bulk of the evidence comprises low level phase I and phase II clinical trials, some of which have been replicated. Those trials suggest that a 70-90% reduction in stuttering severity can be maintained at follow-up. However, a randomised trial with a no treatment group has not been published, so it is not clear how efficacious the treatment is; non-randomised clinical evidence typically overestimates effect sizes. Two phase III randomised trials have evaluated speech restructuring (total n=129) with adults and adolescents. These have shown that a telehealth version of the treatment is not inferior to in-clinic treatment,[32] and that a self modelling procedure added to the treatment improves speech outcomes.[33] Self modelling is a simple procedure where patients regularly watch videos of themselves displaying the required behaviour, in this case stutter-free speech. In contrast to early intervention, this treatment is not suitable for all patients, because many cannot master and sustain the requisite speech pattern for stuttering control. Relapse is common, particularly for those with comorbid mental health problems.[19] Unnatural sounding speech may occur, and for treatment to be successful patients must pay constant attention to speech.

Cognitive behavioural therapy is the most efficacious intervention available for treating social anxiety and has been evaluated extensively in non-stuttering populations.[w14] Historically, speech restructuring treatment has incorporated components of cognitive behavioural therapy. Cognitive behavioural methods specifically aimed at treating the social anxiety of patients who stutter have recently been developed, and a small amount of evidence has emerged from clinical trials. Evidence from a randomised phase II clinical trial suggests that patients who stutter and have social phobia will no longer be diagnosed with social phobia after the intervention.[34] Predictably, that report showed that speech restructuring treatment alone did not control social phobia. Evidence from phase I clinical trials suggests that standalone, internet driven cognitive behavioural therapy may also be a viable treatment.[w15]

The holy grail of research into the treatment of stuttering is a machine that the patient can wear to alleviate stuttering, but for decades efforts to develop one have been disappointing. A recent commercially available device resembling a hearing aid, which distorts the patient's hearing of speech output ("SpeechEasy") is no exception. After a series of encouraging clinical trials a phase I trial of the device reported it not to be efficacious when worn during everyday life.[w16] Some attempts have been made to develop in-clinic machines to alleviate stuttering. Electromyographic feedback showed some promise in a non-randomised trial with adolescent patients,[w17] but again that promise was not sustained, with subsequent trials of adolescents and school age children showing no effect.[w18] A phase I trial of a machine that induces a variant of speech restructuring ("modification of phonation intervals") showed initial promise with five patients,[w19] but no subsequent trials have yet been reported.

The many attempts at alleviating stuttering with the use of drugs have also been disappointing. A review of 31 reports concluded that no worthwhile treatment effects were obtained using a range of drugs.[w20]

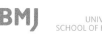

Contributors: Both authors contributed equally to the conceptualisation, drafting, and revision of this manuscript. MO is guarantor.

Competing interests: Both authors have completed the ICMJE uniform disclosure form at www.icmje.org/coi_disclosure.pdf (available on request from the corresponding author) and declare: SO and MO have support from the University of Sydney for the submitted work; no financial relationships with any organisations that might have an interest in the submitted work in the previous three years; no other relationships or activities that could appear to have influenced the submitted work.

Provenance and peer review: Commissioned; externally peer reviewed.

1   Reilly S, Onslow M, Packman A, Wake M, Bavin EL, Prior M, et al. Predicting stuttering onset by the age of 3 years: a prospective, community cohort study. *Pediatrics* 2009;123:270-7.
2   Sommer M, Koch MA, Paulus W, Weiller C, Buchel C. Disconnection of speech-relevant brain areas in persistent developmental stuttering. *Lancet* 2002;360:380-3.
3   Chang SE, Erickson KI, Ambrose NG, Hasegawa-Johnson MA, Ludlow CL. Brain anatomy differences in childhood stuttering. *Neuroimage* 2008;39:1333-44.
4   Felsenfeld S, Kirk KM, Zhu G, Statham DJ, Neale MC, Martin NG. A study of the genetic and environmental etiology of stuttering in a selected twin sample. *Behav Genet* 2000;30:359-66.
5   Cykowski MD, Fox PT, Ingham RJ, Ingham JC, Robin DA. A study of the reproducibility and etiology of diffusion anisotropy differences in developmental stuttering: A potential role for impaired myelination. *Neuroimage* 2010;52:1495-504.
6   Yairi E. The onset of stuttering in two- and three-year-old children: a preliminary report. *J Speech Hearing Disord* 1983;48:171-7.
7   Conture EG, Kelly EM. Young stutterers' nonspeech behaviors during stuttering. *J Speech Hear Res* 1991;34:1041-56.
8   Klein JF, Hood SB. The impact of stuttering on employment opportunities and job performance. *J Fluency Disord* 2004;29:255-73.
9   Hurst MI, Cooper EB. Employer attitudes toward stuttering. *J Fluency Disord* 1983;8:1-12.
10   Langevin M, Packman A, Onslow M. Peer responses to stuttering in the preschool setting. *Am J Speech Lang Pathol* 2009;18:264-76.
11   Ezrati-Vinacour R, Platzky R, Yairi E. The young child's awareness of stuttering-like disfluency. *J Speech Lang Hear Res* 2001;44:368-80.
12   Craig A, Blumgart E, Tran Y. The impact of stuttering on the quality of life in adults who stutter. *J Fluency Disord* 2009;34:61-71.
13   Iverach L, O'Brian S, Jones M, Block S, Lincoln M, Harrison E, et al. Prevalence of anxiety disorders among adults seeking speech therapy for stuttering. *J Anxiety Disord* 2009;23:928-34.
14   De Carle AJ, Pato MT. Social phobia and stuttering. *Am J Psychiatry* 1996;153:1367-8.
15   Blumgart E, Tran Y, Craig A. Social anxiety disorder in adults who stutter. *Depress Anxiety* 2010;27:687-92.
16   Stein MB, Baird A, Walker JR. Social phobia in adults with stuttering. *Am J Psychiatry* 1996;153:278-80.
17   Iverach L, Jones M, O'Brian S, Block S, Lincoln M, Harrison E, et al. Mood and substance use disorders among adults seeking speech treatment for stuttering. *J Speech Lang Hear Res* 2010;53:1178-90.
18   Iverach L, Jones M, O'Brian S, Block S, Lincoln M, Harrison E, et al. Screening for personality disorders among adults seeking speech treatment for stuttering. *J Fluency Disord* 2009;34:173-86.
19   Iverach L, Jones M, O'Brian S, Block S, Lincoln M, Harrison E, et al. The relationship between mental health disorders and treatment outcomes among adults who stutter. *J Fluency Disord* 2009;34:29-43.
20   Yairi E, Ambrose NG. Early childhood stuttering I: persistency and recovery rates. *J Speech Lang Hear Res* 1999;42:1097-112.
21   De Nil LF, Brutten GJ. Speech-associated attitudes of stuttering and nonstuttering children. *J Speech Hear Res* 1991;34:60-6.
22   Langevin M, Bortnick K, Hammer T, Wiebe E. Teasing/bullying experienced by children who stutter: toward development of a questionnaire. *Contemp Issues Commun Sci Disord* 1998;25:12-24.
23   Langevin, M. The peer attitudes toward children who stutter scale: reliability, known groups validity, and negativity of elementary school-age children's attitudes. *J Fluency Disord* 2009;34:72-86.
24   Davis S, Howell P, Cooke F. Sociodynamic relationships between children who stutter and their non-stuttering classmates. *J Child Psychol* 2002;43:939-47.
25   Hayhow R, Cray AM, Enderby P. Stammering and therapy views of people who stammer. *J Fluency Disord* 2002;27:1-17.
26   Hugh-Jones S, Smith PK. Self-reports of short- and long-term effects of bullying on children who stammer. *Br J Educ Psychol* 1999;69:141-58.
27   Kingston M, Huber A, Onslow M, Jones M, Packman A. Predicting treatment time with the Lidcombe program: replication and meta-analysis. *Int J Lang Commun Disord* 2003;38:165-77.
28   Onslow M, Jones M, Menzies R, O'Brian S, Packman A. Stuttering. In: Sturmey P, Hersen M, eds. Handbook of evidence-based practice in clinical psychology. Wiley (forthcoming).
29   Jones M, Onslow M, Packman A, Williams S, Ormond T, Schwarz I, et al. Randomised controlled trial of the Lidcombe programme of early stuttering intervention. *BMJ* 2005;331:659-61.
30   Lattermann C, Euler HA, Neumann K. A randomized control trial to investigate the impact of the Lidcombe program on early stuttering in German-speaking preschoolers. *J Fluency Disord* 2008;33:52-65.
31   Lewis C, Packman A, Onslow M, Simpson JM, Jones M. A phase II trial of telehealth delivery of the Lidcombe program of early stuttering intervention. *Am J Speech Lang Pathol* 2008;17:139.
32   Carey B, O'Brian S, Onslow M, Block S, Jones M, Packman A. Randomized controlled non-inferiority trial of a telehealth treatment for chronic stuttering: the Camperdown program. *Int J Lang Commun Disord* 2010;45:108-20.
33   Cream A, O'Brian S, Jones M, Block S Harrison E, Lincoln M, et al. Randomized controlled trial of video self-modeling following speech restructuring treatment for stuttering. *J Speech Lang Hear Res* 2010;53:887-97.
34   Menzies R, O'Brian S, Onslow M, Packman A, St Clare T, Block S. An experimental clinical trial of a cognitive behavior therapy package for chronic stuttering. *J Speech Lang Hear Res* 2008;51:1451-64.

Related links

bmj.com/blogs
• BMJ blog: Ivan Perry on stammering

bmj.com/archive
• Personal view: The role of role avoidance (2002;324:857)

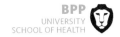

Assessment and management of alcohol use disorders

Ed Day, senior lecturer and consultant in addiction psychiatry[1], Alex Copello, professor[2], Martyn Hull, GP principal and lead GP with a special interest in substance misuse[3]

[1]Addictions Department, Institute of Psychiatry, Psychology & Neuroscience, King's College London, London SE5 8AF, UK

[2]School of Psychology, University of Birmingham, Birmingham, UK

[3]Ridgacre Medical Centres, Quinton, Birmingham, UK

Correspondence to: E Day Edward. Day@kcl.ac.uk

Cite this as: BMJ 2015;350:h715

DOI: 10.1136/bmj.h715

http://www.bmj.com/content/350/bmj.h715

Alcohol can impact on both the incidence and the course of many health conditions, and nearly 6% of all global deaths in 2012 were estimated to be attributable to its consumption.[1] A quarter of the UK adult population drinks alcohol in a way that is potentially or actually harmful to health.[2] Between 2002 and 2012 in England the number of episodes where an alcohol related disease, injury, or condition was the primary reason for hospital admission or a secondary diagnosis doubled.[3] Despite the large numbers of people drinking alcohol at higher risk levels, a relatively low number access treatment.[4] Possible causes for this include missed opportunities to identify problems, limited access to specialist services, and underdeveloped care pathways. International studies have shown that more than 20% of patients presenting to primary care are higher risk or dependent drinkers,[5] yet the problem of alcohol is inadequately addressed. This review focuses on practical aspects of the assessment and treatment of alcohol use disorders from the perspective of the non-specialist hospital doctor or general practitioner.

How are alcohol use disorders defined?

As the level of alcohol consumption goes up, so the risk of physical, psychological, and social problems increases. Alcohol related harm is a public health problem, and strategies that reduce average consumption across the whole population by even a small amount produce considerable health benefits. Increasing the cost of alcohol has been consistently associated with a reduction in alcohol related harm,[6] and a minimum cost for a unit of alcohol has been under consideration in the United Kingdom.[7]

Alcoholic drinks have different strengths, and so alcohol is not measured by number of drinks but by number of "units." In the United Kingdom, 1 unit comprises 8 grams of alcohol (equivalent to 10 mL of pure ethanol), but elsewhere this value is defined differently.[8] Box 1 shows how to calculate the number of units. The terminology used to define alcohol use disorders is currently evolving, with various organisations using slightly different terms.[9][10] However, the general agreement is that there is no such thing as a "safe level" of drinking and that the risk of harm increases with

SOURCES AND SELECTION CRITERIA

We structured this review around a series of clinical guidelines developed by the UK National Institute for Health and Care Excellence. Three separate expert groups considered public health, physical, and psychological and social issues around alcohol use. The guidance is summarised in the form of clinical pathways (http://pathways.nice.org.uk/pathways/alcohol-use-disorders).

either frequency of consumption or amount consumed on a drinking occasion.[8] To plan effective intervention strategies, the categories of alcohol use disorders defined in table 1 are most commonly used. Figure 1 shows the prevalence of these categories in England.

The term "addiction" is not used in current classificatory systems, partly because it has pejorative connotations. The latest version (fifth edition) of the *Diagnostic and Statistical Manual of Mental Disorders* has removed the category of dependence, and instead describes a spectrum of alcohol use disorders of differing severity.[11] The concept of alcohol dependence is, however, important to describe people in whom the ability to control the frequency and extent of consumption has been completely eroded, while recognising that dependence may exist at different levels of severity.[12][13]

How can alcohol use disorders be identified?

Most people with risky patterns of drinking are not dependent on alcohol (fig 1). A few minutes spent systematically identifying drinkers at increased risk of harm and delivering advice about moderating alcohol consumption has been shown to be an effective strategy in various settings,[14][15] and the process of identification and brief advice should be offered as a first step in treatment.[4] In the United Kingdom, the National Institute for Health and Care Excellence recommends that professionals in the National Health Service should carry out alcohol screening as part of routine practice,[4] and all doctors should feel comfortable and confident in raising the topic of alcohol consumption in a consultation. However, the low level of detection and treatment suggests that generalists are not sufficiently proactive in screening groups potentially at risk, including those who have relevant physical conditions (for example, hypertension and gastrointestinal or liver disorders); mental health problems, such as anxiety or depression; been assaulted; are at risk of self harm; regularly experience unintentional injuries or minor trauma; and regularly attend genitourinary medicine clinics or repeatedly seek emergency contraception.

AUDIT, the alcohol use disorders identification test (fig 2), consists of 10 questions about drinking frequency and intensity, experience of alcohol related problems, and signs of possible dependence.[16] It is the ideal screening questionnaire for detecting drinkers at increasing or higher risk.[1] Furthermore, the AUDIT score can guide clinicians as to the best intervention, including brief advice or a referral

THE BOTTOM LINE

- Alcohol use disorders exist across a spectrum, and public health measures to reduce the drinking of a whole population have considerable health benefits
- All front line clinicians should be aware of the potential effects of alcohol consumption and be able to screen for alcohol use disorders using the alcohol use disorders questionnaire test
- Brief interventions are quick and easy to deliver and have a potentially large impact on reducing hazardous and harmful drinking
- Benzodiazepines are the drug of choice for medically assisted alcohol withdrawal
- Relapse to drinking is common in the first year after stopping drinking, but psychological treatments, mutual aid groups, and relapse prevention drugs increase the likelihood of remaining abstinent

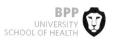

BOX 1: HOW TO CALCULATE UNITS OF ALCOHOL

- The alcohol content of a drink is usually expressed by the standard measure "alcohol by volume," or ABV. This is a measure of the amount of pure alcohol as a percentage of the total volume of liquid in a drink and can be found on the labels of cans and bottles. For example, if the label on a can of beer states "5% ABV" or "alcohol volume 5%," this means that 5% of the volume of that drink is pure alcohol.

- The number of units in any drink can be calculated by multiplying the total volume of a drink (in millilitres) by its ABV (which is measured as a percentage) and dividing the result by 1000. For example, the number of units in a pint (568 mL) of strong lager (ABV 5%) would be calculated:

- This is worth doing, as the increasing strength of many alcoholic drinks and the larger glass sizes served in bars mean that people are often drinking more alcohol than they realise.

Units calculators are available (for example, www.nhs.uk/Tools/Pages/Alcohol-unit-calculator.aspx)

BOX 2: DELIVERING ALCOHOL IDENTIFICATION AND BRIEF ADVICE IN PRACTICE

The rationale

- A large body of international research evidence indicates that 1 in 8 people drinking at increasing risk or higher risk levels who receive structured brief advice reduce their drinking to within lower risk levels.[4] Raising the problem of alcohol consumption with patients often meets with several attitudes, including indifference, confusion about what is and is not healthy, and possibly defensiveness and irritability. Clinicians should ensure that they are aware of the facts about alcohol consumption and health related harms to convey the risks of drinking to patients accurately. It is important to avoid stigmatising terms such as "alcoholic," emphasising the concept of increasing risk with increasing consumption and suggesting trying to cut down to a lower risk level rather than stopping. Clinicians should also be able to detect alcohol dependence and refer to specialist help.

Stage 1: raise the problem

- The most time and resource effective strategy in non-specialist settings is to target those at greatest risk—that is, people with relevant physical (for example, hypertension, gastrointestinal or liver problems) or mental health (anxiety or depression) conditions, at risk of self harm, or who regularly experience unintentional injuries or minor trauma.

- Ask the first three questions on the AUDIT questionnaire (see fig 2) and score the answers (known as AUDIT-C).

- *Score of ≥5*—suggests a high likelihood that the patient is drinking at an increasing risk level, and the full AUDIT questionnaire should be administered (this threshold may be reduced to 3 or more in young people aged less than 18 years or adults older than 65 years)[30] [31]

Stage 2: administer and score the 10 item AUDIT questionnaire

- *Score ≤7*—this result should be fed back in a positive manner—for example, reiterate the sensible drinking guidelines and point out that people who exceed these levels increase their chances of alcohol related health problems such as unintentional injuries, high blood pressure, liver disease, cancer, and heart disease, while congratulating them for adhering to guidance

- *Score 8-19*—this suggests that the patient's drinking pattern is in the increasing risk or higher risk band, and clinicians should move to offering brief advice as described in stage 3

Stage 3: deliver structured brief advice

- Use an open ended "transitional" statement such as "how important is it for you to change your drinking?," possibly accompanied by a simple "readiness ruler"— that is, ask patients to rate between 1 and 10 how confident they feel in making changes. This can be followed by asking what would have to happen to make the number go up.

- A structured episode of brief advice may only last 5-10 minutes and is best guided by a structured advice tool (for example, www.alcohollearningcentre.org.uk/alcoholeLearning/learning/IBA/Module4_v2/pdf/structured_advice_tool.pdf). This makes use of the FRAMES (feedback, responsibility, advice, menu, empathy, self efficacy) structure for brief interventions. The leaflet provides material to use for three of these elements:

- Feedback on patients' level of drinking when compared with others, the common effects of drinking, and the potential benefits of reduction

- A menu of options to support the attainment of their preferred drinking goal

- Advice on units and limits

- Clinicians should aim to be firm enough to ensure that patients realise that it is their responsibility to make the change (restating the need to reduce risk and encouraging patients to begin now), while also showing empathy (for example, "it can be very difficult to make these changes if everyone around you is drinking heavily") and aiming to boost their confidence and self efficacy ("You mentioned you were going to drink a non-alcoholic drink first when you get home in the evening. That sounds like an excellent start. Let's see how you get on and arrange another time to talk to discuss how you get on").

- It is a good idea to offer a follow-up appointment to assess progress. An "extended brief intervention" places greater emphasis on exploring the pros and cons of change and formulating a specific action plan. This approach is often based on the principles of motivational interviewing,[18] and again is best guided by a structured leaflet such as the one available at www.alcohollearningcentre.org.uk/alcoholeLearning/learning/IBA/Module5_v2/extended_intervention_worksheet.pdf.

- Patients should be referred for more specialist alcohol assessment and intervention if they ask for such help, already exhibit major alcohol related harm, have an AUDIT score of >20, or exhibit features of the alcohol dependence syndrome.

A step by step teaching module and full range of materials is available at www.alcohollearningcentre.org.uk/eLearning/.

---

to specialist services (box 2). Owing to the potentially more important effects of alcohol on certain populations, scores should be revised downward when screening young people aged less than 18, or adults aged more than 65 (see box 2). Biochemical measures such as liver function tests are not normally used for screening, but may be helpful in assessing the severity and progress of an established alcohol related problem, or as part of a secondary care assessment.[17]

A guiding style that aims to build motivation and avoid confrontation is recommended, and motivational interviewing

has shown considerable promise in this area. Although a review is beyond the scope of this article, useful materials can be found at www.motivationalinterviewing.org.

What treatments are available for alcohol dependence in the non-specialist setting?

Identification and brief advice is an important public health approach because of the numbers of people drinking at increasing risk or higher risk levels. However, even after gold standard brief interventions in primary care, nearly two

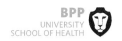

Table 1 Classification and definition of alcohol use disorders

Category of drinking	Definition	AUDIT score
Low risk	No amount of alcohol consumption can be called "safe," but risks of harm are low if consumption is below levels specified in the "increasing risk" category (below)	≤7
Increasing risk (hazardous)	Regularly drinking more than 2 or 3 units a day (women) and more than 3 or 4 units a day (men)	8-15
Higher risk (harmful)	Regularly drinking more than 6 units daily (women) or more than 8 units daily (men), or more than 35 units weekly (women) or more than 50 units weekly (men)	16-19
Dependence, as defined by ICD-10 (international classification of diseases, 10th revision)[9]	A definite diagnosis of dependence should be made only if three or more of the following have been present at the same time during the previous year: (a) a strong desire or sense of compulsion to drink alcohol; difficulties in controlling drinking behaviour in terms of its onset, termination, or levels of consumption; a physiological withdrawal state when drinking has stopped or been reduced, as evidenced by the characteristic alcohol withdrawal syndrome, or use of the same (or a closely related) substance with the intention of relieving or avoiding withdrawal symptoms—for example, benzodiazepines; (d) evidence of tolerance, such that increased quantities of alcohol are required to achieve the effects originally produced by lesser amounts; (e) progressive neglect of alternative pleasures or interests because of alcohol consumption, increased amount of time necessary to obtain or drink alcohol or to recover from its effects; (f) persisting with drinking alcohol despite clear evidence of overtly harmful consequences, such as harm to the liver, depressive mood states, or impaired cognitive functioning. It is an essential characteristic of the dependence syndrome that either alcohol consumption or a desire to drink alcohol is present; the subjective awareness of compulsion to drink alcohol is most commonly seen during attempts to stop or control substance use	≥20

AUDIT=alcohol use disorders identification test.

Table 2 Suggested titrated fixed dose chlordiazepoxide protocol for treatment of alcohol withdrawal. From National Collaborating Centre for Mental Health[19]

Treatment day	15-25 units/day		30-49 units/day		50-60 units/day
	Moderate dependence: SADQ score 15-25		Severe dependence: SADQ score 30-40		Very severe dependence: SADQ score 40-60
Day 1 (starting dose)	15 mg four times/day	25 mg four times/day	30 mg four times/day	40 mg four times/day*	50 mg four times/day†
Day 2	10 mg four times/day	20 mg four times/day	25 mg four times/day	35 mg four times/day*	45 mg four times/day†
Day 3	10 mg three times/day	15 mg four times/day	20 mg four times/day	30 mg four times/day	40 mg four times/day*
Day 4	5 mg three times/day	10 mg four times/day	15 mg four times/day	25 mg four times/day	35 mg four times/day*
Day 5	5 mg twice/day	10 mg three times/day	10 mg four times/day	20 mg four times/day	30 mg four times/day
Day 6	5 mg at night	5 mg three times/day	10 mg three times/day	15 mg four times/day	25 mg four times/day
Day 7	—	5 mg twice/day	5 mg three times/day	10 mg four times/day	20 mg four times/day
Day 8	—	5 mg at night	5 mg twice/day	10 mg three times/day	15 mg four times/day
Day 9	—	—	5 mg at night	5 mg three times/day	10 mg four times/day
Day 10	—	—	—	5 mg twice/day	10 mg three times/day
Day 11	—	—	—	5 mg at night	5 mg three times/day
Day 12	—	—	—	—	5 mg twice/day
Day 13	—	—	—	—	5 mg at night

SADQ=severity of alcohol dependence questionnaire (www.alcohollearningcentre.org.uk/Topics/Latest/Resource/?cid=4615).

*Doses of chlordiazepoxide >30 mg four times/day should be prescribed only in severe alcohol dependence, with response to treatment monitored regularly and closely.

†Doses of chlordiazepoxide >40 mg four times/day should be prescribed only in very severe alcohol dependence. Such doses are rarely necessary in women and children and never in older people or in patients with liver impairment.

thirds of people will still be drinking at an increasing or higher risk level.[15] At the "dependent" end of the drinking spectrum, change is even more difficult to achieve. People with a moderate to severe level of alcohol dependence may benefit from more intensive help from mutual aid groups such as Alcoholics Anonymous or specialist treatment services, or both.[4] Abstinence is the preferred goal for many such people, particularly for those whose organs have already been damaged through alcohol use, or for those who have previously attempted to cut down their drinking without success. In considering the correct level of treatment intensity it is important to consider risks, capacity to consent to treatment, the experience and outcome of previous episodes of treatment, motivation for change, and other existing problems, including harm to others.

Three interventions may assist generalists in altering the drinking trajectory: medically assisted withdrawal, facilitation through mutual aid, and use of drugs to prevent relapse.

Medically assisted withdrawal

The alcohol withdrawal syndrome develops when consumption is abruptly stopped or substantially reduced, and symptoms and signs appear within 6-8 hours. These include anxiety, tremor, sweating, nausea, tachycardia, and hypertension, usually peaking over 10-30 hours and subsiding within two or three days. Seizures may occur in the first 12-48 hours (but rarely after this), and delirium tremens is a serious condition that occurs 48-72 hours after cessation of drinking, characterised by coarse tremor, agitation, fever, tachycardia, profound confusion, delusions (characteristically frightening), auditory and visual hallucinations, and possibly hyperpyrexia, ketoacidosis, and circulatory collapse.

Minor degrees of alcohol withdrawal are common and can be managed with information, reassurance, and adequate fluid intake. However, the alcohol withdrawal syndrome is potentially life threatening; systematic reviews recommend long acting benzodiazepines (chlordiazepoxide or diazepam) as the drug of choice for managing the alcohol withdrawal syndrome and preventing serious complications such as

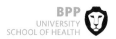

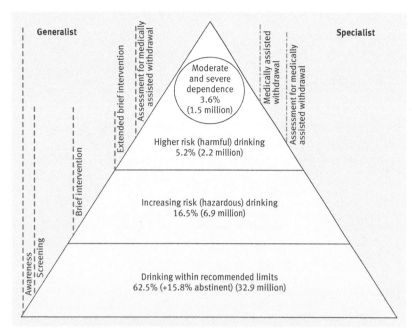

Fig 1 Prevalence of alcohol use disorders in England (taken from general household survey 2009 and psychiatric morbidity survey 2007) and recommended treatment strategies across the spectrum

Alcohol use disorders identification test (AUDIT)

1. How often do you have a drink containing alcohol?
(0) Never
(1) Monthly or less
(2) 2-4 times a month
(3) 2-3 times a week
(4) 4 or more times a week

2. How many units of alcohol do you have on a typical day when you are drinking?
(0) 1 or 2
(1) 3 or 4
(2) 5 or 6
(3) 7, 8, or 9
(4) 10 or more

3. How often do you have 6 or more units if female, or 8 or more units if male, on a single occasion in the past year?
(0) Never
(1) Less than monthly
(2) Monthly
(3) Weekly
(4) Daily or almost daily

4. How often during the past year have you found that you were not able to stop drinking once you had started?
(0) Never
(1) Less than monthly
(2) Monthly
(3) Weekly
(4) Daily or almost daily

5. How often during the past year have you failed to do what was normally expected from you because of drinking?
(0) Never
(1) Less than monthly
(2) Monthly
(3) Weekly
(4) Daily or almost daily

6. How often during the past year have you needed a first drink in the morning to get yourself going after a heavy drinking session?
(0) Never
(1) Less than monthly
(2) Monthly
(3) Weekly
(4) Daily or almost daily

7. How often during the past year have you had a feeling of guilt or remorse after drinking?
(0) Never
(1) Less than monthly
(2) Monthly
(3) Weekly
(4) Daily or almost daily

8. How often during the past year have you been unable to remember what happened the night before because you had been drinking?
(0) Never
(1) Less than monthly
(2) Monthly
(3) Weekly
(4) Daily or almost daily

9. Have you or someone else been injured as a result of your drinking?
(0) No
(2) Yes, but not in the past year
(4) Yes, during the past year

10. Has a relative or friend, doctor, or another health worker been concerned about your drinking or suggested that you cut down?
(0) No
(2) Yes, but not in the past year
(4) Yes, during the past year

Total score: ☐

Fig 2 Alcohol use disorders identification test

seizures or delirium tremens.[19][20] The aim is to titrate the initial dose to the extent of withdrawal symptoms and then slowly to reduce the dose over 7-10 days using a standard fixed dose protocol (table 2). Rating scales such as the clinical institute withdrawal assessment for alcohol (CIWA-Ar) can be used to measure the severity of the withdrawal symptoms and more accurately adjust the dose, but the use of such a regimen triggered by symptoms is only recommended if trained staff are available, such as in an inpatient setting.[21] Prescribing in the community for alcohol dependent patients without adequate assessment and support is not recommended, as successful withdrawal is unlikely and there are considerable associated clinical risks. This is a common scenario facing general practitioners, and expeditious referral to specialist services for support from a specialist alcohol nurse during medicated withdrawal is advised.

Doses of benzodiazepines should be reduced for children and young people aged less than 18 years, adults aged more than 65 years, and those with impaired liver synthetic function, such as reduced albumin or increased prothrombin time (where a benzodiazepine requiring less metabolism within the liver, such as oxazepam, may be preferred). Clinicians should be aware of complications from nutritional deficiency, such as the Wernicke-Korsakoff syndrome. This should be suspected in anyone with a history of alcohol dependence and one or more of ophthalmoplegia, ataxia, acute confusion, memory disturbance, or unexplained hypotension, hypothermia, or unconsciousness. Treatment with intramuscular or intravenous thiamine is important to prevent permanent memory loss and should continue until the symptoms and signs stop improving.[21] Most episodes of medically assisted alcohol withdrawal can take place at home, but inpatient treatment should be considered if patients drink more than 30 units of alcohol daily, have a history of epilepsy, withdrawal related seizures, or delirium tremens, or have comorbid physical or mental health conditions.[19]

Mutual aid facilitation

Treatment of alcohol withdrawal is not sufficient on its own and should be viewed as the precursor to a longer term treatment and rehabilitation process. Research consistently shows that people with alcohol dependence who have stopped drinking are vulnerable to relapse and that they may have unresolved problems that predispose them to it.[22] Mutual aid groups (for example, Alcoholics Anonymous and UK SMART Recovery) are a source of ongoing support for people seeking recovery from alcohol dependence, and for partners, friends, children, and other family members. Long term cohort studies show that people who actively participate in mutual aid are more likely to sustain their recovery,[23] and NICE recommends that treatment staff should routinely provide information about mutual aid groups and facilitate access for those who want to attend.[19]

Clinicians should be aware of the range of mutual aid groups available locally and how to access them. Level of clinician knowledge about Alcoholics Anonymous groups has been positively correlated with levels of referral,[24] and attending a meeting is an invaluable learning experience. Evidence from randomised controlled trials suggests that proactive efforts to engage patients with mutual aid groups increase attendance, particularly introducing the patient to a group member in advance of a meeting.[25] A simple three stage process to guide this is available (www.nta.nhs.uk/uploads/mutualaid-fama.pdf).

Relapse prevention drugs

Interventions based on psychological or social processes of change are the mainstay of treatment for alcohol dependence.[26] Although research suggests that such

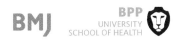

treatments lead to improved outcomes when compared with no treatment, the evidence favouring one type of psychological intervention over another is less clear. Other factors such as therapist characteristics and service variables are also important. The uptake and implementation of psychological approaches in the United Kingdom vary widely,[19][27] and most practice involves an eclectic approach that combines strategies from various psychological approaches and typically lasts 12 weeks. In those who have

---

TIPS FOR NON-SPECIALISTS

- Consider the far reaching effects of alcohol, not only to individual physical and mental health, but to family members and the community as a whole
- Screen for alcohol problems in all healthcare settings, and particularly in high risk populations
- Providing structured brief advice and feedback is an effective strategy in high risk drinkers
- Adopt a positive, motivational approach to managing alcohol use disorders
- Take a long term, stepped care perspective, moving to more intensive interventions when a less intensive option has not worked
- Promote attendance at mutual aid groups such as Alcoholics Anonymous or UK SMART Recovery wherever possible

---

QUESTIONS FOR FUTURE RESEARCH

- What methods are effective for assessing and diagnosing the presence and severity of alcohol use disorders in children and young people?
- What are the most effective strategies for facilitating the delivery of alcohol identification and brief advice in routine clinical practice?
- Is an assertive community treatment model for moderate to severe alcohol dependence clinically and cost effective compared with standard care?
- For people with alcohol dependence, which drug is most likely to improve adherence and thereby promote abstinence and prevent relapse?

ADDITIONAL EDUCATIONAL RESOURCES

Resources for healthcare professionals

- Public Health England Alcohol Learning Resources (www.alcohollearningcentre.org.uk/)—Collates the latest news on evidence based approaches to alcohol use disorders and their implementation in clinical practice. Includes the Alcohol Identification and Brief Advice e-learning project (www.alcohollearningcentre.org.uk/eLearning/IBA), a step by step interactive course on how to deliver identification and brief advice for professionals (free access)
- NICE pathways (http://pathways.nice.org.uk/pathways/alcohol-use-disorders)—Summarises all three NICE guidelines (PH24, CG100, and CG115) in the form of an interactive flowchart, and gathers together other resources such as service improvement audits, advice for commissioners, and information for the public (free access)
- World Health Organization global status report on alcohol and health 2014 (www.who.int/substance_abuse/publications/global_alcohol_report/en/)—A comprehensive perspective on the global consumption of alcohol, patterns of drinking, health consequences, and policy responses (free access)
- National Institute of Alcohol and Alcoholism (http://pubs.niaaa.nih.gov/publications/Practitioner/CliniciansGuide2005/guide.pdf)—A practical guide on alcohol and alcoholism (free access)
- National Institute for Health and Care Excellence. Alcohol-use disorders: diagnosis, assessment and management of harmful drinking and alcohol dependence. (Clinical guideline 115)—Chapter 2 provides a detailed review of the causes and consequences of alcohol use disorders

Resources for patients

- Change 4 Life (www.nhs.uk/Change4Life/Pages/drink-less-alcohol.aspx)—An interactive web based programme to help people drink less
- Alcoholics Anonymous (www.alcoholics-anonymous.org.uk/) and UK SMART Recovery (www.smartrecovery.org.uk)—Mutual aid organisations providing free meetings and support throughout the United Kingdom
- Alcohol Concern (www.alcoholconcern.org.uk/help-and-advice)—Help and advice with finding an alcohol treatment service in the United Kingdom
- Adfam (www.adfam.org.uk/)—A charity aiming to improve support for families affected by drug and alcohol problems

---

decided to become abstinent from alcohol, this treatment is enhanced by both attendance at a mutual aid group and the prescribing of relapse prevention drugs. Several drugs can be prescribed in primary care, although they may all be started and monitored by a specialist.

Acamprosate and the opioid antagonist naltrexone—both these drugs are effective in increasing the time to first drink and to relapse in people with alcohol dependence who have achieved abstinence.[19] Acamprosate may also be neuroprotective and is believed to act by altering the balance between excitatory and inhibitory neurotransmission.[20] Naltrexone seems to reduce cravings by reducing the reinforcing effect of alcohol consumption. Both drugs should only be used in combination with an individual psychological intervention, started as soon as possible after withdrawal, and may be prescribed for six months or more depending on perceived benefit. Systematic reviews suggest a number needed to treat to prevent return to any drinking of between 12 and 20.[28]

Disulfiram—this drug works by interfering with the metabolism of alcohol, causing an accumulation of acetaldehyde in the body and a throbbing headache, facial flushing, palpitations, dyspnoea, tachycardia, nausea, and vomiting within 10 minutes of alcohol consumption. Its use as a deterrent is most suited to people who have abstinence as a goal and who have someone to supervise consumption each day. Treatment should be started at least 24 hours after the last alcoholic drink and should be used with caution in the context of pregnancy, liver disease, severe mental illness, stroke, heart disease, or hypertension. Patients need to know about the symptoms caused by the interaction between alcohol and disulfiram and the rare and unpredictable onset of hepatotoxicity, which is unrelated to dose.

Nalmefene—is an opioid antagonist that is indicated for the reduction of alcohol consumption in adults with alcohol dependence who have a high risk drinking level (>7.5 units/day in men and >5 units/day in women), but without physical withdrawal symptoms and who do not need immediate medically assisted withdrawal. The drug should be started only in patients who continue to have a high risk drinking level two weeks after initial assessment, and it should only be prescribed in conjunction with continuous psychosocial support focused on treatment adherence and reducing alcohol consumption. Such psychosocial support can be delivered in primary care, and this seems to be a cost effective approach to dealing with higher risk drinking.[29] The recommended dose is one tablet on each day the patient perceives a risk of drinking, ideally 1-2 hours before the anticipated time of drinking.

When should people with alcohol use disorders be referred?

Referral for specialist treatment should be considered if patients have failed to benefit from a brief intervention or an extended brief intervention and want to receive further help, show signs of moderate or severe alcohol dependence (see table 1), or have severe alcohol related physical impairment or a related comorbid condition (for example, liver disease or mental health problems). General practitioners should actively encourage patients to attend local mutual aid groups such as Alcoholics Anonymous, as well as access local specialist services for full assessment and management. The general practitioner's role in supporting patients and their family is crucial, as in any long term chronic disorder.

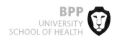
Contributors: ED was approached to write this review and produced the first draft. ED and AC were part of the guideline development group that produced the NICE clinical guideline 115, and used the searches conducted as part of the NICE process as the basis for the review. AC and MH commented on the initial draft and contributed sections on brief interventions (AC, MH), specialist treatment (AC), and drug treatment in primary care (MH). ED is the guarantor.

Competing interests: We have read and understood the BMJ policy on declaration of interests and declare: ED is a member of the Addictions Department at the Institute of Psychiatry, Psychology and Neuroscience, King's College London. The department is in receipt of or has received grants from the Medical Research Council (MRC) and the National Institute for Health Research (NIHR) to research both drug and psychosocial treatments for alcohol use disorders. He is currently a coinvestigator on NIHR Health Technology Assessment grant (13/86/03) to investigate the effectiveness of adjunctive medication management and contingency management in enhancing adherence to drugs for relapse prevention in alcohol dependence. He is a trustee of the charities Action on Addiction and Changes UK. AC is an honorary member of the School of Psychology at the University of Birmingham, and his department is in receipt or has received grants from the MRC and the NIHR to research psychosocial treatments for alcohol use disorders. He is chief investigator on a randomised controlled trial of a family and social network intervention for young people who misuse alcohol and drugs (HTA grant 11/60/01) and principal investigator on a pilot study to assess the feasibility and impact of a motivational intervention on problem drug and alcohol use in adult mental health inpatient units (NIHR—PB-PG-1010-23138). He is an expert advisor to the charity Action on Addiction. MH is a member of SMMGP (Substance Misuse Management in General Practice) and has been funded through SMMGP by Lundbeck to complete and tutor on the SMMGP advanced certificate in the community management of alcohol disorders.

Provenance and peer review: Commissioned; externally peer reviewed.

1 World Health Organization. Global status report on alcohol and health 2014. WHO, 2014.
2 Office for National Statistics. General lifestyle survey overview: a report on the 2009 general lifestyle survey. In: Dunstan S, ed. ONS, 2011.
3 Health and Social Care Information Centre. Statistics on alcohol: England, 2013. HSCIC, 2013.
4 National Institute for Health and Care Excellence. Alcohol-use disorders: preventing harmful drinking. (Public health guidance 24.) 2010. www.nice.org.uk/guidance/ph24.
5 Funk M, Wutzke S, Kaner E, Anderson P, Pas L, McCormick R, et al. A multicountry controlled trial of strategies to promote dissemination and implementation of brief alcohol intervention in primary health care: findings of a World Health Organization collaborative study. J Stud Alcohol 2005;66:379-88.
6 Babor T, Caetano R, Casswell S, Edwards G, Giesbrecht N, Graham K, et al. Alcohol: no ordinary commodity: research and public policy. 2nd ed. Oxford University Press, 2010.
7 Rice P, Drummond C. The price of a drink: the potential of alcohol minimum unit pricing as a public health measure in the UK. Br J Psychiatry 2012;201:169-71.
8 House of Commons Science and Technology Committee. Alcohol guidelines: 11th report of session 2010-2012. Stationery Office, 2012.
9 World Health Organization. The ICD-10 classification of mental and behavioural disorders. Geneva: WHO, 1992.
10 American Psychiatric Association. Diagnostic and statistical manual of mental disorders, fifth edition. American Psychiatric Publishing, 2013.
11 Hasin DS, O'Brien CP, Auriacombe M, et al. DSM-5 Criteria for Substance Use Disorders: Recommendations and Rationale. Am J Psychiatry 2013;170:834-51.
12 Heather N. A radical but flawed proposal: comments on Rehm et al. defining substance use disorders: do we really need more than heavy use? Alcohol Alcohol 2013;48:646-7.
13 Rehm J, Marmet S, Anderson P, Gual A, Kraus L, Nutt DJ, et al. Defining substance use disorders: do we really need more than heavy use? Alcohol Alcohol 2013;48:633-40.
14 Jackson R, Johnson M, Campbell F, Messina J, Guillaume L, Meier P, et al. Screening and brief intervention for prevention and early identification of alcohol use disorder in adults and young people. School of Health and Related Research (ScHARR) Public Health Collaborating Centre, 2010.
15 Kaner E, Bland M, Cassidy P, Coulton S, Dale V, Deluca P, et al. Effectiveness of screening and brief alcohol intervention in primary care (SIPS trial): pragmatic cluster randomised controlled trial. BMJ 2013;346:e8501.
16 Babor TF, Higgins-Biddle JC, Saunders JB, Monteiro MG. AUDIT: the alcohol use disorder identification test. Guidelines for use in primary health care. World Health Organization, 2001. http://whqlibdoc.who.int/hq/2001/WHO_MSD_MSB_01.6a.pdf?ua=1.
17 Drummond C, Ghodse H, Chengappa S. Use of investigations in the diagnosis and management of alcohol use disorders. In: Day E, ed. Clinical topics in addiction. RCPsych Publications, 2007:113-29.
18 Rollnick S, Butler CC, Kinnersley P, Gregory J, Mash B. Motivational interviewing. BMJ 2010;340:1242-5.
19 National Collaborating Centre for Mental Health. Alcohol-use disorders: the NICE guideline on diagnosis, assessment and management of harmful drinking and alcohol dependence. British Psychological Society and Royal College of Psychiatrists, 2011.
20 Lingford-Hughes AR, Welch S, Peters L, Nutt DJ; British Association for Psychopharmacology, Expert Reviewers Group. BAP updated guidelines: evidence-based guidelines for the pharmacological management of substance abuse, harmful use, addiction and comorbidity: recommendations from BAP. J Psychopharmacol 2012;26:899-952.
21 National Institute for Health and Care Excellence. Alcohol-use disorders: diagnosis and clinical management of alcohol-related physical complications. (Clinical guideline 100.) 2010. http://guidance.nice.org.uk/CG100.
22 Marlatt GA, Gordon JR. Relapse prevention: maintenance strategies in the treatment of addictive behaviors. Guilford Press, 1985.
23 Moos RH, Moos BS. Participation in treatment and Alcoholics Anonymous: a 16-year follow-up of initially untreated individuals. J Clin Psychol 2006;62:735-50.
24 Wall R, Sondhi A, Day E. What influences referral to 12-step mutual self-help groups by treatment professionals. Eur Addict Res 2014;20:241-7.
25 Timko C, DeBenedetti A. A randomized controlled trial of intensive referral to 12-step self-help groups: one-year outcomes. Drug Alcohol Depend 2007;90:270-9.
26 Raistrick D, Heather N, Godfrey C. Review of the effectiveness of treatment for alcohol problems. National Treatment Agency for Substance Misuse, 2006. www.nta.nhs.uk/uploads/nta_review_of_the_effectiveness_of_treatment_for_alcohol_problems_fullreport_2006_alcohol2.pdf.
27 Drummond C, Oyefeso A, Phillips T, Cheeta S, Deluca P, Perryman K, et al. Alcohol needs assessment research project (ANARP). The 2004 national alcohol needs assessment for England. Department of Health, 2004:1-31.
28 Jonas DE, Amick HR, Feltner C, Bobashev G, Thomas K, Wines R, et al. Pharmacotherapy for adults with alcohol use disorders in outpatient settings: a systematic review and meta-analysis. JAMA 2014;311:1889-900.
29 National Institute for Health and Care Excellence. Nalmefene for reducing alcohol consumption in people with alcohol dependence. (Technology appraisal guidance TA325). 2014. www.nice.org.uk/guidance/ta325.
30 Public Health England. Young people's hospital alcohol pathways: support pack for A&E departments. PHE, 2014.
31 Center for Substance Abuse Treatment. Alcohol use among older adults: pocket screening for health and social care providers. Substance Abuse and Mental Health Services Administration, 2001.

Related links

thebmj.com
- Access this article online to hear a linked podcast interview with the authors

bmj.com/archive
Previous articles in this series

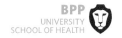

Assessment and management of cannabis use disorders in primary care

Adam R Winstock, clinical senior lecturer, honorary consultant psychiatrist[1],
Chris Ford, clinical director[2], general practice principal[3],
John Witton, research coordinator[1]

[1]National Addiction Centre, Institute of Psychiatry, King's College London, London SE5 8AF

[2]Substance Misuse Management in General Practice (SMMGP), c/o NTA, Skipton House, London SE1 6LH

[3]24 Lonsdale Road, London NW6 6SY

Correspondence to: A R Winstock
Adam.winstock@kcl.ac.uk

Cite this as: BMJ 2010;340:c1571

DOI: 10.1136/bmj.c1571

http://www.bmj.com/content/340/bmj.c1571

About a third of adults in the UK have tried cannabis, and 2.5 million people, mostly 16-29 year olds, have used it in the past year.[1] Although most people who smoke cannabis will develop neither severe mental health problems nor dependence, regular use of cannabis may be associated with a range of health, emotional, behavioural, social, and legal problems, particularly in young, pregnant, and severely mentally ill people.[2][3] The past decade has seen a shift in available cannabis preparations from resinous "hash" to intensively grown high potency herbal preparations, often referred to as skunk, which now dominates the UK market.[4] Compared with traditional cannabis preparations, skunk tends to have higher levels of tetrahydrocannabinol, the main psychoactive constituent of cannabis, and lower levels of the anxiolytic cannabinoid cannabidiol. In January 2009 cannabis was returned to its original class B classification (from class C) under the UK Misuse of Drugs Act.

Despite high levels of use, only 6% of those seeking treatment for substance misuse in England cite cannabis as their major drug of concern, and most of those with cannabis use disorders do not have cannabis use as their presenting complaint (box 1).[5] Low levels of treatment seeking may reflect a lack of awareness of the associated harms of cannabis.[w1] This review highlights the adverse health outcomes associated with cannabis and outlines optimal approaches to assessing and managing cannabis use in primary care.

Methods

We searched electronic databases, including Medline and PsycINFO; the Cochrane Library; specialist websites; databases of England's National Treatment Agency for Substance Misuse and of the UK centre DrugScope; the US National Institute on Drug Abuse; the European Monitoring Centre for Drugs and Drug Addiction; and Australia's National Cannabis Prevention and Information Centre. We also consulted primary care providers and specialists in addiction treatment.

SUMMARY POINTS

- Cannabis use is common, especially among young people
- The greatest risk of harm from cannabis use is in young people and those who are pregnant or have serious mental illness
- A tenth of cannabis users develop dependence, with three quarters of them experiencing withdrawal symptoms on cessation
- Most dependent users have concurrent dependence on tobacco, which increases the health risks and worsens outcomes for cannabis treatment
- Brief interventions and advice on harm reduction can improve outcomes
- Psychoeducation (for a better understanding of dependence), sleep hygiene, nicotine replacement therapy (where indicated), and brief symptomatic relief form the mainstay of withdrawal management
- Dependent users may present with symptoms suggestive of depression, but diagnosis and treatment should be deferred until two to four weeks after withdrawal to improve diagnostic accuracy

How does cannabis exert its effect?

Metabolites of cannabis act on the body's endogenous cannabinoid system via type 1 cannabinoid receptors (CB1 receptors) in the central nervous system and CB2 receptors peripherally. They may modulate mood, memory, cognition, sleep, and appetite.[w2]

What are the effects of intoxication?

Most people smoke cannabis for its relaxant and euphoriant effects (box 2). The impact of higher potency cannabis will depend partly on its ratio of tetrahydrocannabinol to cannabidiol and whether users are able and willing to titrate their consumption as they might alcohol.[3][6] The authors of a recent review suggested that more potent forms may increase the risk of dependence and adverse psychological experiences.[3]

Routes of use

Cannabis is often rolled in a cigarette paper and smoked with tobacco in a "joint" or "spliff," and it produces inhaled carcinogens. Most carcinogens in tobacco are present in cannabis. Typical cannabis use results in a larger volume of smoke being inhaled than with ordinary tobacco products and a fivefold increase in concentrations of carboxyhaemoglobin.[7] Tetrahydrocannabinol is fat soluble and is absorbed from the gastrointestinal tract. Although oral ingestion of cannabis avoids the risks associated with smoking, secondary active metabolites are formed and dose titration is difficult.[w3] Oral use may lead to intense, unpredictable prolonged intoxication.[w4]

Harms and risks associated with the use of cannabis

Table 1 (table 1) outlines the harms and risks associated with cannabis use, such as acute and chronic effects and possible risks in specific populations.

Associations with use at young age

Large population based longitudinal studies have shown that the earlier the age of first use of cannabis, the greater the risk of dependence, other problems of substance misuse, mental health problems, and poor emotional, academic, and social development.[3][w5] Vulnerability to the reinforcing positive effects of cannabis use and to dependence, has a heritable component.[w6]

Pulmonary harms

Cannabis smoking shows a dose-response relation with pulmonary risk in the same way that tobacco smoking does. A longitudinal study of young cannabis smokers showed that regular heavy use can produce chronic inflammatory changes in the respiratory tract, resulting in increased symptoms of chronic bronchitis such as coughing, shortness of breath, production of sputum, and wheezing.[8] A study comparing results of pulmonary function tests and computed tomography scans across different smoking groups estimated

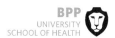

BOX 1 WHAT PROBLEMS MIGHT CANNABIS USERS PRESENT WITH IN PRIMARY CARE?

- Respiratory problems, such as exacerbation of asthma, chronic obstructive airways disease, wheeze or prolonged cough, or other chest symptoms
- Mental health symptoms, such as anxiety, depression, paranoia, panic, depersonalisation, exacerbation of an underlying mental health condition
- Problems with concentration while studying or with employment and relationships
- Difficulties stopping cannabis use
- Legal or employment problems (arising from use of cannabis)

BOX 2 PHYSIOLOGICAL AND PSYCHOLOGICAL EFFECTS OF CANNABIS*

Psychological (mood/perceptual) effects

- A sense of euphoria and relaxation
- Perceptual distortions, time distortion, and the intensification of sensory experiences
- Impairment of attention, concentration, short term memory, information processing, and reaction time
- Feelings of greater emotional and physical sensitivity
- Anxiety, panic, and paranoia

Physiological effects

- Increase in appetite
- Increase in heart rate, decrease in blood pressure
- Conjunctival injection and suffusion
- Dry mouth
- Impaired psychomotor coordination and sedation

*The effects peak after 30 minutes and last for two to four hours

Table 1 Harms and risks associated with cannabis use. Adapted from the 2009 guidelines from Australia's National Cannabis Prevention and Information Centre[w7] and from Hall and Degenhardt[3]

Acute intoxication risks	Impaired attention, memory, and psychomotor performance while intoxicated
	Increased risk of road traffic crashes, especially if cannabis is mixed with alcohol
	Psychotic symptoms at high doses
Most probable chronic effects	Dependence (1 in 10 users)
	Subtle cognitive impairment in attention, verbal memory, and the organisation and integration of complex information in daily user (with >10 years' use). Some evidence of reversibility with prolonged abstinence
	Pulmonary disease and respiratory symptoms such as chronic obstructive pulmonary disease and chronic cough (synergistic harm with tobacco)
	Malignancy of the oropharynx
Possible chronic effects	Xerostomia (dry mouth) and consequent dental health problems
	Some evidence that cannabis may affect female fertility
	In utero exposure to cannabis may lead to low birthweight babies and later behavioural, problem solving, and attention difficulties
	Increased rate of lung cancer
Probable risks in specific populations	Impaired personal and educational attainment
	Adolescent cannabis use is associated with: higher rates of truancy, delinquency, and criminality; higher rates of problems of other substance misuse, including alcohol; poorer academic achievement and educational attainment, with more unemployment; lower levels of relationship satisfaction; possible exacerbation of mental health conditions such as depression, anxiety, and psychotic conditions
Limited or no evidence	Birth defects (except low birth weight, for which good evidence exists)

that one cannabis joint caused the equivalent airflow obstruction associated with smoking two and a half to five cigarettes.[9] A recent cross sectional study examining an older population of smokers suggests that concurrent smoking of cannabis and tobacco leads to synergistic respiratory harm, whereas smoking cannabis alone probably does not lead to chronic obstructive pulmonary disease.[10] However, a large case-control study from New Zealand does suggest that cannabis smoking is an independent risk factor for lung malignancy; heavy smokers (more than 10 years of smoking cannabis joints) had a relative risk of 5.7 after adjustment for age, tobacco use, and family history of lung cancer.[11] A large prospective study found that cannabis use may be a risk for coronary events, especially in those with pre-existing cardiovascular disease.[w8]

Mental health and cognition

Observational evidence associates cannabis use and psychotic disorders, but causality is not established.[w9] Cannabis use is associated with double the risk of schizophrenia (from 0.7 in 1000 to 1.4 in 1000), and some evidence exists that starting use under the age of 16 years increases the risk.[12] A cross sectional study showed that a family history of psychotic illness and a personal history of unusual experiences raised the risk of psychotic illness associated with cannabis use.[13] A recent review highlighted consistent evidence that onset of schizophrenia presents earlier (by 1.9-6.7 years) in male cannabis smokers.[14] A recent systematic review found that cannabis use was associated with increased relapse and non-adherence to medication in patients with schizophrenia.[15]

Cross sectional and cohort studies have found higher levels of depressive symptoms in cannabis users than in non-users.[w10] However, a systematic review concluded that cannabis use does not cause affective disorders.[12] Rates of cannabis use are higher in those with anxiety disorders than in those without, and heavy users of cannabis have higher levels of anxiety, but the nature of this relation is not clear.[16]

Differentiating between chronic cannabis intoxication and psychiatric disorders

The presenting symptoms of chronic cannabis use and intoxication can sometimes be confused with those of depression (lethargy, sleep and appetite disturbance, social withdrawal, problems at work or at home, cognitive impairment). Symptoms may improve or resolve outside periods of intoxication or withdrawal. Psychiatric disorders that are unrelated to cannabis use may have been present before the onset of use and their symptoms are likely to persist with abstinence from cannabis. If symptoms resolve when cannabis use ceases, the likelihood of a primary psychiatric diagnosis diminishes. In a small inpatient withdrawal study of 20 heavy users of cannabis, mean baseline depression symptom scores reduced to normal levels after four weeks of abstinence.[17] The diagnosis of a depressive disorder and start of antidepressants should therefore usually be deferred until after a period or two to four weeks of abstinence. Resolution of affective symptoms after cessation may act as a good motivator for maintaining abstinence (fig 1).

Recent imaging studies have identified reductions in the volumes of the amygdala and hippocampus that are related to cannabis use,[18] consistent with studies that have identified duration of use and dose related impairments in memory and attention in long term heavy users of cannabis.[19]

Identifying the cannabis user for whom use is a problem

Although problems of cannabis use can arise at any level of use, however low, cannabis use disorders and other problems are more likely to arise in long term, heavy daily users than in casual, infrequent users. Screening questions about cannabis use and other substance use can accompany other lifestyle questions about tobacco and alcohol use and can be raised during consultations on smoking, mental health, and sleep disturbances (fig 2). Some patients may try to avoid such questions or they may ask subtle questions to check that drug use is OK to talk about. Others will be relieved to be asked. Questions should focus on frequency of use and amount used. If a patient's cannabis use is not impairing any aspect of psychosocial functioning, and he or she seems to control

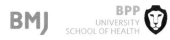

the use and recognise the risks and when use might be considered a problem, then the intervention can be restricted to giving health information and discussing risks.

Box 3 lists questions that may be useful in quantifying the level of use and confirming the presence of a cannabis use disorder. Both ICD-10 (the international classification of diseases, 10th revision) and the DSM-IV-TR (*Diagnostic and Statistical Manual of Mental Disorders*, fourth edition, text revision) recognise cannabis as a substance that causes dependence. About 1 in 10 users develops dependence.[20] Dependence is defined by a cluster of symptoms, including loss of control, inability to cut down or stop, preoccupation with use, neglecting activities unrelated to use, continued use despite experiencing problems related to use, and the development of tolerance and withdrawal (which results from the body requiring (but not receiving) more of the drug to achieve the same effect).

BOX 3 QUESTIONS TO ASK CANNABIS USERS TO IDENTIFY PROBLEMS, INCLUDING WITHDRAWAL

- How long does a gram (or an eighth of an ounce (3.5 g)) last you? How many joints a day do you smoke? How many joints do you make from a gram?
- On how many days a week or month do you smoke?
- Do you mix it with tobacco? Do you smoke cigarettes as well?
- Does your cannabis use cause you any problems, such as anxiety, cough, interference with your sleep or appetite?
- Does your smoking ever interfere with what you want to do or what you have to do, such as working or studying?
- Have you ever thought about cutting down or stopping?
- Have you ever tried to cut down or stop? What happened? Were you able to sleep? Do you get irritable or moody?
- If you managed to stop for a while, how did you feel afterwards?

BOX 4 MANAGEMENT OF WITHDRAWAL

- Advise gradual reduction in amount of cannabis used before cessation
- Suggest that the patient delays first use of cannabis till later in the day
- Suggest that the patient considers use of nicotine replacement therapy if he or she plans to stop separate tobacco use at the same time
- Advise the patient on good sleep hygiene, including avoidance of caffeine, which may exacerbate irritability, restlessness, and insomnia
- Suggest relaxation, progressive muscular relaxation, distraction
- Suggest psychoeducation sessions for the user and family members on the nature, duration, and severity of withdrawal, to help with a better understanding of dependence and reduce likelihood of relapse
- Advise the patient to avoid the cues and triggers associated with cannabis use
- Prescribe short term analgesia and sedation for withdrawal symptoms if required
- If irritability and restlessness are marked, consider prescribing very low dose diazepam for three to four days

---

BOX 5 ADVICE FOR PATIENTS ON REDUCING THEIR RISK OF HARM FROM CANNABIS*

- Do not mix cannabis with tobacco
- Avoid daily and binge use
- Do not use a cigarette filter—this will reduce the ratio of cannabis to tar (30% less cannabis, 60% more tar)
- Do not hold smoke in your lungs—this will not get you more stoned but will increase tar and carcinogens coming into contact with your lungs
- Do not inhale too deeply—most tetrahydrocannabinol is absorbed from the upper airways
- Do not mix cannabis with alcohol and/or other drugs such as cocaine
- Remove stalks and leaves
- Do not use too many papers
- Avoid using a bong (water pipe)—pulling on a bong or using a bucket may cool smoke but will also force smoke deeper into your lungs and may filter out more tetrahydrocannabinol than tar
- Avoid plastic bottles/pipes/aluminium foil as these can increase toxic fumes
- If you do use pipes and/or bongs clean them thoroughly
- Avoid cannabis use if you have a history of serious mental illness
- Do not drive while intoxicated especially if you have consumed alcohol as well as cannabis

*Adapted from 1999-2005 HIT UK[w16]

What if assessment suggests problematic use or dependency?

Although some dependent users recognise their use as problematic, others may not, and in such cases a motivational approach may be appropriate: to raise awareness of the consequences of use, explore and resolve ambivalence, and subsequently motivate change.[21] Asking the patient to draw up a pros and cons table can be good way to get them to think about their use (table 2). Although abstinence may be an optimal outcome, a reduction in use may be a more attainable initial goal.[22]

No intervention to date has proved consistently effective for the majority of those with dependence on cannabis. Trials in the United States and Australia support four methods of behavioural based interventions: motivational interviewing, motivational enhancement therapy, cognitive behavioural therapy, and contingency management.

Cognitive behavioural therapy and contingency management have the most evidence for reduction in cannabis use and maintaining abstinence.[22] For younger users, family based interventions may be more effective.[22] Brief, behaviourally based interventions suitable for delivery by general practitioners may be effective. One randomised study of a brief motivational intervention in young users showed a reduction in cannabis use from 15 days to five days a month, and at three months one in six were abstinent.[23] Extended abstinence can be supported through maintaining motivation and the use of relapse prevention techniques.[22] A randomised trial that enrolled members of the general public who fulfilled criteria for dependency explored contingency management (money vouchers for continued abstinence) and motivational and cognitive behavioural therapy interventions for maintaining abstinence. Contingency management alone led to the highest rates of initial abstinence in adult cannabis smokers, but longer term abstinence was helped by the use of coping skills and post-treatment self efficacy training.[24] A computer based intervention to treat comorbid depression and cannabis dependence tested in a randomised controlled trial seemed to have potential in managing this group.[w11]

Figure 2 outlines in an algorithm how to identify and respond to cannabis use disorders.

How to manage withdrawal

Symptoms of withdrawal (table 2) may be a barrier to abstinence as they may be of similar intensity to those accompanying tobacco cessation. As many as 85% of users experience withdrawal.[20] A cross sectional survey of treatment seekers found that concurrent use of cannabis and tobacco makes it harder to quit either substance[25]

Table 2   Pros and cons of cannabis use—a decisional matrix

	Good things	Bad things
Continuing cannabis use	Feeling relaxed; rolling a joint; socialising with friends; sleeping well	Cost; partner unhappy; need to stop going out as much; health worries; smell of smoke on clothes
Stopping/reducing cannabis use	Save money; go out more; get healthier; partner happy	Not being able to relax; not seeing some old friends; not sleeping as well

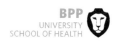

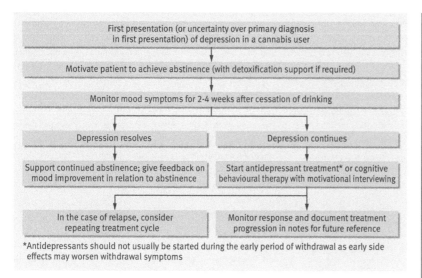

First presentation (or uncertainty over primary diagnosis in first presentation) of depression in a cannabis user

↓

Motivate patient to achieve abstinence (with detoxification support if required)

↓

Monitor mood symptoms for 2-4 weeks after cessation of drinking

↓

Depression resolves

Support continued abstinence; give feedback on mood improvement in relation to abstinence

In the case of relapse, consider repeating treatment cycle

Depression continues

Start antidepressant treatment* or cognitive behavioural therapy with motivational interviewing

Monitor response and document treatment progression in notes for future reference

*Antidepressants should not usually be started during the early period of withdrawal as early side effects may worsen withdrawal symptoms

Fig 1 Decision pathway for assessing affective symptoms in cannabis users

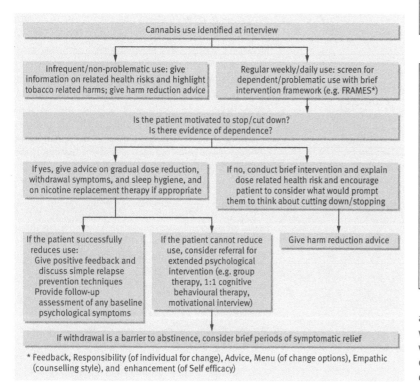

Cannabis use identified at interview

Infrequent/non-problematic use: give information on related health risks and highlight tobacco related harms; give harm reduction advice

Regular weekly/daily use: screen for dependent/problematic use with brief intervention framework (e.g. FRAMES*)

↓

Is the patient motivated to stop/cut down?
Is there evidence of dependence?

If yes, give advice on gradual dose reduction, withdrawal symptoms, and sleep hygiene, and on nicotine replacement therapy if appropriate

If no, conduct brief intervention and explain dose related health risk and encourage patient to consider what would prompt them to think about cutting down/stopping

If the patient successfully reduces use:
Give positive feedback and discuss simple relapse prevention techniques
Provide follow-up assessment of any baseline psychological symptoms

If the patient cannot reduce use, consider referral for extended psychological intervention (e.g. group therapy, 1:1 cognitive behavioural therapy, motivational interview)

Give harm reduction advice

If withdrawal is a barrier to abstinence, consider brief periods of symptomatic relief

* Feedback, Responsibility (of individual for change), Advice, Menu (of change options), Empathic (counselling style), and enhancement (of Self efficacy)

Fig 2 Identifying and responding to cannabis use disorders

ONGOING RESEARCH

- A multicentre European trial is examining risk and protective factors and multidimensional family therapy for adolescents
- US trials are investigating effective interventions to manage withdrawal and to support abstinence in otherwise healthy populations, including the use of computerised treatments, contingency management with adolescents, and cannabis patches
- The UK MIDAS trial is examining whether an integrated intervention that combines motivational interviewing and cognitive behavioural therapy can effectively reduce use in those with severe mental illness

UNANSWERED QUESTIONS

- What is the precise nature of the association between cannabis use and development of schizophrenia?
- How do higher potency strains of cannabis affect the physical and psychological risks of individuals and the population as a whole?
- What is the degree of recovery in cognitive functioning with prolonged abstinence?
- What is the neurobiological mechanism underlying cannabis withdrawal?

TIPS FOR NON-SPECIALISTS

- Most cannabis users will not develop dependence or severe mental health problems. Concerns should be highest for daily smokers, adolescents, those who are pregnant, and those with coexisting severe mental illness
- A gradual reduction in tolerance and levels of use among daily smokers can be helped by getting users to delay the time of first use in the day and to engage in other daytime activities
- The insomnia, irritability, and craving that can occur for a few days on cessation of cannabis can be a barrier to attaining abstinence. Cessation is less likely to result in serious withdrawal symptoms if use has fallen to lower levels before quit attempts
- If users are reluctant to accept the possibility of a causal relation between cannabis use and an adverse psychological experience or state, encouraging a period of abstinence and self monitoring using a diary and feedback from trusted friends or family members can be useful
- Consider discussing concurrent tobacco dependence with patients even if they only use tobacco when they use cannabis

ADDITIONAL EDUCATIONAL RESOURCES

- Know Cannabis (www.knowcannabis.org.uk)—Self help website
- Talk to Frank (www.talktofrank.com/section.aspx?ID=110)—Self help website, with helpline (phone/online)
- Young Minds (youngminds.org.uk)—Self help website focusing on young people's mental wellbeing
- Marijuana Anonymous (www.marijuana-anonymous.org)—Online support group for users wishing to quit
- Connexions (www.connexions.gov.uk)—Website for young people aged 13-19 years that offers support and links them with a practitioner or personal adviser
- Helpfinder, DrugScope (www.drugscope.org.uk/resources/databases/helpfinder.htm)—DrugScope's database of drug treatment services

and withdrawal tends to be more severe in cannabis users who are also heavy users of tobacco and in cannabis users with mental illness. Withdrawal symptoms peak on day 2 or 3, and most are over by day 7. Sleep problems and vivid dreams can continue for two to three weeks.[20]

No evidence based pharmacological intervention exists for managing cannabis withdrawal.[26] Some small studies exploring the utility of oral tetrahydrocannabinol show promise in reducing withdrawal and craving.[27] If bupropion is used in nicotine dependence it must begin at least one week before cessation of both substances, as starting treatment on day 1 of cannabis cessation may exacerbate withdrawal symptoms.[28] Our experience is that providing a patient with information about withdrawal symptoms may help them to prepare for discomfort, which if severe can be alleviated with a few days of symptomatic relief. Most dependent users, however, probably do not require any drug intervention to manage their withdrawal. Box 4 outlines what advice to give to patients on managing withdrawal.

Cessation of use can be monitored with urine tests over several weeks for the inactive metabolite of cannabis (carboxy-tetrahydrocannabinol); heavy smokers may continue to be positive for cannabis for up to six weeks.[W12]

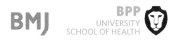

Harm minimisation for those who choose to continue using cannabis

Initial assessment and feedback could focus on the pulmonary harms of smoking, citing strategies that target both tobacco and cannabis (for example, Health Scotland's publication *Fags 'n' Hash*[29]).

Water pipes (also known as bongs), which cool and filter smoke, are not a safer way of smoking. They filter out more tetrahydrocannabinol than they do tar, resulting in greater tar delivery to the lungs.[W13] The role of vaporisers (which heat the plant material, releasing the tetrahydrocannabinol as a vapour but avoiding combustion) as an effective harm reduction intervention is uncertain.[W13, W15] Box 5 outlines advice for patients on how they can reduce their risk of harm from cannabis use.

When to refer to a specialist

Persistent use despite recognition of harms and unsuccessful attempts to reduce use should lead to specialist referral; consider specialist referral also for those with severe comorbid mental health problems and those who are pregnant.

Contributors: ARW conceived the review, wrote the initial draft, prepared the final draft, and is the guarantor; CF helped with conception of the review and wrote the screening and assessment sections; JW helped with the literature search and the preparation of the final draft for submission.

Competing interests: All authors have completed the Unified Competing Interest form at www.icmje.org/coi_disclosure.pdf (available on request from the corresponding author) and declare (1) no support from any company for the submitted work; (2) no relationships with any companies that might have an interest in the submitted work in the previous 3 years; (3) their spouses, partners, or children have no financial relationships that may be relevant to the submitted work; and (4) no non-financial interests that may be relevant to the submitted work.

Provenance and peer review: Not commissioned; externally peer reviewed.

1 Hoare J. Drug misuse declared: findings from the 2008/09 British Crime Survey. Home Office, 2009.
2 Dennis M, Babor TF, Roebuck MC, Donaldson J. Changing the focus: the case for recognizing and treating cannabis use disorders. *Addiction* 2002;97:4-15.
3 Hall W, Degenhardt L. Adverse health effects of non-medical cannabis use. *Lancet* 2009;374:1383-91.
4 Hardwick S, King L. Home Office Potency Study 2008. Home Office, 2008.
5 Department of Health, National Treatment Agency. Statistics from the National Drug Treatment Monitoring System (NDTMS) 1 April 2008-31 March 2009. NTA, 2009.
6 Smith N. High potency cannabis: the forgotten variable. *Addiction* 2005;100:1558-9.
7 Henry JA, Oldfield WLG, Kon OM. Comparing cannabis with tobacco. *BMJ* 2003;326:942-3
8 Taylor DR, Fergusson DM, Milne BJ, Horwood LJ, Moffitt TE, Sears MR, et al. A longitudinal study of the effects of tobacco and cannabis exposure on lung function in young adults. *Addiction* 2002;97:1055-61.
9 Aldington S, Williams M, Nowitz M, Weatherall M, Pritchard A, McNaughton A, et al. Effects of cannabis on pulmonary structure, function and symptoms. *Thorax* 2007;62:1058-63.
10 Tan WC, Lo C, Jong A, FitzGerald MJ, Vollmer WM, Buis SA, et al. Marijuana and chronic obstructive lung disease: a population-based study. *CMAJ* 2009;180:814-20.
11 Aldington S, Harwood M, Cox B, Weatherall M, Beckert L, Hansell A, et al. Cannabis use and risk of lung cancer: a case-control study. *Eur Respir J* 2008;31:280-6.
12 Moore THM, Zammit S, Lingford-Hughes A, Barnes TRE, Jones PB, Burke M, et al. Cannabis use and risk of psychotic or affective mental health outcomes: a systematic review. *Lancet* 2007;370:319-28.
13 Verdoux H, Ginde C, Sorbora F, Tournier M, Swendsen J. Effects of cannabis and psychosis vulnerability in daily life: an experience sampling study. *Psychol Med* 2003;33:3-6.
14 Sugranyes G, Flamarique I, Parellada E, Baeza I, Goti J, Fernandez-Egea E, et al. Cannabis use and age of diagnosis of schizophrenia. *Eur Psychiatry* 2009;24:282-6.
15 Zammit S, Moore TH, Lingford-Hughes A, Barnes TR, Jones PB, Burke M, et al. Effects of cannabis use on outcomes of psychotic disorders: systematic review. *Br J Psychiatry* 2008;193:357-63.
16 Crippa JA, Zuardi AW, Martín-Santos R, Bhattacharyya S, Atakan Z, McGuire P, et al. Cannabis and anxiety: a critical review of the evidence. *Hum Psychopharmacol* 2009;24:515-23.
17 Winstock AR, Lea T, Copeland J. Lithium carbonate in the management of cannabis withdrawal. *J Psychopharmacol* 2009;23:84-93.
18 Yücel M, Solowij N, Respondek C, Whittle S, Fornito A, Pantelis C, et al. Regional brain abnormalities associated with long-term heavy cannabis use. *Arch Gen Psychiatry* 2008;65:694-701.
19 Solowij N, Stephens RS, Roffman RA, Babor T, Kadden R, Miller M, et al. Cognitive functioning of long-term heavy cannabis users seeking treatment [published correction: JAMA 2002;287:1651]. *JAMA* 2002;287:1123-31.
20 Budney AJ, Hughes JR, Moore BA, Vandrey R. Review of the validity and significance of cannabis withdrawal syndrome. *Am J Psychiatry* 2004;161:1967-77.
21 Miller WR, Rollnick S. Motivational interviewing: preparing people for change. Guilford Press, 2002.
22 Copeland J, Frewen A, Elkins K. Management of cannabis use disorder and related issues. A clinician's guide. National Cannabis Prevention and Information Centre, 2009.
23 McCambridge J, Strang J. The efficacy of single-session motivational interviewing in reducing drug consumption and perceptions of drug-related risk and harm among young people: results from a multi-site cluster randomised trial. *Addiction* 2006;99:39-52.
24 Litt MD, Kadden RM, Kabela-Cormier E, Petry NM. Coping skills training and contingency management treatments for marijuana dependence: exploring mechanisms of behaviour change. *Addiction* 2008;103:638-48.
25 Moore BA, Budney AJ. Tobacco smoking in marijuana dependent outpatients. *J Subst Abuse* 2001;3:585-8.
26 Vandrey R, Haney M. Pharmacotherapy for cannabis dependence: how close are we? *CNS Drugs* 2009;23:543-53.
27 Budney AJ, Vandrey RG, Hughes JR, Moore BA, Bahrenburg B. Oral delta-9-tetrahydrocannabinol suppresses cannabis withdrawal symptoms. *Drug Alc Depend* 2007;86:22-9.
28 Haney M, Ward AS, Comer SD, Hart CL, Foltin RW, Fischman MW. Bupropion SR worsens mood during marijuana withdrawal in humans. *Psychopharmacology* 2001;155:171-9.
29 ASH Scotland, Health Scotland, Scottish Drugs Forum, West Lothian Drug and Alcohol Service. Fags 'n' hash: the essential guide to cutting down the risks of using tobacco and cannabis. Health Scotland, 2008.

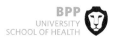

Supporting smoking cessation

Nicholas A Zwar, professor of general practice[1],
Colin P Mendelsohn, tobacco treatment specialist[2],
Robyn L Richmond, professor of public health[1]

[1]School of Public Health and Community Medicine, University of New South Wales, Sydney 2052, Australia

[2]Brain and Mind Research Institute, University of Sydney, Level 2, Camperdown, NSW 2050, Australia

Correspondence to: N Zwar n.zwar@unsw.edu.au

Cite this as: BMJ 2014;348:f7535

DOI: 10.1136/bmj.f7535

http://www.bmj.com/content/348/bmj.f7535

Despite the decrease in prevalence of tobacco use in developed countries, smoking remains the most common preventable cause of disease and death in the world today.

Advice on smoking cessation from doctors and other health professionals has been shown to improve quit rates and is highly cost effective.[1] Given the importance to health of tobacco use and the benefits of cessation, every doctor should encourage attempts to stop, be able to provide brief smoking cessation intervention, and be aware of referral options (see box 1).

Over the past decade there have been advances in the science and practice of smoking cessation support. These include new medicines to treat nicotine dependence, new ways of using existing medicines, and increasing use of technology to support behavioural change. This review provides an update on evidence based approaches to maximise the effectiveness of the treatment of tobacco dependence.

Who smokes?

The prevalence of tobacco use varies around the world. Of the more than one billion smokers worldwide, 80% live in low and middle income countries, where the burden of tobacco related illness is heaviest.[3]

As smoking rates fall in developed countries, tobacco use is increasingly concentrated in certain groups who have greater difficulty in quitting than other smokers. These include people with mental illnesses, especially schizophrenia, those with substance use problems, people from lower socioeconomic groups, and some indigenous people. There is also some evidence that those who present for treatment have higher levels of nicotine dependence than those presenting 10 or more years ago.[4]

As with other addictions, there is a strong genetic component to smoking behaviour. The estimated mean heritability for starting smoking has been calculated at 50% and for developing nicotine dependence at 56%.[5] Genetic factors also have a substantial role in nicotine withdrawal symptoms, cigarette consumption, difficulty in quitting, and response to smoking cessation therapies.[6] Most smokers are nicotine dependent and for these people smoking can be thought of as a chronic medical illness that requires ongoing care.[7]

Why is stopping tobacco use so important?

There is considerable urgency about providing effective smoking cessation treatment; after the age of about 35, on average three months of life are lost for each year of continued smoking.[8] Fortunately the health benefits of cessation are substantial and rapid. The excess risk of death from smoking begins to decrease shortly after cessation and continues to decline for at least 10 to 15 years.[9] The British doctors' study found that male doctors who stopped smoking before the age of 35 survived about as well as those who had never smoked.[8] [9] More recent data have shown that this benefit also occurs for women.[10]

How can health professionals help patients to quit?

Most smokers want to stop smoking, and about 40% try to stop at least once each year.[11] Only 3-5% of unaided attempts, however, are successful 6-12 months later.[12] Brief advice from doctors (defined as advice provided in a consultation lasting up to 20 minutes plus up to one follow-up visit) increases cessation rates by about two thirds (relative risk 1.66, 95% confidence interval 1.42 to 1.94) compared with no advice or usual care (an absolute increase of 1-3%) at 12 months, and more intensive treatment nearly doubles the chances of quitting.[1] The 5As approach originally proposed by the US Clinical Practice Guidelines[13] provides health professionals with an evidence based framework for structuring smoking cessation support. The elements of the 5As are:

- Ask: Regularly ask all patients if they smoke and record the information in the medical record
- Advise: Advise all smokers to quit in a clear, unambiguous way such as "the best thing you can do for your health is to stop smoking"
- Assess: Assessment of interest in quitting helps to tailor advice to each smoker's needs and stage of change.[14] Nicotine dependence should also be assessed and helps to guide treatment. Assessment of other relevant problems such as mental health conditions, other drug dependencies, and comorbidities is necessary to develop a comprehensive treatment plan
- Assist: All smokers should be offered help to quit
- Arrange: Follow-up visits have been shown to increase the likelihood of long term abstinence[15] and are especially useful in the first few weeks after quitting.

In the United Kingdom the National Centre for Smoking Cessation and Training approach of "very brief advice" is increasingly used. The steps are:

- Establish smoking status (ASK)
- ADVISE that the best way of quitting is with a combination of behavioural support and drug treatment
- Provide a referral or offer behavioural support and follow-up appointments (ASSIST).

SOURCES AND SELECTION CRITERIA

This review is based on evidence synthesis from relevant Cochrane systematic reviews; review and distillation of clinical practice guidelines from Australia, the United States, and New Zealand; information from UK National Centre for Smoking Cessation and Training (www.ncsct.co.uk); and other evidence from the authors' personal libraries. We have focused on developments since the review by Aveyard and West in 2007.[2]

SUMMARY POINTS

- Throughout the world tobacco smoking is the leading cause of preventable death and illness
- As smoking rates in the general population fall in developed countries, a greater proportion of smokers have coexisting problems such as mental illness
- Cessation support from doctors and other health professionals increases quit rates
- Tobacco dependence is most effectively treated with a comprehensive approach involving behavioural support and pharmacotherapy
- Effective medicines include nicotine replacement therapy, varenicline, bupropion, nortriptyline, and cytisine. The availability and registration of these medicines varies between countries

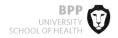

A recent Cochrane meta-analysis found that reducing the number of cigarettes smoked before quit day and quitting abruptly produced comparable quit rates. Patients can be given the choice of quitting in either of these ways.[16] There is a range of options for referring patients for cessation support (box 1).

How is nicotine dependence assessed?

Most smokers are nicotine dependent, and the level of dependence is a predictor of withdrawal symptoms and the intensity of treatment required. Smoking within 30 minutes of waking is a reliable indicator of nicotine dependence. Smoking within five minutes of waking indicates more severe dependence.[18] Cravings and withdrawal symptoms experienced in previous quit attempts are also a useful guide. The number of cigarettes smoked a day is less predictive; smoking more than 10 cigarettes a day, however, is associated with a higher likelihood of dependence (see box 2).

What are evidence based approaches to counselling and behavioural therapy?

Cochrane meta-analyses have found that cognitive and behavioural therapy delivered by health professionals has a significant effect on quit rates. Individual counselling improves long term quit rates by 39% compared with minimal behavioural intervention (relative risk 1.39, 95% confidence interval 1.24 to 1.57)[18] and group programmes double success rates compared with self help programmes (1.98, 1.6 to 2.46).[19]

Aspects of counselling and behavioural advice include:
- Building rapport and boosting motivation
- Assisting with choice of drugs and ensuring that patients have a realistic expectation of how they can aid quit attempts—for example, by reducing withdrawal symptoms
- Describing withdrawal symptoms and cravings and exploring ways of managing these such as distraction strategies (for example, doing exercise)
- Agreeing on a quit date and promoting the "not-a-puff" rule
- Dealing with barriers to quitting such as stress and weight gain. Stress management strategies include breathing and progressive muscle relaxation techniques. Drinking water and choosing low fat foods can help to minimise weight gain
- Discussing strategies for coping with smoking triggers. For example, minimal or no alcohol in the early weeks of a quit attempt is advised
- Getting support from family and friends, patient support services, and printed materials
- Promoting lifestyle changes such as exercise and avoiding high risk situations
- Relapse prevention.

Interventions can also be delivered by telephone, text message, and the internet. A meta-analysis of five trials of mobile phone based interventions found an increase in the long term quit rates compared with control programmes (relative risk 1.71, 95% confidence interval 1.47 to 1.99).[19] Internet based programmes have the advantage of being low cost and can be individualised to meet the smoker's needs. There is evidence from three trials that interactive and individually tailored internet based interventions are more effective than usual care or written self help (1.48, 1.11 to 2.78).[20] Motivational interviewing has a role in encouraging ambivalent smokers to try to quit. A meta-analysis of motivational interviewing versus brief advice or usual care yielded a modest but significant increase in quitting (1.27, 1.14 to 1.42).[21] The four guiding principles[22] that underlie motivational interviewing are:
- Express empathy
- Develop discrepancy (the gap between goals or values and actual behaviour)
- Roll with resistance
- Support self efficacy.

What is the role of pharmacotherapy in smoking cessation?

In meta-analyses of randomised clinical trials, several drug treatments have been shown to assist smoking cessation. Pharmacotherapy is appropriate in patients who are found to be nicotine dependent (see box 2 on assessment of nicotine dependence). Medicines are most effective when given in combination with behavioural support. The most widely available preferred pharmacotherapy options are nicotine replacement therapy, varenicline, and bupropion. All these drugs have been shown to be effective in a range of patient populations including smokers with depression, schizophrenia, and cardiac and respiratory diseases. Figure 1 summarises the effect of these medicines compared with placebo.

A Cochrane network analysis concluded that combinations of nicotine replacement therapy and varenicline are the most effective quitting aids and are of similar efficacy.[22] Head to head comparisons between bupropion and nicotine replacement monotherapy showed equal efficacy.[23] Clinical suitability and patient preference are important in guiding the choice of pharmacotherapy or combination of therapies (see fig 2).

Nicotine replacement therapy

Nicotine replacement therapy is available in a long acting form (nicotine patch) and in several short acting products (nicotine gum, inhalator, mouth spray, lozenge, microtablet, nasal spray). Other forms are in development. A Cochrane systematic review found that nicotine replacement therapy

---

BOX 1: REFERRAL OPTIONS FOR SMOKING CESSATION SUPPORT

- Telephone quitlines are available in many countries. Proactive telephone counselling is preferred as it has been shown to be more effective than reactive counselling[17]
- In the UK, the National Health Service (NHS) provides a range of services including telephone and online support, quit kits, and a mobile phone application through http://smokefree.nhs.uk/
- Specialised services are available in some countries either in hospitals or community settings. In the UK specialised support is available through local stop smoking services. Information is available at http://smokefree.nhs.uk/. In the US there are a growing number of dedicated providers. Details are available on the Association for the Treatment of Tobacco Use and Dependence website www.attud.org. In Australia the number of smoking cessation professionals is also increasing. Information is available at www.aascp.org.au

---

BOX 2: NICOTINE DEPENDENCE

Assessment of nicotine dependence
Nicotine dependence can be briefly assessed by asking about:
- Minutes after waking to first cigarette?
- Number of cigarettes a day?
- Cravings or withdrawal symptoms in previous quit attempts?

Indication of nicotine dependence
- Smoking within 30 minutes of waking
- Smoking more than 10 cigarettes a day
- History of withdrawal symptoms in previous quit attempts

During the assessment of need for drug treatment, consider also the patient's previous experience and views on pharmacotherapy for smoking cessation

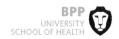

is an effective aid to long term cessation (relative risk 1.60, 95% confidence interval 1.53 to 1.68), and the efficacy is similar between all available forms.[24] Combination nicotine replacement therapy (nicotine patch combined with a rapid delivery form) should be recommended to smokers who are unable to quit or who experience cravings or withdrawal symptoms with monotherapy.[25] There is evidence from nine trials that this type of combination nicotine replacement therapy is more effective than a single type (1.34, 1.18 to 1.51).[24] Pre-cessation treatment with a nicotine patch (usually started two weeks before quit day) can increase the rate of successful quitting compared with starting treatment on quit day (1.34, 1.08 to 1.65; six trials).[24] Nicotine replacement therapy is generally safe and well tolerated. Side effects, which can include nausea, headache, and dizziness, are generally mild and improve over time. Nicotine patches can cause skin irritation and disturbed sleep, and oral preparations can cause hiccups, sore mouth, and heartburn. Nicotine replacement therapy can be safely used in people with stable cardiovascular disease (fig 2).

Varenicline

Varenicline is a partial nicotine agonist that acts centrally to relieve cravings and withdrawal symptoms as well as reducing the rewarding effect of smoking. A Cochrane meta-analysis of 14 trials of varenicline found it more than doubled sustained abstinence rates at six months' follow-up (risk ratio 2.27, 95% confidence interval 2.20 to 2.55).[25] The most common adverse effect is nausea, affecting about 30% of users; but this is mild to moderate and leads to discontinuation of treatment in only about 3%.[25] Nausea is reduced by gradual up-titration of the dose and by taking the drug with food. There have been post-marketing reports of depression, agitation, changes in behaviour, and suicidal ideation, although a causal association with varenicline has not been established.[25] A recent meta-analysis of data from 17 trials found no evidence of higher rates of suicidal events, depression, or aggression/agitation in participants taking varenicline compared with placebo. This was the case in participants both with and without a history of psychiatric disorders.[26]

Bupropion

Bupropion was originally developed as an antidepressant. It reduces both the urge to smoke and symptoms of nicotine withdrawal. A meta-analysis of 36 trials of bupropion found that it substantially increases quit rates over placebo (relative risk 1.69, 95% confidence interval 1.53 to 1.85).[27] There is a further modest increase in efficacy when it is combined with nicotine replacement therapy.[14 23] Bupropion is contraindicated in patients with a history of seizures and eating disorders and patients taking monoamine oxidase inhibitors. It should be used with caution in people taking drugs that can lower seizure threshold, such as antidepressants and oral hypoglycaemic agents (fig 2).[28]

Second line options

The tricyclic antidepressant nortriptyline doubles cessation rates compared with placebo treatment at six months (relative risk 2.03, 95% confidence interval 1.48 to 2.78).[27] Side effects include dry mouth, constipation, nausea, sedation, and headaches. Nortriptyline is not licensed for smoking cessation. It is dangerous in overdose and can increase the risk of arrhythmia in patients with cardiovascular disease.

Cytisine is an inexpensive plant derived partial nicotine agonist that is available for smoking cessation in parts of eastern Europe but is not licensed in the UK. In a Cochrane meta-analysis of two recent trials comparing cytisine with placebo, the risk ratio was 3.98 (95% confidence interval 2.01 to 7.87).[25]

Effects of smoking and smoking cessation on drug metabolism

Chemicals in tobacco smoke accelerate the metabolism of many common drugs by inducing the cytochrome P450 enzyme, CYP1A2. This can substantially lower the serum concentrations and effectiveness of these drugs in smokers (table 1). Conversely, blood levels of these drugs might rise when smoking is stopped. Patients should be monitored for adverse effects, and dose reductions might be required. Immediate dose reductions should be considered for drugs with a narrow therapeutic index—such as olanzapine, clozapine, and warfarin—to avoid drug toxicity.[29] Patients should also be advised to reduce caffeine intake.

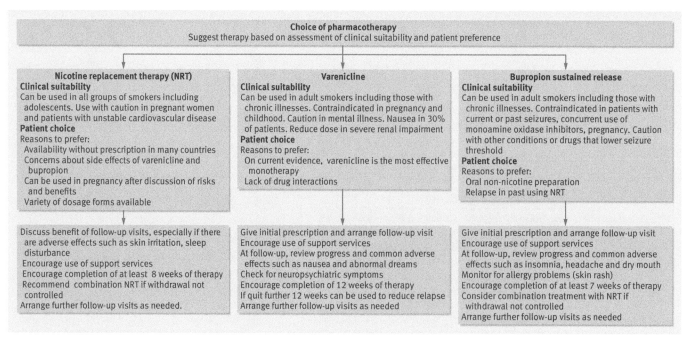

Fig 2 Pharmacotherapy treatment algorithm for nicotine dependent smokers. Adapted and reproduced with permission from the Royal Australian College of General Practitioners[28]

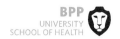

Table 1 Drugs that interact with smoking. Blood concentrations rise after cessation of smoking

Class	Drug
Antipsychotics	Olanzapine, clozapine. Haloperidol, chlorpromazine, fluphenazine
Antidepressants	Duloxetine, fluvoxamine, tricyclic antidepressants, mirtazapine
Anti-anxiety agents	Alprazolam, oxazepam, diazepam
Cardiovascular drugs	Warfarin, propranolol, verapamil, flecainide. Clopidogrel (efficacy increased in smokers)
Diabetes	Insulin, metformin
Other	Naratriptan, oestradiol, ondansetron, theophylline, dextropropoxyphene
Others	Caffeine, alcohol

Table 2 Suitability of preferred pharmacotherapy in special populations. Quitting smoking can alter the metabolism of several drugs. Adapted and reproduced with permission from the Royal Australian College of General Practitioners[28]

	Varenicline	Bupropion	NRT
Pregnant and lactating women	ND	ND	Yes*
Children and adolescents (age 12-18)	ND	ND	Yes
People with smoking related diseases:			
Cardiovascular disease	Yes†	Yes	Yes‡
Chronic obstructive pulmonary disease	Yes	Yes§	Yes
Diabetes	Yes§	Yes§	Yes§
Severe renal impairment	Yes¶	Yes¶	Yes
Moderate to severe hepatic impairment	Yes	Yes¶	Yes
People with mental illness:			
Any	Yes**	Yes	Yes
Depression	Yes**	Yes	Yes
Schizophrenia	Yes**	Yes	Yes
People with substance misuse disorders	Yes	Yes††	Yes
Existing contraindications to use	Yes‡‡	Yes‡‡§§	Yes‡‡

NRT=nicotine replacement therapy; ND=lack of safety data.

*There is currently inconclusive evidence to determine whether or not NRT is effective or safe when used in pregnancy for smoking cessation, if it is used risks and benefits should be discussed with patient; intermittent dosing products preferable.

†Association between varenicline use and non-fatal cardiac events has been suggested, Subsequent studies and meta-analysis have not found association.

‡Caution is advised for people in hospital for acute cardiovascular events such as myocardial infarction, unstable or progressive angina, severe cardiac arrhythmias, or acute phase stroke. NRT can be used under medical supervision, where the clinician should balance risk of using nicotine replacement against risk of smoking.

§Closely monitor blood sugar concentrations as insulin or other drug requirements might change.

¶Dosing adjustment required.

**Close follow-up required. Check for any unusual or serious changes in mood or behaviour at two-three week follow-up visit and after treatment is completed. Careful monitoring required for mood changes, depression, behaviour disturbance, and suicidal thoughts.

††Caution with alcohol abuse.

‡‡Hypersensitivity to active substance or any excipients.

§§Contraindications: seizures, anorexia, bulimia, central nervous system tumours, monoamine oxidase inhibitor treatment within 14 days.

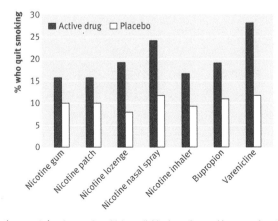

Fig 1 Long term (≥6 months) quit rates for widely available drugs for smoking cessation. Data adapted from Cochrane Database of Systematic Reviews[24] [25] [27]

How do I treat special groups?

Pregnant women

Smoking in pregnancy has important adverse effects on the fetus and increases complications in pregnancy, including low birth weight, preterm birth, miscarriage, and placental abruption. A Cochrane systematic review found smoking cessation interventions in pregnancy reduce the proportion of women who continue to smoke in late pregnancy by about 6%.[30] There is inconclusive evidence of the effectiveness and safety of nicotine replacement therapy during pregnancy and other forms of pharmacotherapy are contraindicated.[31] If nicotine replacement therapy is used, the benefits and risks should be discussed with the patient. Although nicotine is presumed to have some risk, clinical trials of therapeutic nicotine have not generally reported adverse fetal effects.[31] Available data and expert opinion suggest that it is less harmful than continued smoking.[28] [32] Intermittent (oral) nicotine replacement therapy is generally recommended as this delivers a lower total nicotine dose.

Adolescents

Adolescence is the primary time when people start smoking and transition from experimentation to dependence occurs. A meta-analysis of interventions shows some benefit from interventions based on motivational enhancement or tailored to stage of change.[33] There is currently insufficient evidence to determine whether pharmacotherapy is effective for adolescent smokers. It is, however, reasonable to offer nicotine replacement therapy and behavioural support after assessment of nicotine dependence and motivation to quit. In many countries nicotine replacement therapy is now licensed for use in this age group.[28]

People with mental health problems

The rate of smoking in people with mental illness is about twice the rate in those without mental illness. In general, the more severe the psychiatric diagnosis, the higher the prevalence of smoking. People with mental illness also smoke more heavily than other smokers, are more nicotine dependent, and might need more intensive or prolonged support to quit. There is evidence, however, that they are just as motivated to quit as the general population.[34]

The doses of medicines used to treat depression and psychotic disorders might also require adjustment after smoking cessation (table 1). Contrary to common perceptions smoking cessation is not associated with worsening of psychiatric illnesses and in fact improvement is more common.[35]

Table 2 provides a summary of the use of smoking cessation pharmacotherapy in special populations.

What are the emerging approaches in smoking cessation?

Nicotine vaccines have been researched, but a Cochrane meta-analysis of four trials found no benefit in long term cessation compared with placebo.[23]

Electronic cigarettes (e-cigarettes) are battery powered devices that deliver nicotine in a vapour without tobacco or smoke. E-cigarettes can relieve cravings and symptoms of nicotine withdrawal as well as simulating the behavioural and sensory aspects of smoking.[36] A small number of randomised controlled trials have suggested that e-cigarettes could have a role in cessation and harm reduction, though further research is needed before recommendations for their use can be confidently made.[36] [37] Concerns about e-cigarettes include a lack of evidence for long term safety, a lack of regulation, the possibility of

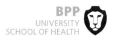

use acting as a gateway to smoking, potential for dual use while a person is still smoking, and the renormalisation of smoking behaviour.[38]

Physical activity is routinely recommended as an aid to quitting. Short bursts of moderate exercise, such as brisk walking, rapidly reduce cigarette cravings and symptoms of withdrawal.[39] Regular exercise also attenuates post-cessation weight gain for up to two years, improves mental wellbeing, and has general health benefits. The clinical trials so far have not shown an effect of exercise on cessation rates.[40]

Mindfulness is increasingly being explored to assist smoking cessation, especially in smokers with mental illness. Mindfulness involves being aware of present moment experiences such as cravings, withdrawals, and negative affect, instead of responding automatically with a cigarette. Focusing on and accepting these uncomfortable sensations can cause them to diminish.[41] Several studies to date have found that a course of mindfulness training (usually eight weeks) can help reduce cravings, withdrawal symptoms, and cigarette intake and might improve rates of abstinence.[42] [43] [44]

Which strategies have not been shown to work?

Meta-analyses of trials of acupuncture and hypnotherapy have not shown either to be effective.[45] [46]

How do I help patients avoid relapse?

Relapse is a return to regular smoking. Most smokers relapse in the first eight days after a quit attempt.[12] Common triggers for relapse are alcohol, negative emotional states, and exposure to smoke. There is currently no evidence from randomised trials of effective behavioural interventions to prevent relapse.[47] In terms of pharmacological

interventions, extended treatment with varenicline (defined as an additional 12 weeks) had a significant benefit in one trial, but pooled results of six studies with bupropion showed no effect. There have been mixed results with nicotine replacement therapy, with two studies of orally administered therapy showing a benefit.[48]

Is there a role for harm reduction?

Smokers who are not willing or able to quit in the short term can use nicotine replacement therapy to reduce their tobacco intake. The health benefits of long term reduction in smoking are uncertain, though cutting down with nicotine replacement therapy nearly doubles the odds of quitting altogether.[48]

For smokers who have quit, the long term use of nicotine replacement therapy might help to reduce the harm from smoking. Evidence from studies with up to five years' follow-up suggests that nicotine replacement products do not pose a significant health risk.[48] Most of the health effects of tobacco are caused by the toxins and carcinogens in tobacco smoke, not nicotine. The exception to this is in pregnancy, when nicotine reduces fetal growth and animal studies suggest that it is toxic to the fetal brain and lungs.[48]

Comments on the article from Andy McEwen, executive director, National Centre for Smoking Cessation and Training, are gratefully acknowledged.

Contributors: All authors contributed to the decisions on content of the article. NAZ led the writing process and developed the first draft. All authors provided comments on drafts and contributed to the decisions on the final submission. NAZ is guarantor.

Competing interests: We have read and understood the BMJ Group policy on declaration of interests and declare the following interests: NAZ has received honorariums for providing advice on smoking cessation programmes to Pfizer and GlaxoSmithKline Australia and has received support to attend smoking cessation conferences; CPM has received honorariums for teaching, consulting and travel from Pfizer, GlaxoSmithKline, and Johnson and Johnson Pacific.

Provenance and peer review: Commissioned; externally peer reviewed.

TIPS FOR NON SPECIALISTS

- Identify and document smoking and offer support for smoking cessation at every opportunity
- Provide support based on the 5As or refer, depending on the clinical context
- Encourage comprehensive treatment consisting of behavioural support and pharmacotherapy for smokers addicted to nicotine

---

ADDITIONAL EDUCATIONAL RESOURCES

- UK National Centre for Smoking Cessation and Training (www.ncsct.co.uk/)—delivers training and assessment programmes, support services for local and national providers and conducts research into behavioural support for smoking cessation. This includes the "very brief advice" training module
- Society for Research on Nicotine and Tobacco and the Society for the Study of Addiction (www.treatobacco.net)—provides information on treatment of tobacco dependence. The website has links to clinical practice guidelines for cessation from around the world
- United States Smoking Cessation Guidelines (www.ahrq.gov/professionals/clinicians-providers/resources/tobacco/treating-tobacco-use.html#.UrJWcieRNSY)—http:///literature review and meta-analysis of intervention and clinical practice guidelines based on the 5As approach
- Australian Smoking Cessation Guidelines (www.racgp.org.au/your-practice/guidelines/smoking-cessation/)—clinical practice guidelines aimed at a wide range of health professionals
- New Zealand Smoking Cessation Guidelines (www.health.govt.nz/publication/new-zealand-smoking-cessation-guidelines)—clinical practice guidelines based on the ABC approach: Ask about smoking status; give Brief advice to stop smoking to all smokers; and provide evidence based Cessation support for those who want to stop smoking)

QUESTIONS FOR FUTURE RESEARCH

- What is the role of e-cigarettes in cessation and harm reduction and how should their use be regulated?
- Does exercise increase smoking cessation rates?
- Can pharmacogenetics guide personalised choices of drug treatment and, if so, is it more effective?

1 Stead LF, Buitrago D, Preciado N, Sanchez G, Hartmann-Boyce J, Lancaster T. Physician advice for smoking cessation. *Cochrane Database Syst Rev* 2013;5:CD000165.
2 Aveyard P, West R. Managing smoking cessation. *BMJ* 2007;335:37-41.
3 Tobacco Fact Sheet No 339. World Health Organization, 2013 July 2013.
4 Hughes JR. The hardening hypothesis: is the ability to quit decreasing due to increasing nicotine dependence? A review and commentary. *Drug Alcohol Depend* 2011;117:111-7.
5 Li MD, Cheng R, Ma JZ, Swan GE. A meta-analysis of estimated genetic and environmental effects on smoking behavior in male and female adult twins. *Addiction* 2003;98:23-31.
6 Ho MK, Goldman D, Heinz A, Kaprio J, Kreek MJ, Li MD, et al. Breaking barriers in the genomics and pharmacogenetics of drug addiction. *Clin Pharmacol Ther* 2010;88:779-91.
7 Foulds J, Schmelzer AC, Steinberg MB. Treating tobacco dependence as a chronic illness and a key modifiable predictor of disease. *Int J Clin Pract* 2010;64:142-6.
8 Doll R, Peto R, Boreham J, Sutherland I. Mortality in relation to smoking: 50 years' observations on male British doctors. *BMJ* 2004;328:1519.
9 Doll R, Peto R, Wheatley K, Gray R, Sutherland I. Mortality in relation to smoking: 40 years' observations on male British doctors. *BMJ* 1994;309:901-11.
10 Jha P, Ramasundarahettige C, Landsman V, Rostron B, Thun M, Anderson RN, et al. 21st-century hazards of smoking and benefits of cessation in the United States. *N Engl J Med* 2013;368:341-50.
11 Cooper J, Borland R, Yong HH. Australian smokers increasingly use help to quit, but number of attempts remains stable: findings from the International Tobacco Control Study 2002-09. *Aust N Z J Public Health* 2011;35:368-76.
12 Hughes JR, Keely J, Naud S. Shape of the relapse curve and long-term abstinence among untreated smokers. *Addiction* 2004;99:29-38.
13 Fiore MC, Jaen CR, Baker TB, Bailey WC, Benowitz NL, Curry SJ, et al. for the Guideline Panel. Treating tobacco use and dependence: 2008 update. Clinical Practice Guideline. Department of Health and Human Services. Public Health Service, 2008.
14 Prochaska JO, Velicer WF. The transtheoretical model of health behavior change. *Am J Health Promot* 1997;12:38-48.

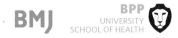

15 Richmond RL, Makinson RJ, Kehoe LA, Giugni AA, Webster IW. One-year evaluation of three smoking cessation interventions administered by general practitioners. *Addict Behav* 1993;18:187-99.

16 Lindson N, Aveyard P, Hughes JR. Reduction versus abrupt cessation in smokers who want to quit. *Cochrane Database Syst Rev* 2010;3:CD008033.

17 Stead LF, Hartmann-Boyce J, Perera R, Lancaster T. Telephone counselling for smoking cessation. *Cochrane Database Syst Rev* 2013;8:CD002850.

18 Fagerstrom K. Time to first cigarette; the best single indicator of tobacco dependence? *Monaldi Arch Chest Dis* 2003;59:91-4.

19 Whittaker R, McRobbie H, Bullen C, Borland R, Rodgers A, Gu Y. Mobile phone-based interventions for smoking cessation. *Cochrane Database Syst Rev* 2012;11:CD006611.

20 Civljak M, Stead LF, Hartmann-Boyce J, Sheikh A, Car J. Internet-based interventions for smoking cessation. *Cochrane Database Syst Rev* 2013;7:CD007078.

21 Lai DT, Cahill K, Qin Y, Tang JL. Motivational interviewing for smoking cessation. *Cochrane Database Syst Rev* 2010;1:CD006936.

22 Miller WR, Rollnick S. Motivational interviewing: preparing people for change. 2nd ed. Guidlford Press, 2002.

23 Cahill K, Stevens S, Perera R, Lancaster T. Pharmacological interventions for smoking cessation: an overview and network meta-analysis. *Cochrane Database Syst Rev* 2013;5:CD009329.

24 Stead LF, Perera R, Bullen C, Mant D, Hartmann-Boyce J, Cahill K, et al. Nicotine replacement therapy for smoking cessation. *Cochrane Database Syst Rev* 2012;11:CD000146.

25 Cahill K, Stead LF, Lancaster T. Nicotine receptor partial agonists for smoking cessation. *Cochrane Database Syst Rev* 2012;4:CD006103.

26 Gibbons RD, Mann JJ. Varenicline, smoking cessation, and neuropsychiatric adverse events. *Am J Psychiatry* 2013;170:1460-7.

27 Hughes JR, Stead LF, Lancaster T. Antidepressants for smoking cessation. *Cochrane Database Syst Rev* 2007;1:CD000031.

28 Zwar N, Richmond R, Borland R, Peters M, Litt J, Bell J, et al. Supporting smoking cessation: a guide for health professionals. Royal Australian College of General Practitioners, 2011.

29 Schaffer SD, Yoon S, Zadezensky I. A review of smoking cessation: potentially risky effects on prescribed medications. *J Clin Nurs* 2009;18:1533-40.

30 Lumley J, Chamberlain C, Dowswell T, Oliver S, Oakley L, Watson L. Interventions for promoting smoking cessation during pregnancy. *Cochrane Database Syst Rev* 2009;3:CD001055.

31 Coleman T, Chamberlain C, Davey MA, Cooper SE, Leonardi-Bee J. Pharmacological interventions for promoting smoking cessation during pregnancy. *Cochrane Database Syst Rev* 2012;9:CD010078.

32 Dempsey DA, Benowitz NL. Risks and benefits of nicotine to aid smoking cessation in pregnancy. *Drug Saf* 2001;24:277-322.

33 Stanton A, Grimshaw G. Tobacco cessation interventions for young people. *Cochrane Database Syst Rev* 2013;8:CD003289.

34 Siru R, Hulse GK, Tait RJ. Assessing motivation to quit smoking in people with mental illness: a review. *Addiction* 2009;104:719-33.

35 Prochaska JJ, Hall SM, Tsoh JY, Eisendrath S, Rossi JS, Redding CA, et al. Treating tobacco dependence in clinically depressed smokers: effect of smoking cessation on mental health functioning. *Am J Public Health* 2008;98:446-8.

36 Caponnetto P, Russo C, Bruno CM, Alamo A, Amaradio MD, Polosa R. Electronic cigarette: a possible substitute for cigarette dependence. *Monaldi Arch Chest Dis* 2013;79:12-9.

37 Caponnetto P, Campagna D, Cibella F, Morjaria JB, Caruso M, Russo C, et al. EffiCiency and Safety of an eLectronic cigAreTte (ECLAT) as tobacco cigarettes substitute: a prospective 12-month randomized control design study. *PloS One* 2013;86:e66317.

38 Pepper JK, Brewer NT. Electronic nicotine delivery system (electronic cigarette) awareness, use, reactions and beliefs: a systematic review. *Tob Control* 2013 doi:10.1136/tobaccocontrol-2013-051122

39 Roberts V, Maddison R, Simpson C, Bullen C, Prapavessis H. The acute effects of exercise on cigarette cravings, withdrawal symptoms, affect, and smoking behaviour: systematic review update and meta-analysis. *Psychopharmacology* 2012;222:1-15.

40 Ussher MH, Taylor A, Faulkner G. Exercise interventions for smoking cessation. *Cochrane Database Syst Rev* 2012;1:CD002295.

41 Brewer JA, Elwafi HM, Davis JH. Craving to quit: psychological models and neurobiological mechanisms of mindfulness training as treatment for addictions. *Psychol Addict Behav* 2013;27:366-79.

42 Cropley M, Ussher M, Charitou E. Acute effects of a guided relaxation routine (body scan) on tobacco withdrawal symptoms and cravings in abstinent smokers. *Addiction* 2007;102:989-93.

43 Davis JM, Fleming MF, Bonus KA, Baker TB. A pilot study on mindfulness based stress reduction for smokers. *BMC Complement Altern Med* 2007;7:2.

44 Brewer JA, Mallik S, Babuscio TA, Nich C, Johnson HE, Deleone CM, et al. Mindfulness training for smoking cessation: results from a randomized controlled trial. *Drug Alcohol Depend* 2011;119:72-80.

45 White AR, Rampes H, Liu JP, Stead LF, Campbell J. Acupuncture and related interventions for smoking cessation. *Cochrane Database Syst Rev* 2011;1:CD000009.

46 Barnes J, Dong CY, McRobbie H, Walker N, Mehta M, Stead LF. Hypnotherapy for smoking cessation. *Cochrane Database Syst Rev* 2010;10:CD001008.

47 Hajek P, Stead LF, West R, Jarvis M, Hartmann-Boyce J, Lancaster T. Relapse prevention interventions for smoking cessation. *Cochrane Database Syst Rev* 2013;8:CD003999.

48 NICE. Tobacco: harm reduction approaches to smoking. National Institute for Health and Care Excellence, June 2013. www.guidance.nice.org.uk/ph45.

Related links

bmj.com
- Get Cleveland Clinic CME credits for this article

bmj.com/archive
Previous articles in this series
- Abortion (BMJ 2014;348:f7553)
- Diagnosis, management, and prevention of rotavirus gastroenteritis in children (BMJ 2013;347:f7204)
- Tick bite prevention and tick removal (BMJ 2013;347:f7123)
- Polymyalgia rheumatica (BMJ 2013;347:f6937)
- Diagnosis and management of hyperhidrosis (BMJ 2013;347:f6800)

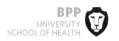

The assessment and management of insomnia in primary care

Karen Falloon, PhD candidate[1], Bruce Arroll, professor and head of department[1],
C Raina Elley, associate professor[1], Antonio Fernando III, senior lecturer[2]

[1]Department of General Practice and Primary Health Care, University of Auckland, Private Bag 92109, Auckland 1142, New Zealand

[2]Department of Psychological Medicine, University of Auckland

Correspondence to: B Arroll b.arroll@auckland.ac.nz

Cite this as: *BMJ* 2011;342:d2899

DOI: 10.1136/bmj.d2899

http://www.bmj.com/content/342/bmj.d2899

Insomnia affects about a third of the general population according to a recent longitudinal study in the UK[1] and cross sectional studies estimate the prevalence in patients attending primary care to be between 10% and 50%.[2] [3] According to the American Sleep Disorders Association International Classification of Sleep Disorders coding manual, insomnia refers to "a repeated difficulty with sleep initiation, duration, consolidation, or quality that occurs despite adequate time and opportunity for sleep and results in some form of daytime impairment and lasting for at least one month."[4] Although some patients who have this problem may not report it as such, inadequate sleep has been associated with reduced physical health[3] [4] [5] [6] and mental health.[7] [8] [9] The continued widespread use of sedative medication to treat insomnia raises concern about the potential for long term tolerance and addiction, particularly where insomnia is the presenting complaint of missed diagnoses such as depression, or when adverse effects might be a problem—for example, falls in older adults.[10] [11] [12] The normal range of sleep is seven to nine hours per night,[13] although some individuals claim they can function on as little as four hours, whereas others need up to 10 hours. This article reviews the causes of insomnia and its treatment, focusing on the many non-drug options that may be suitable for use by general clinicians. This review is based on evidence from randomised trials for interventions and guidance from the American Academy of sleep medicine guidelines (www.aasmnet.org).

What is insomnia and who gets it?

Patients with insomnia may report difficulty with falling asleep, trouble staying asleep or frequent waking, waking too early and being unable to get back to sleep, or still feeling tired after waking up. As many as 40% of patients in primary care will report these symptoms if asked.[2] Insomnia is either primary, in which case no other contributing cause is present, or secondary, in which case it is caused or affected by an underlying condition (table 1). Patients can have more than one underlying diagnosis. Depression and anxiety underpin insomnia in as many as half of cases and they frequently co-exist.[2] Physical health problems are also present in about a third of cases.[2] Excessive alcohol consumption and illicit drug use may also be associated with reports of poor sleep (about 8% and 6% of cases, respectively).[2] About 12% of those who report difficulty in sleeping have delayed sleep phase disorder, a circadian rhythm disorder in which the person has trouble getting to sleep at the time most people do.[2] They tend to go to bed very late and have difficulty in waking up when most others get up. People with insomnia function better on weekends when they can sleep late and wake up late. Obstructive sleep apnoea is a relatively common cause of sleep disturbance and can have a profound effect on daily functioning (box 1).

Sleep requirements may fall with age. A recent review summarises the literature on normal and abnormal sleep in older people.[17] A mean sleep duration of seven hours per night was found among 1000 older adults interviewed in a French study.[17] Another study found that total sleep time decreased on average by 27 minutes per decade from midlife to the eighth decade of life. Older people "spend more time in bed but have deterioration in both the quality and quantity of sleep."[17]

How is insomnia diagnosed?

Taking a good history is important for diagnosing insomnia and identifying any underlying causes. Box 2 outlines the questions posed and information gained when asking about insomnia.

Considering secondary causes

Case finding for depression or anxiety using brief questions may identify an underlying mental illness.[18] [19] [20] Enquiry about other secondary causes shown in table 1 is warranted. For people with bipolar disorder, insomnia may herald a manic episode. Several tools are available for assessing depression and anxiety, including the patient health questionnaire (PHQ)-9, hospital anxiety and depression scale (HADS-7), or PHQ-4.[14] [20] [21] The alcohol use disorders identification test (AUDIT) or CAGE may be used to assess alcohol use[22] [23] and the alcohol, smoking and substance involvement screening test (ASSIST) to assess drug use.[24]

Sleep diaries

General practitioners can make use of sleep diaries in which patients record their sleep pattern for one to two weeks; however, using them makes the consultation more involved. Several diary templates are available on the internet (for example, www.sleepeducation.com/pdf/sleepdiary.pdf). Sleep diaries can provide patients with insight into their actual sleep habits. They often reflect sleep trends,

---

SOURCES AND SELECTION CRITERIA

As well as using our personal reference collections, we searched the Cochrane database (www.cochrane.org), *Clinical Evidence* (http://clinicalevidence.bmj.com), and Best Practice (http://bestpractice.bmj.com). We also reviewed guidelines from the National Institute for Health and Clinical Excellence, the American Academy of Sleep Medicine, and the International Classification of Sleep Disorders. We selected systematic reviews and meta-analyses and when these were not available we used large randomised controlled trials.

SUMMARY POINTS

- Insomnia affects a third of people and is a common cause of consultation in primary care
- History is the main diagnostic tool
- There are many causes of secondary insomnia, which should be ruled out and treated first
- Excessive daytime sleepiness should raise questions about obstructive sleep apnoea
- Primary insomnia is diagnosed after excluding other causes of insomnia. It can be treated effectively by sleep hygiene techniques, by restricting time in bed, or with behavioural interventions
- Sedatives should be used as a last resort when other approaches have failed because of risks of tolerance and adverse effects

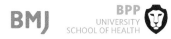

such as erratic schedules, or identify predominant sleep patterns, such as taking a long time to fall asleep, frequent awakenings, early morning awakenings, or a mixture. They can provide a starting point for the management of sleep problems in a personalised manner and can be used to monitor progress of certain treatments.

Physical examination

Although a physical examination cannot diagnose insomnia, it may be useful to help identify or exclude obvious underlying causes of sleep disorder such as obstructive sleep apnoea or a neurological condition such as Parkinson's disease. High body mass index (.30) and neck circumference of 40 cm or greater increase the risk of obstructive sleep apnoea.[25] Usually the primary care doctor will be aware of other co-morbidities. Blood tests for hyperthyroidism and low ferritin levels, which can cause restless legs, may be warranted. A full blood count may rule out anaemia.

Polysomnography (overnight sleep study)

Patients can be referred for polysomnography to confirm sleep apnoea and limb movement disorders or restless legs syndrome. Polysomnography measures brain and muscle activity and assesses oxygen saturation overnight.

BOX 1 OBSTRUCTIVE SLEEP APNOEA

- Affects about 9% of those reporting poor sleep in primary care[2]
- More common in people who are obese
- Episodic partial or complete upper airway obstruction is usually associated with oxygen desaturations in the blood and arousals from sleep
- Symptoms include chronic snoring, insomnia, gasping and breath holding, un-refreshing sleep, and daytime sleepiness. Be alert to this as a possible diagnosis if the patient reports falling asleep during the day including as a passenger in a car on short trips, in waiting rooms, or in lectures
- Bed partners may report the patient's snoring and gasping[14]
- If a patient answers yes to all or most of the following questions they will have a significant pre-test probability of obstructive sleep apnoea and will require further investigation and/ or treatment.[4] Do you: experience excessive sleepiness during the day?; experience frequent episodes of breathing pauses? (or gasping for air) during sleep. Or has someone told you that while you are asleep you: stop breathing?; snore very loudly? Do you: get morning headaches?; have a dry mouth on awakening?
- There may be a legal obligation for health professionals to advise professional drivers and machine operators of falling asleep at work.
- The diagnosis can be confirmed with polysomnography or nocturnal pulse oximetry.[15]
- The initial treatment is for patients to use a continuous positive airways pressure (CPAP) machine at night[16]; if this is unsuccessful consider surgical options. Level A evidence from meta-analysis supports CPAP.[16]

Table 1 Secondary causes of insomnia and appropriate treatments

Secondary cause	Treatment
Depression	Treat depression (for example, antidepressants, cognitive behavioural therapy)
Anxiety	Treat anxiety (drug or cognitive behavioural therapy)
Physical health problem (such as pain or dyspnoea)	Treat pain and other symptoms
Obstructive sleep apnoea	Continuous positive airways pressure or devices to improve airway (such as mandibular advancement splint in mild cases); consider referral to a respiratory doctor or sleep physician
Excess alcohol	Interventions to reduce alcohol intake or promote abstinence
Delayed sleep phase disorder (a circadian rhythm disorder)	Change work hours; melatonin in the evening and light exposure (via sunlight or artificial light box) in the morning
Illicit drug use	Interventions to reduce drug use
Parasomnias (restless legs, sleep talking, sleep walking, sleep terrors, periodic limb movements, bruxism (teeth grinding), nightmare disorder, sleep related eating disorder, sleep sex	For restless legs check ferritin, consider non-drug based measures or non-ergot dopamine antagonist drugs for severe cases; for other parasomnias consider referral

How can insomnia be managed in primary care without medication?

For all patients following the principles of basic sleep hygiene may be beneficial (table 2).

Secondary insomnia

For patients in whom a cause of the insomnia is identified (secondary insomnia) we recommend beginning with treatment of the underlying condition (see table 1). For all patients following the principles of basic sleep hygiene may be beneficial (table 2). In our experience patients may have several contributing diagnoses. Addressing some of these issues may solve other problems. For example, advising patients to reduce their use of drugs and alcohol along with treating pain or breathing difficulty may resolve depression and anxiety as well as improving the insomnia.

Delayed sleep phase disorder and parasomnias

The use of melatonin at night and light boxes in the morning are helpful; at least two randomised trials have shown a benefit for those with delayed sleep phase disorder.[26][27]

For most cases of restless legs, non-drug treatments such as massage, exercise, stretching, and warm baths before bedtime are recommended.[28] For more severe cases, non-ergot dopamine antagonists are recommended, on the basis of evidence from randomised controlled trial.[28] Advice should be sought for other parasomnias, such as sleep walking and other nocturnal behaviours that are not common in primary care (box 3).

Primary insomnia

About 30% of patients with primary insomnia will improve with basic sleep hygiene alone (table 2).[29]

Restriction of time in bed

Recommendations developed and published by the American Academy of Sleep Medicine in 2006 have concluded from the available evidence that psychological and behavioural interventions are effective in the treatment of chronic primary insomnia.[30] Empirically-supported treatments include: cognitive behavioural therapy, bedtime restriction (sleep restriction), stimulus control therapy, relaxation training, and paradoxical intention (instructions to remain passively awake and avoid any effort to sleep).[31]

Cognitive behavioural therapy has been shown to be an effective treatment for insomnia in meta-analyses of randomised trials.[32][33] It aims to address the various cognitive and behavioural aspects of insomnia using a combination of interventions such as behavioural strategies (such as bedtime restriction, stimulus control therapy, and relaxation), education (for example, about sleep hygiene), and cognitive strategies (cognitive therapy). Importantly, it is not designed to be administered by a general practitioner (typically administered in six to eight sessions, as shown in a randomised controlled trial)[34] and thus it remains underused in primary care. Therefore, a simple starting point for treatment of primary insomnia is to address sleep hygiene and to try a behavioural intervention such as bedtime restriction or stimulus control.

Bedtime restriction involves curtailing time spent in bed to closely match actual time spent asleep (box 4).[35] Evidence from a randomised controlled trial suggests that this method is effective for some patients with primary insomnia.[w1] Restricting time in bed often forms part of cognitive behavioural therapy interventions. This is

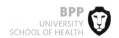

potentially a very simple treatment that can be used in primary care and is useful for people who spend a lot of time in bed but not sleeping.

Stimulus control refers to a set of instructions designed to reassociate the bed and bedroom with sleep and re-establish a regular sleep-wake routine (box 5).[w2]

What is the role of medication in primary insomnia?

Hypnotic drugs are often used to manage insomnia in general practice.[w3] Different classes of sleep medications are prescribed (table 3) or purchased over the counter (for example, sedating antihistamines, melatonin, and natural supplements such as valerian), although this approach is

---

BOX 2 HISTORY TAKING AND INFORMATION GAINED

Question

Can you describe your problem with sleeping?

- Does it interfere with your function the next day (for example, feeling unrefreshed in the morning, fatigued, having poor concentration or irritability)?
- Can you tell me about your bedtime routine starting with the time you get into bed?
- Time that you go to bed
- Time to fall asleep
- Awakenings (number, duration, do you know what causes you to awaken? Do you have any associated symptoms, such as heartburn, coughing, shortness of breath, pain, anxiety, or full bladder?)
- Last awakening time in the morning
- Time of rising from bed
- Usual duration of sleep
- How is your routine different at the weekends or during holidays? Do you have the same bedtime?
- Do you do vigorous activity late in the evening?

Information gained

- Some patients think they do not get enough sleep but function well the next day. Technically they do not have insomnia because the definition of insomnia includes "results in some form of daytime impairment"[4]
- Frequent changes in routine and vigorous activity just before bedtime can cause sleep problems
- Physical health problems are a significant cause (43%) of insomnia in primary care and will require attention[2]
- If the time in bed greatly exceeds the time asleep (for example, by a few hours), the patient may have primary insomnia if no other causes are present. Spending less time in bed can lead to a dramatic improvement in sleep quality and may decrease the fragmentation of sleep. Exposure to computer screens in the hours before bed can delay sleep onset.

Question

How do you feel on awakening?

- Unrefreshed and still sleepy?
- Any symptoms such as headaches or dry mouth?
- Daytime sleepiness—falling asleep in waiting rooms, as a passenger in a car, or during lectures

Information gained

- Need to consider obstructive sleep apnoea. Consider asking the patient to fill out the Epworth sleepiness scale,[16] which measures levels of daytime sleepiness

Question

Are there any symptoms of obstructive sleep apnoea (ask bed partner too if possible)?

- Such as heavy snoring, pauses in breathing, and gasping

Information gained

- Provides information on obstructive sleep apnoea

Question

What other factors may interfere with sleeping?

- Use of stimulants (such as caffeine, alcohol, cigarettes, drugs)
- Other drugs that may interfere with sleep
- Important recent life events (such as bereavement)

Information gained

- Ideally avoid use of stimulants after 6 pm
- Oral decongestants, such as pseudoephedrine; asthma, drugs such as long and short acting sympathomimetics; amphetamines; antidepressants, such as selective serotonin reuptake inhibitors can all cause insomnia, and a trial without them is simple and potentially diagnostic

Question

Do you take any naps?

- Ask about frequency, timing, and duration
- Where are you sleeping when you have the problem? Is the problem persistent when you sleep elsewhere (for example, when on holiday?) Is it persistent throughout the week and year?

Information gained

- Long naps during the day can affect the quality of sleep at night
- If the patient sleeps better when on holiday or at weekends, think of delayed sleep phase disorder, especially if he or she goes to bed after midnight

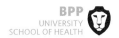

BOX 2 HISTORY TAKING AND INFORMATION GAINED (CONTINUED)

Question

Do you experience any of the following?

- Low mood or lack of pleasure in some or most activities or worrying a lot; nocturnal panic attacks
- Restless sleep
- Leg or body twitching
- Leg jerking (consider restless legs syndrome)
- Shaking fits
- Sleep walking or talking
- Waking up in terror
- Unusual night time behaviours

Information gained

- Patients who answer yes to the first question may have depression and anxiety; consider using the formal inventories for case finding
- The other symptoms may be related to parasomnias

Table 2 "Sleep hygiene" instructions and rationale

Instruction	Rationale
Limit use of caffeine to 1 cup of coffee in the morning (if at all), avoid alcohol and cigarettes at night, and limit other substances that can affect sleep	Caffeine and nicotine are stimulants that can delay sleep onset and impair sleep quality; people vary in their ability to metabolise these substances from their system; some people use alcohol to help them get to sleep because it relaxes them, but it may cause awakenings and reduce sleep quality later in the sleep period
Avoid going to bed until you are drowsy and ready to sleep	People do not fall asleep if their brain is wide awake, so going to bed before they are sleepy leads to frustration at not being able to sleep, which can further delay sleep onset; people's sleep patterns and needs may not match those of their bed partners
Avoid napping during the day	Napping reduces the "sleep pressure" that builds up during the day to the point where a threshold is reached and we are ready to sleep; napping may delay the time of readiness for sleep and lead to erratic bedtimes, especially if the person can sleep in to compensate for a later bedtime (leading to a "domino" effect for the day after); if naps have been taken during the day, and the "usual" bedtime is kept, sleep onset may be delayed, leading to frustration and anxiety, which further prolongs sleep onset
Regular daily exercise can help improve sleep, but avoid exercise late in the evening	Exercise too close to a sleep period can serve as an arousal stimulus, delaying sleep onset
Ensure that the bedtime environment is comfortable and conducive to sleep	The bed should be comfortable, the temperature not too hot or cold, the room dark, and noise minimised; discomfort, being too hot or cold, noise, and light can disrupt sleep
Think about computer screens, clocks, and co-sleepers	Looking at a computer screen in the hours before bed may delay sleep onset (the light waves emitted are thought to reduce the production of melatonin, a hormone that is secreted by the pineal gland to promote sleep); looking at a clock during awakenings can delay sleep onset by contributing to frustration at being awake (lit clocks may also contribute arousal stimuli to the brain); if co-sleepers are disturbing sleep (by excessive movements or snoring) they probably warrant their own assessment for sleep disorders
If not asleep within 15-20 minutes, get out of bed and return only when drowsy	The thought behind this idea is that bed needs to be associated with being asleep not with being awake and having difficulty getting to sleep

BOX 3 PARASOMNIAS (NEUROLOGICAL CONDITIONS, RARE IN PRIMARY CARE)

- Restless legs syndrome
- Sleep talking
- Sleep walking
- Sleep terrors
- Periodic limb movements
- Bruxism (teeth grinding)
- Nightmare disorder
- Sleep related eating disorder
- Sleep sex

sleep medications will depend on whether the clinician or the patient raises medication as an option. Patients who raise the matter must be informed of the benefits of non-drug based treatment. They may eventually need drugs, but optimal practice should include a trial of non-drug based treatment. If the clinician raises the matter then presumably the patient has completed a trial of non-drug treatment or the situation is extreme and urgent.

Concerns about hypnotics

Hypnotic drugs (benzodiazepines or "z-drugs" such as zopiclone) are associated with perceived tolerance, dependence, and withdrawal syndrome and with "rebound insomnia" on cessation.[w7-w9] They can also have side effects, and in rare cases can be associated with unusual sleep behaviours (such as "sleep driving" or making phone calls, with no remembrance of the events), especially if taken with alcohol.[w8] There is also the risk of misuse—hypnotics can enhance the "high" from other drugs[w9] and have been used in overdose attempts. Further problems include drug interactions, issues around driving under the influence of psychotropics, and potential risks when prescribing to the elderly (falls, cognitive impairment, and fatigue).[w10]

Despite these potential problems, benzodiazepine receptor agonists are often prescribed for insomnia.[w11] Tolerance and dependence are common concerns despite the contradictory evidence in many clinical studies. A six month double blind placebo controlled study of eszopiclone in hundreds of patients showed sustained response and no tolerance.[w12] Benzodiazepines have been consistently shown to improve sleep latency and increase total sleep time,[w11] and they have significantly fewer side effects than sedating antidepressants and sedating antipsychotics.[w13] Shorter acting benzodiazepines (zolpidem, triazolam) are preferred for insomnia with delayed sleep latency (long onset of

not evidence based as a treatment of chronic insomnia.[w4] [w5] Recent reviews have shown that pharmacotherapy and psychological or behavioural interventions result in similar short term (up to four weeks) improvements, but that psychological and behavioural treatments have persisting benefits that can also improve with time.[w4] [w5] Furthermore, the use of sleep medication as monotherapy may not result in the quality of sleep that can be achieved by other methods and may not deal with the underlying sleep problem. A randomised comparison between zopiclone and cognitive behavioural therapy found better sleep efficiency in the cognitive behavioural therapy group, along with fewer awakenings.[w6] The total sleeping time did not differ between the groups.

A high level of suspicion is warranted if an unknown or new patient asks for a hypnotic by name because he or she may want the drug for illicit purposes. The discussion about

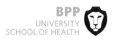

Table 3 Drugs commonly used for insomnia

Drug	Class	Usual hypnotic dose	Half life	
Temazepam	Benzodiazepine receptor agonist	10-20 mg	5-15 hours[w16]	Sedation, confusion, amnesia, impaired coordination, disinhibition
Triazolam	Benzodiazepine receptor agonist	0.125-0.25 mg	2-3 hours[w16]	Same as above
Zolpidem	Benzodiazepine receptor agonist	5-10 mg	1.5-2.4 hours[w11]	Same as above
Zopiclone	Benzodiazepine receptor agonist	7.5 mg	5-6 hours [w11]	Same as above
Doxepin	Sedating antidepressant	25-50 mg	8-24 hours[w11]	Sedation, falls, dizziness, dry mouth (and other anticholinergic side effects) headache, nausea, lightheadedness
Quetiapine	Sedating antipsychotic	25-200 mg	6 hours[w11]	Sedation, weight gain, hypotension
Promethazine	Sedating antihistamine	10-20 mg	5-15 hours[w16]	Sedation, urinary retention, dizziness

---

BOX 4 BED TIME RESTRICTION FOR PRIMARY INSOMNIA

- Ensure the diagnosis is most likely to be primary insomnia (no other conditions)
- Advise workers who drive vehicles or operate heavy machinery to consider treatment during their vacation, because there is a short term risk of sleep deprivation
- Estimate time spent in bed versus time spent asleep, with use of a sleep diary if necessary. A common scenario is that a patient stays in bed around 8-9 hours but only sleeps for a total of 6 hours. Advise the patient to restrict their total time in bed to their estimated total sleep time. We find it best for the patient to get up at the usual (household) time and go to bed later. For example, if the usual getting up time is 0600, suggest that they go to bed at 2400 instead of their usual 2200. Advise the patient to do only quiet, relaxing activities before bedtime. These activities have to be done outside of bed and not lying down to avoid naps, which can disrupt the routine. We recommend patients keep their bedtime allowance for two weeks before making any adjustments. The patient usually reports that the quality of their sleep improves as they feel they are starting to have deep sleep and the sleep period is consolidated.
- After two weeks:
- If the patient is sleeping better and functioning well nothing else is needed. Many patients prefer to continue on the bed restriction schedule as they find it very effective
- If they are sleeping better but feel sleep deprived the next day they may wish to add 30 minutes to their time allowed in bed every week and continue doing so until the feelings of sleep deprivation disappear, while still maintaining continuous sleep at night
- If they are not sleeping better, they may wish to reduce their time in bed by 30 minutes (but not to less than five hours at night). Ensure that the patient tries each option for at least two weeks before making another change. If they are not sleeping better on five hours per night you may wish to get some advice from a sleep specialist
- The bedtime allowance is never set at less than the estimated average time spent asleep or five hours (whichever is longer)

BOX 5 STIMULUS CONTROL INSTRUCTIONS

- (1) Go to bed only when sleepy
- (2) Get out of bed if unable to sleep after 15-20 minutes, returning to bed only when sleepy (repeat as necessary)
- (3) Use the bed/bedroom only for sleep
- (4) Arise at the same time each day
- (5) No naps

primary insomnia,[w14] although it does affect the circadian rhythm and is used to treat insomnia caused by jet lag,[w15] circadian rhythm disorders, and shift work.

Although drugs have their place, they should be considered only in patients who do not improve after cognitive behavioural therapy or other non-drug based interventions.

When and to whom to refer?

If any uncertainty exists about the diagnosis or if any safety concerns have been identified (such as excessive daytime sleepiness or parasomnias causing injuries) referral to and assessment by a sleep specialist is indicated. If a sleep specialist is unavailable, discussion with neurology, general medical, or psychiatry services may help determine the appropriate avenue for referral.

Contributors: BA had the idea for the review and KF wrote the first draft. The subsequent drafts were written by all authors, CRE contributed to the draft and provided the primary care input, AF wrote the section on medication and provided the sleep specialist input, and all authors read all drafts. BA is the guarantor.

Competing interests: All authors have completed the ICMJE uniform disclosure form at www.icmje.org/coi_disclosure.pdf (available on request from the corresponding author) and declare: no support from any organisation for the submitted work; no financial relationships with any organisations that might have an interest in the submitted work in the previous three years; no other relationships or activities that could appear to have influenced the submitted work.

Provenance and peer review: Not commissioned, externally peer reviewed.

1. Morphy H, Dunn KM, Lewis M, Boardman HF, Croft PR, Morphy H, et al. Epidemiology of insomnia: a longitudinal study in a UK population. *Sleep* 2007;30:274-80.
2. Arroll B, Fernando A, Falloon K, Warman G, Goodyear-Smith F. Sleepless in Seattle? Finding patients with primary insomnia using the Auckland Sleep Questionnaire. North American Primary Care Research Group Seattle, 2010.
3. Simon GE, VonKorff M. Prevalence, burden, and treatment of insomnia in primary care. *Am J Psychiatry* 1997;154:1417-23.
4. American Sleep Disorders Association. International Classification of Sleep Disorders, second edition: diagnostic and coding manual. American Sleep Disorders Association, 2005.
5. Kuppermann M, Lubeck D, Mazonson P, Patrick D, Stewart A, Buesching D, et al. Sleep problems and their correlates in a working population. *J Gen Int Med* 1995;10:25-32.
6. Marshall NS, Bolger W, Gander PH. Abnormal sleep duration and motor vehicle crash risk. *J Sleep Res* 2004;13:177-8.
7. Breslau N, Roth T, Rosenthal L, Andreski P. Sleep disturbance and psychiatric disorders: a longitudinal epidemiological study of young adults. *Biological Psychiatry* 1996;39:411-8.

getting to sleep). Medium acting ones like temazepam and zopiclone are preferred for patients who wake in the middle of the night. Long acting drugs like clonazepam are preferred for patients with insomnia and daytime anxiety. To limit the risk of dependence or tolerance, prescribers can tell patients to use benzodiazepines "as needed," with a maximum frequency per week (no more than three nights).

Non-benzodiazepine drugs used as hypnotics
Sedating antidepressants and sedating antipsychotics generally do not result in physical dependence, tolerance, or misuse. Because of this, many doctors prefer to prescribe these groups of drugs instead of benzodiazepines. This is despite their common adverse effects including daytime sedation, weight gain, and anticholinergic side effects. Sedating antidepressants are more toxic than benzodiazepines in overdose. There is also less evidence for the efficacy of sedating antidepressants than benzodiazepines in insomnia. Sedating antipsychotics also carry the risk of tardive dyskinesia and weight gain. Sedating antidepressants may be useful if there are anxious or depressive components to the clinical picture.

Melatonin is a pineal hormone that is naturally secreted during darkness. It is thought to signal sleep onset and has some sleep promoting effects. However, most clinical trials have shown that exogenous melatonin is not effective in

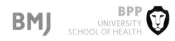

8   Ford DE, Kamerow DB. Epidemiologic study of sleep disturbances and psychiatric disorders. An opportunity for prevention? *JAMA* 1989;262:1479-84.

9   Mallon L, Broman JE, Hetta J, Mallon L, Broman J-E, Hetta J. High incidence of diabetes in men with sleep complaints or short sleep duration: a 12-year follow-up study of a middle-aged population. *Diabetes Care* 2005;28:2762-7.

10 Panneman MJ, Goettsch WG, Kramarz P, Herings RM. The costs of benzodiazepine-associated hospital-treated fall injuries in the EU: a Pharmo sudy. *Drugs Aging* 2003;20:883-9.

11 Campbell SS, Broughton RJ. Rapid decline in body temperature before sleep: fluffing the physiological pillow? *Chronobiol Int* 1994;11:126-31.

12 Curran HV, Collins R, Fletcher S, Kee SC, Woods B, Illife S. Older adults and withdrawal from benzodiazepine hypnotics in general practice: effects on cognitive function, sleep, mood and quality of life. *Psychological Med* 2003;33:1223-37.

13 Shapiro CM, Dement WC. Impact and epidemiology of sleep disorders. *BMJ* 1993;306:1604-7.

14 Johns MW. A new method for measuring daytime sleepiness: the Epworth sleepiness scale. *Sleep* 1991;14:540-5.

15 Rofail LM, Wong KH, Unger G, Marks GB, Grunstein RR. Comparison between a single-channel nasal airflow device and oximetry for the diagnosis of obstructive sleep apnea. *Sleep* 2010;33:1106-14.

16 National Institute for Health and Clinical Excellence. Continuous positive airway pressure for the treatment of obstructive sleep apnoea/hypopnoea syndrome. NICE, 2008. http://guidance.nice.org.uk/TA139.

17 Cooke JR, Ancoli-Israel S. Normal and abnormal sleep in the elderly. *Handb Clin Neurol* 2011;98:653-5.

18 Arroll B, Goodyear-Smith F, Kerse N, Fishman T, Gunn J. Effect of the addition of a "help" question to two screening questions on specificity for diagnosis of depression in general practice: diagnostic validity study. *BMJ* 2005;331:884.

19 Puddifoot S, Arroll B, Goodyear-Smith FA, Kerse NM, Fishman TG, Gunn JM. A new case-finding tool for anxiety: a pragmatic validity study in primary care. *I J Psychiatry Med* 2007;4:371-81.

20 Kroenke K, Spitzer RL, Williams BW, Lowe B. A ultra-brief screening scale for anxiety and depression: the PHQ 4. *Psychosomatics* 2009;50:613-21.

21 Zigmond AS, Snaith RP. The hospital anxiety and depression scale. *Acta Psychiatr Scand* 1983;67:361-70.

22 Mayfield D, McLeod G, Hall P. The CAGE questionnaire: validation of a new alcoholism screening instrument. *Am J Psychiatry* 1974;131:1121-3.

23 Wennberg P, Escobar F, Espi F, Canteras M, Lairson DR, Harlow K, et al. The alcohol use disorders identification test (AUDIT): A psychometric evaluation. *Reports Dept Psychol U Stockholm* 1996;811:1-14.

24 WHO. The ASSIST project—Alcohol, Smoking and Substance Involvement Screening Test. 2011. www.who.int/substance_abuse/activities/assist/en/index.html.

25 Chung F, Yegneswaran B, Liao P, Chung SA, Vairavanathan S, Islam S, et al. Stop questionnaire. A tool to screen patients for obstructive sleep apnea. *Anesthesiology* 2008;108:812-21.

26 Kayumov L, Brown, G, Jindal R, Buttoo K, Shapiro CM. A randomized, double-blind, placebo-controlled crossover study of the effect of exogenous melatonin on delayed sleep phase syndrome. *Psychosom Med* 2001;63:40-8.

27 Rosenthal NE, Joseph-Vanderpool JR, Levendosky AA, Johnston SH, Allen R, Kelly KA, et al. Phase-shifting effects of bright morning light as treatment for delayed sleep phase syndrome. *Sleep* 1990;13:354-61.

28 Best Practice. Insomnia. http://bestpractice.bmj.com/best-practice/monograph/227.html.

29 Edinger JD, Olsen MK, Stechuchak KM, Means MK, Lineberger MD, Kirby A, et al. Cognitive behavioral therapy for patients with primary insomnia or insomnia associated predominantly with mixed psychiatric disorders: a randomized clinical trial. *Sleep* 2009;32:499-510.

30 Morgenthaler T, Kramer M, Alessi C, Friedman L, Boehlecke B, Brown T, et al. Practice parameters for the psychological and behavioral treatment of insomnia: an update. An American academy of sleep medicine report. *Sleep* 2006;29:1415-9.

31 Morin CM, Bootzin RR, Buysse DJ, Edinger JD, Espie CA, Lichstein KL, et al. Psychological and behavioral treatment of insomnia: update of the recent evidence (1998-2004). *Sleep* 2006;29:1398-414.

32 Irwin MR, Cole JC, Nicassio PM. Comparative meta-analysis of behavioral interventions for insomnia and their efficacy in middle-aged adults and in older adults 55+ years of age. *Health Psychology* 2006;25:3-14.

33 Smith MT, Perlis ML, Park A, Smith MS, Pennington J, Giles DE, et al. Comparative meta-analysis of pharmacotherapy and behavior therapy for persistent insomnia. *Am J Psychiatry* 2002;159:5-11.

34 Edinger JD, Sampson WS, Edinger JD, Sampson WS. A primary care "friendly" cognitive behavioral insomnia therapy. *Sleep* 2003;26:177-82.

35 Spielman AJ, Saskin P, Thorpy MJ. Treatment of chronic insomnia by restriction of time in bed. *Sleep* 1987;10:45-56.

Related links

bmj.com/archive
Previous articles in this series
- The management of tennis elbow (2011;342:d2687)
- Diagnosis and management of schistosomiasis (2011;342:d2651)
- Advising on travel during pregnancy (2011;342:d2506)
- Laser refractive eye surgery (2011;342:d2345)
- Management of paracetamol poisoning (2011;342:d2218)

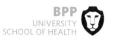

Subjective memory problems

Steve Iliffe, professor of primary care for older people[1], chief investigator [2],
Louise Pealing, general practitioner[3]

[1]University College London, London WC1E 6BT

[2]Evidence-based Interventions in Dementia (EVIDEM) programme

[3]London School of Hygiene and Tropical Medicine, London

Correspondence to: S Iliffe
s.iliffe@ucl.ac.uk

Cite this as: *BMJ* 2010;340:c1425

DOI: 10.1136/bmj.c1425

http://www.bmj.com/content/340/bmj.c1425

The National Dementia Strategy for England, published in 2009,[1] urges general practitioners to become skilled at recognising dementia at an early stage and to promptly refer those at risk to specialist memory services. The implementation of the strategy includes a public awareness campaign to reduce the stigma of dementia and encourage people to approach their GP if they have concerns about their memory. Subjective memory loss, which is seen as the cardinal symptom of dementia by the public, is likely to be the main problem reported by those who consult their doctor. However, the findings of the Kungsholmen cohort study, which included 1435 people aged 75-95 years without dementia, suggest that only 18% of future cases of dementia will be identified in the preclinical phase by investigating those who screen positive for memory problems.[2]

What evidence is available to guide GPs in management and referral decisions for patients with subjective memory loss? This clinical review is based on the findings of five systematic reviews, three of which[3][4][5] investigated the association between subjective memory problems and concurrent objective memory impairment (mild cognitive impairment, dementia, or objective impairment meeting neither clinical diagnosis criteria) or the risk for subsequent memory impairment or dementia. These three reviews included 21, 26, and 10 studies, respectively. The other two reviews investigated patients' quality of life associated with subjective memory problems (five studies)[6] and methods used to ascertain subjective memory impairment (44 studies).[7] In addition to exploring factors associated with subjective memory symptoms, we describe tools and "rules of thumb" that could assist GPs in managing patients who report such problems.

How common are subjective memory problems in older people?

The prevalence of memory problems in people aged 65 and older ranges from 25% to 50%[3] dependent on the method of measuring or eliciting symptoms and on the characteristics of study populations.[7] The prevalence of subjective memory problems increases with age,[8] from 43% in people aged 65-74 to as high as 88% in those older than 85. In a postal survey of nearly 2000 Dutch people aged 25 to 85, 52% of those aged 70 to 85 reported forgetfulness and 23% of this age group reported impairment in everyday living because of memory problems.[9] In a recent systematic review a pooled analysis from eight community studies of people aged 50 and over found the prevalence of dementia to be 8.8%, whereas in a pooled analysis from seven community studies 16.8% of people aged 60 and older had mild cognitive impairment.[5] Because a large proportion of patients with mild cognitive impairment later develop dementia, such impairment is assumed to be the prodrome of dementia syndrome (loss of memory and one other aspect of cognition sufficient to cause impairment).[10]

Are subjective memory problems associated with concurrent objective memory impairment?

In the most recent review, eight studies with a pooled population of 9148[5] reported the rate of subjective memory problems in patients with dementia, seven reported the rate in those with mild cognitive impairment, and of these four compared the rates in dementia and mild cognitive impairment head to head. Subjective memory problems were reported by 43% of those with known dementia and 38% of those with known mild cognitive impairment. Across the spectrum of cognitive impairment (mild cognitive impairment or dementia) 40% of patients had subjective memory problems compared with 17% in healthy adult controls.[5] In this review the pooled sensitivity of subjective memory problems for prediction of dementia was 43% and the specificity was 86%. For mild cognitive impairment, the pooled sensitivity was 37% and specificity was 87%. In cross sectional community studies people with subjective memory problems only had 20-30% probability of concurrently having either dementia or mild cognitive impairment.[5]

Even with direct questioning, 60% of those with dementia and 62% of those with mild cognitive impairment do not report simple memory problems,[5] suggesting that loss of awareness of change occurs early in cognitive impairment. If general practitioners asked directly about problems with memory the majority of the patient group they were trying to identify would deny any difficulty, whereas 17% of healthy adults would answer positively.[5]

SOURCES AND SELECTION CRITERIA

We did a systematic review of published work in three databases—Embase, Medline, and PsycINFO—using 17 search categories that cover the breadth of patient demographics and health thought to have a possible association with memory problems. We searched for reviews of studies in human beings that were published in the English language between January 1989 and May 2009. We excluded cognitive science studies, studies in animals, studies of people with learning difficulties or HIV infection, trials of interventions, correspondence, and commentaries.

SUMMARY POINTS

- Subjective memory problems are much more common in later life than the objective problems that suggest minor cognitive impairment or dementia
- Subjective memory problems are not simply a characteristic of the "worried well" and should be taken seriously
- Depression is associated with subjective memory problems, as are older age, female sex, and low educational attainment
- Depression is itself a risk factor for dementia, making the diagnostic task even more difficult
- Subjective memory problems are a poor predictor of dementia syndrome (loss of memory and one other aspect of cognition sufficient to cause impairment)
- When deciding whether to refer to specialist services, practitioners need to rely on rules of thumb to evaluate the extent and possible significance of symptoms or subjective memory loss

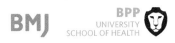

Are subjective memory problems a symptom of depression?

Cross sectional studies do not show a consistent association between subjective memory problems and current objective memory impairment[4] until adjustment is made for depression.[3] Depression may mimic dementia, as memory loss is reported in both conditions, and there is a view that subjective memory problems are the chief complaint in older adults with depression.[11] Although loss of awareness is a feature of dementia, awareness of memory loss is increased in patients with dysthymia and anxiety, but it is not in those with major depression.[12] Some epidemiological evidence from longitudinal studies suggests that depression increases the likelihood of developing dementia syndrome independently[13] and synergistically with diabetes, itself a risk factor for dementia syndrome (fully adjusted hazard ratio 2.69, 95% confidence interval 1.77 to 4.07).[14] In depressed patients with and without mild cognitive impairment, however, findings on increased risk of incident mild cognitive impairment or its progression to dementia are conflicting.[15] The study design, the sample population, the length of follow-up, and methodological differences may affect the detection of an association between baseline depression and subsequent development of mild cognitive impairment or dementia. Depressive symptoms may be an early manifestation of, rather than a risk factor for dementia, and in some subsets of elderly patients late life depression, mild cognitive impairment, and dementia might represent a clinical continuum.[15]

Are subjective memory problems a risk factor for developing dementia?

Most longitudinal studies have shown that patients with subjective memory problems have an increased risk of future cognitive decline or dementia. The risk of developing dementia if subjective memory problems are present varies, and studies use different methods to ascertain subjective and objective impairment. For example, in the Adult Changes of Thought study of 1883 people aged 65 and older, a subset with normal cognition at baseline but high levels of subjective memory problems were nearly three times more likely to develop dementia than their asymptomatic peers (odds ratio 2.7, 95% CI 1.45 to 4.98).[16]

Baseline cognitive impairment may be an important factor for progression to dementia in patients with subjective memory problems.[4] In a study of 364 community dwelling older people without dementia,[17] those who reported subjective memory problems at follow-up and not at baseline were nearly five times more likely to have significant cognitive impairment than those without subjective memory problems at follow-up (odds ratio 4.5, 95% CI 1.3 to 15.4). However, not all longitudinal studies support the view that subjective memory problems are associated with an increased risk of developing dementia. The Maastricht Aging Study, which involved 557 participants aged 55 to 85 years, showed that although being forgetful might indicate slower general information processing and delayed recall at baseline, it did not predict cognitive change over six years.[18]

Do subjective memory symptoms indicate other problems?

Older age, female sex, and low education level are more commonly associated with subjective memory problems in cross sectional community studies.[3] In studies where participants were volunteers or had referred themselves to memory clinics, those with subjective memory problems tended to be younger and their symptoms correlated with depression rather than objective memory problems on cognitive tests.[3] Subjective memory problems were strongly associated with depression, neurotic personality trait, or both, even when there was no association with objective cognitive performance, in 26 studies in one review.[4]

All five studies included in a systematic review reported an association between subjective memory problems and poorer quality of life.[6] The Maastricht Aging Study also reported such an association that persisted over a period of nine years.[19] These findings suggest that even if subjective memory problems are not a direct risk factor for dementia, they are not simply a characteristic of the "worried well" and should be taken seriously.

How should general practitioners approach patients with concerns about their memory?

History and examination

As asking non-specific questions about subjective memory loss is not helpful, practitioners need other tools to assess concerns about forgetfulness. Box 1 lists the types of cognitive loss to consider in a patient with subjective memory loss. This list is not exhaustive but may help practitioners to assess the extent of change in cognitive function.

The categories in the global assessment of early dementia take the clinical inquiry away from memory into function and behaviour, changes that may overshadow memory loss (box 2).[20]

Box 3 lists the "questions for informants" from the GPCog (GP assessment of cognition) test,[21] a brief assessment tool designed for general practice that includes the clock drawing test and a checklist for informants that may provide information on some of the forms of memory shown in box 1.

Use of a brief cognitive function test, as recommended in the dementia clinical guidelines of the National Institute for Health and Clinical Excellence and Social Care Institute for Excellence, may reveal cognitive losses.[22] As the guideline points out, however, the tests do not perform well enough to always detect mild cognitive impairment. One new instrument, the memory alteration test (M@T), distinguished between subjective memory impairment, mild cognitive impairment, and Alzheimer's disease in a Spanish study, but further evaluation is needed.[23]

BOX 1 TYPES OF MEMORY AND OTHER COGNITIVE IMPAIRMENTS TO CONSIDER

- Episodic memory—memory of specific past events that involved the person; forgetting a wedding anniversary is qualitatively different from forgetting that you are married.
- Semantic memory—the store of facts and general knowledge (for example, knowing the answer to the question "who is the monarch?" in the abbreviated mental test score)
- Implicit memory—the non-conscious part of memory that uses past experience to shape current behaviour. Inhibitions may be lost and much offence caused by someone whose manners and social behaviour had been impeccable
- Executive functioning—the forms of thinking necessary for goal directed behaviour. Anticipation of and adaptability to new situations are reduced when executive function is impaired, and thinking becomes concrete rather than conceptual and abstract. For example, driving on an unfamiliar route becomes problematic, and proverbs lose their meaning

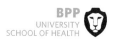

BOX 2 SIMPLIFIED VERSION OF GLOBAL ASSESSMENT OF EARLY DEMENTIA, BASED ON CLINICAL DEMENTIA RATING SCALE[20]

- The patient is impaired by their loss of memory for recent events (for example, they may forget that they have already collected their repeat prescription and argue with the receptionist about it)
- Some variable disorientation occurs in time and place, but not in relation to people (the individual gets lost easily or turns up for an appointment days late or early)
- Some difficulty with complex problems (such as understanding what a letter or official form is telling them or requiring them to do)
- Engagement in some social activities, but not independently (the individual may appear normal because they retain the ability to conduct "small talk," but they cannot sustain a serious conversation)
- More difficult tasks and hobbies are abandoned (bills go unpaid, the garden is neglected)
- Some prompting is needed for personal care (clothes are not washed or baths are missed)

BOX 3 QUESTIONS FOR INFORMANTS FROM THE GPCOG TEST[21]

- Does the patient have more trouble remembering things that have happened recently?
- Does he or she have more trouble recalling conversations a few days later?
- When speaking, does the patient have more difficulty in finding the right word or tend to use the wrong words more often?
- Is the patient less able to manage money and financial affairs (for example, paying bills, budgeting)?
- Is the patient less able to manage his or her medication independently?
- Does the patient need more assistance with transport (either private or public)?

Referral

Publicity campaigns suggesting that memory loss is a sign of dementia may result in increasing pressure from patients for referral to specialist services. In the absence of simple, well validated reliable tests for mild objective cognitive impairment[22] GPs need to rely on "rules of thumb" to guide referral.[24] When referring patients with subjective memory loss it is helpful to note possible causes of impaired memory and to identify potential associated factors. In box 4 we suggest a list of important factors to remember for patients concerned about forgetfulness; the acronym "MIMIC" captures the themes that arise from the synthesis of published reviews and from our workshops with general practitioners, in which we discussed the complexities of early diagnosis of dementia.[25] This is not a validated tool, but we suggest that it may help GPs to characterise forgetful patients when considering or making a referral.

Contributors: Both authors were responsible for the conception and design of this review, the analysis and interpretation of data, and the drafting, revising, and final approval of the version submitted for publication. SI is the guarantor.

BOX 4 MIMIC—A MNEMONIC PROPOSED FOR CHARACTERISATION OF PATIENTS WITH MEMORY PROBLEMS

- Memory loss—what type? (box 1)
- Informant history—use GPCog checklist (box 3) or global assessment of early dementia (box 2)
- Mood—depressed mood, now or in the past; PHQ-9 (patient health questionnaire) score
- Individual—age, sex, education, other long term psychological problems (anxiety, personality type)
- Cognitive function test results—from, for example, the minimental state examination, the six item cognitive impairment test (6CIT), or the GPCog score

QUESTIONS FOR FUTURE RESEARCH

- What symptoms predict the onset of dementia syndrome, and how important is memory loss as a herald symptom? The clinical problem of distinguishing those patients with subjective memory concerns who will develop dementia syndrome is made worse by the wide variation in the definition and measurement of subjective memory problems.[7]
- What is included under the heading of subjective memory impairment and how is it assessed? As most research has been conducted with selected populations, community based longitudinal studies are needed to explore the context in which memory problems are ascertained. We may suspect that an individual with a cognitively demanding lifestyle is more likely to notice memory loss than someone in a less demanding environment, but we do not yet know this. Longer follow-up studies will allow the risk of conversion to dementia to be estimated more reliably and also to measure help seeking behaviour and service use in those reporting memory problems.
- How exactly is depression associated with dementia? If depression is a risk factor for dementia then treatment for depression may affect the incidence of dementia syndrome. If, on the other hand, depression is one part of a continuum towards dementia then treatment would be for symptom relief alone.

ADDITIONAL EDUCATIONAL RESOURCES FOR PATIENTS

- *Worried About Your Memory?* (www.alzheimers.org.uk/memoryworry)—Information, including a factsheet and booklet, from the Alzheimer's Society
- *Memory Loss and Dementia* (www.patient.co.uk/health/Memory-Loss-and-Dementia.htm)—Memory loss, age associated memory impairment, and dementia are discussed on the Patient UK website

Competing interests: SI is chief investigator of the EVIDEM programme (Evidence-based Interventions in Dementia) and has received financial support from the Department of Health's National Institute for Health Research Programme Grants for Applied Research funding scheme (RP-PG-0606-1005). The views and opinions expressed in this article are those of the authors and not necessarily those of the NHS, the National Institute for Health Research (NIHR), or the Department of Health. SI is also associate director of the coordinating centre for the Dementias and Neurodegenerative Diseases research network (DeNDRoN), funded by the NIHR. He has received speaker's fees from pharmaceutical companies with an interest in dementia but has no other conflicting financial academic or personal interests relevant to this paper.

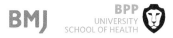

Provenance and peer review: Commissioned, externally peer reviewed.

1   Department of Health. Living well with dementia: National Dementia Strategy. DH, 2009.

2   Palmer K, Bäckman L, Winblad B, Fratiglioni L. Detection of Alzheimer's disease and dementia in the preclinical phase: population based cohort study. *BMJ* 2003;326:245.

3   Jonker C, Geerlings MI, Schmand B Are memory complaints predictive for dementia? A review of clinical and population-based studies. *Int J Geriatr Psychiatry* 2000;15:983-91.

4   Reid LM, Maclullich AM. Subjective memory complaints and cognitive impairment in older people. *Dement Geriatr Cogn Disord* 2006;22:471-85.

5   Mitchell AJ. The clinical significance of subjective memory complaints in the diagnosis of mild cognitive impairment and dementia: a meta-analysis. *Int J Geriatr Psychiatry* 2008;23:1191-202.

6   Mol M, Carpay M, Ramakers I, Rozendaal N, Verhey F, Jolles J. The effect of perceived forgetfulness on quality of life in older adults; a qualitative review. *Int J Geriatr Psychiatry* 2007;22:393-400.

7   Abdulrab K, Heun R. Subjective memory impairment. A review of its definitions indicates the need for a comprehensive set of standardised and validated criteria. *Eur Psychiatry* 2008;23:321-30.

8   Larrabee GJ, Crook TH III. Estimated prevalence of age-associated memory impairment derived from standardised tests of memory function. *International Psychogeriatrics* 1994;6:95-104.

9   Commissaris CJ, Pondson RW, Jolles J. Subjective forgetfulness in a normal Dutch population: possibilities for health education and other interventions. *Patient Education and Counselling* 1998;34:25-32.

10 Panza F, Capurso C, D'Introno A, Colacicco AM, Zenzola A, Menga R, et al. Impact of depressive symptoms on the rate of progression to dementia in patients affected by mild cognitive impairment. The Italian Longitudinal Study on Aging. *Int J Geriatr Psychiatry* 2008;23:726-34.

11 American Psychiatric Association. *Diagnostic and statistical manual* . 4th ed. American Psychiatric Association Press, 1994.

12 Aalten P, Van Valen E, Clare L, Kenny G, Verhey F. Awareness in dementia: a review of clinical correlates. *Aging Mental Health* 2005;9:414-22.

13 Leonard BE, Myint A. Inflammation and depression: is there a causal connection with dementia? *Neurotox Res* 2006;10:149-60.

14 Katon WJ, Lin EH, Williams LH, Ciechanowski P, Heckbert SR, Ludman E, et al. Comorbid depression is associated with an increased risk of dementia diagnosis in patients with diabetes: a prospective cohort study. *J Gen Intern Med* 2010; published online 18 January.

15 Panza F, Frisardi V, Capurso C, D'Introno A, Colacicco AM, Imbimbo BP, et al. Late-life depression, mild cognitive impairment, and dementia: possible continuum? *Am J Geriatr Psychiatry* 2010;18:98-116.

16 Wang L, van Belle G, Crane PK, Kukull WA, Bowen JD, McCormick WC, et al. Subjective memory deterioration and future dementia in people aged 65 and older. *J Am Geriatr Soc* 2004;52:2045-51.

17 Schofield PW, Jacobs D, Marder K, Sano M, Stern Y. The validity of new memory complaints in the elderly. *Arch Neurol* 1997;54:756-9.

18 Mol ME, van Boxtel MP, Willems Mol ME, van Boxtel MP, Willems D, Jolles J. Do subjective memory complaints predict cognitive dysfunction over time? A six-year follow-up of the Maastricht Aging Study. *Int J Geriatr Psychiatry* 2006;21:432-41.

19 Mol ME, van Boxtel MP, Willems D, Verhey FR, Jolles J. Subjective forgetfulness is associated with lower quality of life in middle-aged and young-old individuals: a 9-year follow-up in older participants from the Maastricht Aging Study. *Aging Ment Health* 2009;13:699-705.

20 Hughes CP, Berg L, Danziger WL, Coben LA, Martin RL. A new clinical scale for the staging of dementia. *Br J Psychiatry* 1982;140:566-72.

21 Brodaty H, Pond D, Kemp N, Luscombe G, Harding L Berman K, et al. The GPCOG: a new screening test for dementia designed for general practice. *J Am Geriatr Soc* 2002;50:530-4.

22 National Institute for Health and Clinical Excellence/Social Care Institute for Excellence guidelines. Dementia—supporting people with dementia and their carers in health and social care. London: National Institute for Health and Clinical Excellence, 2006.

23 Rami L, Bosch B, Sanchez-Valle R, Molinuevo JL. The memory alteration test (M@T) discriminates between subjective memory complaints, mild cognitive impairment and Alzheimer's disease. *Arch Gerontol Geriatr* 2010;50:171-4.

24 Andre M, Borgquist L, Foldevi M, Molstad S. Asking for 'rules of thumb': a way to discover tacit knowledge in general practice. *Family Practice* 2002;19:617-22.

25 Iliffe S, Jain P, Wong G, Lefford F, Gupta S, Warner A, et al. Dementia diagnosis in primary care: looking outside the educational box. *Aging Health* 2009;5:51-59.

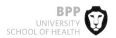

Diagnosis and management of premenstrual disorders

Shaughn O'Brien, professor of academic obstetrics and gynaecology[1],
Andrea Rapkin, professor of obstetrics and gynaecology[2],
Lorraine Dennerstein, professorial fellow[3],
Tracy Nevatte, postdoctoral research associate[4]

[1]Keele University and University Hospital of North Staffordshire, Staffordshire, UK

[2]David Geffen School of Medicine at UCLA, Department of Obstetrics and Gynecology, Box 951740, Los Angeles, CA, USA

[3]National Aging Research Institute, Department of Psychiatry, University of Melbourne, Vic, Australia

[4]Keele University, Institute of Science and Technology in Medicine, Guy-Hilton Research Centre, Stoke on Trent, Staffordshire ST4 7QB, UK

Correspondence to: T Nevatte
t.nevatte@pmed.keele.ac.uk

Cite this as: BMJ 2011;342:d2994

DOI: 10.1136/bmj.d2994

http://www.bmj.com/content/342/bmj.d2994

Premenstrual disorders have a substantial social, occupational, academic, and psychological effect on the lives of millions of women (from menarche to menopause) and their families.[1] Published criteria for diagnosis vary greatly between authoritative bodies, so the true prevalence rates are unknown. A new classification from the International Society for Premenstrual Disorders (ISPMD) will allow this to be resolved.[2] It will also enable clinicians to provide accurate diagnosis and effective management.[2] Little is known about what causes premenstrual syndromes, and the few treatments that are licensed are ineffective,[3][4][5] although treatment can, however, be provided for most women with good effect using unlicensed approaches. In this article, we discuss the classification of premenstrual disorders, how to measure symptoms and diagnose the condition, and effective management strategies. This review is based on evidence from randomised placebo controlled trials where available, recent Cochrane reviews, Royal College of Obstetricians and Gynaecologists' evidence based guidelines and published consensus statements and textbooks by internationally recognised experts.

How should symptoms be measured?

Women usually present with their own retrospective diagnosis of premenstrual syndrome, which is based on the symptoms of previous cycles; however, a large comprehensive study that compared retrospective diagnosis with a prospective assessment of symptoms showed retrospective diagnosis to be unreliable.[6] There is no objective diagnostic test and diagnosis depends on the woman prospectively recording symptoms over two cycles, as recommended in Royal College of Obstetricians and Gynaecologists' (RCOG) guidelines,[7] which can delay the start of treatment. The RCOG recommends the daily record of severity of problems tool,[7] the completion and

analysis of which is laborious. More patient friendly internet based systems are now available (www.symptometrics.com). Some form of screening (patient history or structured questionnaire, such as the premenstrual syndrome screening tool[8]) would avoid patients unnecessarily embarking on two months of data collection when diagnosis of a premenstrual disorder seems unlikely.

How are premenstrual disorders diagnosed?

The ISPMD recently defined precise criteria for diagnosing the core premenstrual disorder (box 1). Symptoms occur regularly in ovulating women during the luteal phase of the cycle, resolve by the end of menstruation, and are followed by a symptom-free interval. Substantial impairment of daily activities at work or school, social activities and hobbies, and interpersonal relationships is a key feature. The criteria do not require specific symptoms to be present and, although well over 200 have been reported, some are considered key or characteristic symptoms (box 2).

Symptoms may be predominantly physical, predominantly psychological, or both. A proportion of patients with severe psychological symptoms will also fulfil American Psychiatric Association (APA) criteria for premenstrual dysphoric disorder.[10] The restrictive diagnostic criteria for this disorder reduce its usefulness in clinical practice. For instance, in the United States, severely affected women who do not quite fit the specific criteria would not be eligible for treatment (and reimbursement). The American Congress of Obstetricians and Gynecologists (ACOG) and the RCOG have outlined criteria for premenstrual syndrome that are more liberal.[7][11] The criteria for premenstrual syndrome and premenstrual dysphoric disorder fulfil the ISPMD criteria for core premenstrual disorder.[2]

Variants of the core premenstrual disorder include premenstrual exacerbation of an underlying physiological, somatic, or medical condition[12]; premenstrual symptoms in the absence of menstruation (after hysterectomy with ovarian conservation, endometrial ablation, or with a levonorgestrel releasing intrauterine system); progestogen induced premenstrual syndrome occurring during progestogen treatment (cyclical hormonal replacement therapy, hormonal contraception); and symptoms of premenstrual disorder with unspecified non-ovulatory ovarian activity. The table summarises the characteristics of the premenstrual disorders.

How are premenstrual disorders managed?

The consultation and treatment planning

Box 3 outlines an approach to careful history taking. Bearing in mind available treatment options, it is important to review the patient's previous treatment and her future plans for pregnancy or contraception. Ask the woman whether psychotropic therapy, endocrine agents, surgery, or an intrauterine system are acceptable. The severity of symptoms and the degree of impairment will usually

SUMMARY POINTS

- Premenstrual disorders can considerably impair functioning at work or school and affect interpersonal relationships
- The cause of premenstrual disorders is not understood but symptoms are clearly related to ovulation
- Precise diagnosis and classification are key to successful treatment of most patients
- Severity of symptoms, pregnancy and contraceptive needs, and the patient's wishes will dictate the invasiveness of treatment
- Patients may be treated effectively using non-drug based interventions, suppression of ovulation, or specific psychotropics, often in general practice
- Given the disorder's complexity, a tailored empirical approach, based on evidence and good clinical judgment, is preferable

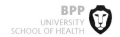

dictate the level of invasiveness of any intervention used. The condition can be treated by psychotropic drugs or suppression of ovulation with a hormonal agent that does not reinstitute the symptoms, and it is important to communicate this clearly to the patient.

Which treatments can be effective without suppressing ovulation?

Non-drug based treatments

Box 4 summarises non-drug based approaches to management that are supported by some research evidence and expert consensus. These approaches may be more effective for women with less severe symptoms. Dietary recommendations and herbal supplements have not been studied robustly. The only herbal supplement that has been shown to be effective in small placebo controlled trials is fruit extract of *Vitex agnus castus*.[13] Placebo controlled studies show that calcium, vitamin B-6, and exercise may be superior to placebo. A programme of 10 cognitive behavioural therapy sessions that included relaxation, stress management, and assertiveness training, has been reported to be effective and comparable to treatment with fluoxetine over six months, with cognitive behavioural therapy possibly having a longer duration of effect when assessed at 12 months.[14]

Diuretics

Spironolactone 100 mg/day given in the luteal phase has been shown in randomised placebo controlled studies to reduce abdominal bloating, swelling, breast discomfort, and mood symptoms.[15]

Psychotropic drugs

Meta-analyses of placebo controlled trials have found that selective serotonin reuptake inhibitors (SSRIs; fluoxetine, paroxetine, citalopram, sertraline) or serotonin and noradrenaline reuptake inhibitors (SNRIs; venlafaxine) are effective in reducing mood and physical symptoms when used continuously or 14 days before menses (usually at a lower dose than that recommended to treat a mood disorder).[16] [17] [18] Symptoms may improve within 48 hours of beginning treatment. Irritability is particularly responsive. SSRIs are licensed in the US, but not in the United Kingdom, for the management of premenstrual dysphoric disorder.

The reversible side effects of SSRIs seem to be less common with intermittent treatment. These include fatigue, insomnia, nausea, gastrointestinal disturbance, headache, sweating, and tremor. Continuous use has been associated with decreased libido and difficulty achieving orgasm. Dizziness, lethargy, nausea, irritability, low mood, and vivid dreams are all symptoms of serotonin withdrawal and are rarely reported with intermittent treatment.[18] SSRIs and oral contraceptives can be given concurrently without decreasing the efficacy of either class of drug. Obviously, some patients

may become pregnant while taking SSRIs, however, these drugs have been shown to be teratogenic.[19]

Continuous treatment with SSRIs or SNRIs may be a more logical approach for patients with premenstrual exacerbation of an affective disorder.

No studies have directly compared the psychotropic agents so there is no evidence to suggest that one preparation works better than another. Moreover, the response to one SSRI does not predict the efficacy, side effects, or outcomes of another. Different drugs, doses, and timings should be tried empirically in individual patients.

Certain anxiolytics (alprazolam, buspirone) have been shown in placebo controlled studies to be superior to placebo[18] [20] [21] but seem to be less effective than SSRIs. The side effect profiles of these agents and risks of dependence make them less desirable options than SSRIs.

How can we treat premenstrual disorders using hormones?

Hormonal treatment that does not suppress ovulation

Progesterone and progestogens (norethisterone, medroxyprogesterone acetate, levonorgestrel) administered in the luteal phase are the only hormonal agents licensed for managing premenstrual syndrome in the UK. However, a systematic review showed that they are ineffective and often restimulate the symptoms.[4] These agents are useful only for endometrial protection during treatment with oestrogen to suppress ovulation.

Treatment by suppression of ovulation

Ovulation can be suppressed with oral contraceptives, gonadotrophin releasing hormone (GnRH) agonists, the gonadotrophin inhibitor danazol, oestrogen, and by removal of the ovaries (box 5).

BOX 2 SYMPTOMS[9]

Physical symptoms

- Joint pain, muscle pain, back pain
- Breast tenderness or pain
- Abdominal swelling or bloating
- Headaches
- Skin disorders
- Weight gain
- Swelling of extremities (hands or feet, or both)

Psychological and behavioural symptoms

- Changes in appetite, overeating, or specific food cravings
- Fatigue, lethargy, or lack of energy
- Mood swings (for example, feeling suddenly sad or crying, increased sensitivity to rejection)
- Irritability
- Anger
- Sleep disturbances
- Restlessness
- Poor concentration
- Social withdrawal
- Not in control
- Lack of interest in usual activities
- Loneliness
- Anxiety
- Depressed mood
- Confusion
- Tension
- Hopelessness

BOX 1 CRITERIA FOR DIAGNOSING THE CORE PREMENSTRUAL DISORDER

- It is precipitated by ovulation
- Symptoms are not defined, although typical symptoms exist
- Any number of symptoms can be present
- Physical and psychological symptoms are important
- Symptoms recur in the luteal phase
- Symptoms disappear by the end of menstruation
- A symptom-free week occurs between menstruation and ovulation
- Symptoms must be prospectively rated
- Symptoms are not an exacerbation of an underlying psychological or physical disorder
- Symptoms cause substantial impairment

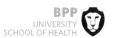

Oral contraception

Oral contraceptive agents suppress ovulation but introduce a new exogenous endocrine cycle that can lead to progestogen induced symptoms. A newer oral contraceptive that contains drospirenone and 20 μg of ethinylestradiol, consisting of 24 active followed by four placebo pills, may counteract this effect. This regimen is not currently available in the UK. Drospirenone has antidiuretic and antiandrogenic properties, and, in combination with the lower dose of ethinylestradiol administered in the above 24/4 regimen, suppresses ovulation and treats symptoms

effectively without regenerating physical or psychological symptoms, according to two randomised controlled trials.[22] [23] The 20 μg pills do have higher rates of breakthrough bleeding, as noted in a recent Cochrane review. The benefits for premenstrual disorders may still apply using a 30 μg ethinylestradiol and drospirenone oral contraceptive pill in the standard 21/7 regimen.[24]

GnRH agonist analogues

Several randomised controlled trials have shown that GnRH agonists are effective in relieving symptoms of premenstrual disorders.[25] Long acting GnRH suppresses ovarian steroid production, resulting in a "medical menopause" and hence relief of premenstrual syndrome. The induced hypo-oestrogenic state can cause hot flushes and night sweats, low mood, insomnia, and eventually osteoporosis. "Add back" treatment with combinations of oestrogen and progesterone or tibolone ameliorates side effects and prolongs treatment, without reducing efficacy. There are few long term safety data for GnRH agonists with add back treatment. GnRH agonist analogues do not prevent pregnancy, so contraception must be used. Tibolone appears less likely to reintroduce premenstrual symptoms than cyclical oestrogen and progestogen according to a recent meta-analysis.[25]

It may be useful to consider a "trial" of GnRH agonists to establish the relative contributions of endocrine related pathology versus underlying psychopathology in patients with premenstrual exacerbation, or to mimic the effect of a bilateral oophorectomy to determine the potential benefit of surgery.

Danazol

Danazol is androgenic, and a randomised placebo controlled crossover trial found considerable benefit over placebo in the treatment of patients with premenstrual syndrome.[26] Administration during the luteal phase only is beneficial for cyclical mastalgia but no other symptoms of the syndrome. Its side effects are predominantly androgenic and include acne, hirsutism, weight gain, voice change and deepening, adverse lipid profile, and teratogenesis.

BOX 3 MINIMUM INFORMATION TO BE OBTAINED IN FIRST TWO CLINIC OR SURGERY APPOINTMENTS

- Menstrual history: frequency, duration, heaviness, pain, regularity, amenorrhoea, last menstrual period
- Premenstrual symptom history: character, timing, absence or presence after menstruation, symptom-free follicular phase week, when they begin, how long they have been occurring
- Has there been any suicidal ideation?
- Impairment: effect on work, school, hobbies, social activities, family, partner, work colleagues. Level of distress caused
- Is there an underlying problem (psychological, physical, medical) that worsens before menstruation? Is this reduced during the follicular phase?
- Amenorrhoea: has the patient undergone a procedure that has resulted in amenorrhoea (hysterectomy with ovarian conservation, levonorgestrel releasing intrauterine system, endometrial ablation) but symptoms persist?
- Is the patient being treated with hormones? For example, combined or progestogen-only contraception, progestogens, hormonal replacement therapy
- What are the patient's contraceptive needs and current contraception? Is her family complete, is she trying to become pregnant?
- Does she have other medical diagnoses, particularly gynaecological diagnoses like heavy menstrual bleeding, endometriosis, pelvic pain, dyspareunia, cervical smear abnormalities?
- What treatment approaches—non-medical, behavioural therapy, psychotropics, hormones, intrauterine hormones, surgical interventions—would she find acceptable?
- Is she willing to receive unlicensed drugs? Is she prepared to receive treatment that will usually prevent her getting pregnant and is she happy to use barrier methods of contraception during treatment?
- What treatments have been self administered or prescribed by doctors and what have been the positive or negative effects? Have they been used appropriately and failed or inappropriately and been unsuccessful?

Possible diagnoses in women presenting with premenstrual symptoms

Diagnosis	Cyclical symptoms	Symptoms in luteal phase	Symptoms in follicular phase	Impairment	Comment
Physiological premenstrual symptoms*	Present	Present	Absent	None	Although symptoms are cyclical and there is a symptom-free week, they are of insufficient severity to cause serious impairment
Core premenstrual disorder*	Present	Present	Absent	Present	This is the typical or core premenstrual disorder: symptoms are cyclical, relieved by the end of menstruation with a follicular phase symptom-free week; they cause serious impairment
Premenstrual exacerbation	Present	Present	Remain high but reduced compared with luteal phase	Present	Symptoms are cyclical, cause serious impairment but are only partially alleviated by menstruation because of an underlying psychological, physical, or medical condition
Premenstrual disorder, menstruation absent*	Present	Present	Absent	Present	Essentially the same as core premenstrual disorder but without menstruation as a reference event as a result of iatrogenic amenorrhoea (hysterectomy with ovarian conservation, endometrial ablation, levonorgestrel intrauterine system)
Progestogen induced premenstrual disorder†	Present	Present during progestogen treatment	Absent during progestogen-free phase of HRT or variably during exposure to hormonal contraceptives	Present	Symptoms are generated without ovulation by the cyclical administration of progestogen for therapeutic (HRT) or contraception purposes
Mis-attribution	Absent	Present	Present	Present	Although symptoms may be severe they are non-cyclical; this suggests the presence of a continuous and serious psychological disorder

*Symptoms probably result from ovulation and endogenous progesterone or its metabolites.
†Symptoms are iatrogenic and result from treatment with exogenous progestogens.
HRT=hormone replacement therapy.

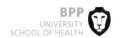
Estradiol

Transdermal patches and subcutaneous implants of estradiol are effective in suppressing ovulation.[27] The use of unopposed oestrogen may lead to endometrial hyperplasia

---

BOX 4 TREATMENTS

The following treatments are supported by evidence based studies and expert consensus reports. The doses that have shown efficacy in randomised trials are given in parenthesis.

Non-drug based treatments

Lifestyle

- Education about premenstrual syndrome
- Cognitive behavioural therapy
- Relaxation techniques
- Regular aerobic exercise (at least 20-30 minutes, three times a week)

Supplements

- Calcium carbonate
- Magnesium oxide
- Vitamin B-6 supplements (dose not to exceed 100 mg/day)
- Fruit extract of *Vitex agnus castus*

Non-hormonal agents

Diuretics

- Spironolactone (100 mg/day during luteal phase)

Psychotropic drugs

- Fluoxetine (selective serotonin reuptake inhibitor (SSRI); 10-20 mg/day continuously or luteal phase only; can be increased to 40 mg/day)
- Paroxetine (SSRI; 10-30 mg/day)
- Citalopram (SSRI; 10-30 mg/day)
- Sertraline (SSRI; 25-50 mg/day initially, can be increased to 150 mg/day)
- Venlafaxine (serotonin and noradrenaline reuptake inhibitor; 75-112.5 mg/day)

Anxiolytics

- Alprazolam (0.25-4.0 mg two to three times a day)
- Buspirone (10-60 mg/day)

Hormone based treatments

Progesterone and progestogens: not recommended

- Norethisterone
- Medroxyprogesterone acetate
- Levonorgestrel

Ovulation suppression

Oral contraception

- Drospirenone and lower doses of ethinylestradiol

Gonadotrophin releasing hormone agonist

- Goserelin (one off injection of 3.6 mg for one month or 10.8 mg for three months), with or without add back with gonadotrophin releasing hormone treatment (tibolone 2.5 mg/day)

Gonadotrophin inhibitor

- Danazol (200-400 mg/day)

Estradiol

- Transdermal patches (100 mg; increase to 200 mg if ovulation is not suppressed)
- Subcutaneous implants (50 mg; increase to 75 mg or 100 mg if ovulation is not suppressed)

Surgery

- Bilateral oophorectomy and hysterectomy

BOX 5 SUPPRESSION OF OVULATION

- Oral contraceptives containing ethinylestradiol and drospirenone
- Estradiol patch or implant with cyclical oral or intrauterine progestogen
- Gonadotrophin releasing hormone agonist with or without oestrogen and progestogen or tibolone add back treatment
- Danazol continuously (luteal phase for breast symptoms)
- Bilateral salpingo-oophorectomy and hysterectomy with unopposed oestrogen replacement

---

and increases the risk of endometrial cancer. Providing endometrial protection with progestogen is important, but if administered orally progesterone may induce premenstrual symptoms. Using a levonogestrel releasing uterine system theoretically avoids this problem because the progesterone effects of this system are intended to be local, although some women experience premenstrual symptoms and breast tenderness in the early months of treatment. The combination of oestrogen administration and the levonogestrel releasing intrauterine system will protect the endometrium, provide contraception, and reduce menstrual flow in women who also have heavy menstrual bleeding. Although not recent, randomised controlled trials have shown the efficacy of oestrogen in suppressing ovulation and managing symptoms.[27] [28] However, the suppression of ovulation is not sufficiently assured for contraceptive purposes and patients should be advised appropriately.

Is surgery a reasonable option?

Endometrial ablation or hysterectomy will eliminate menstruation but not premenstrual symptoms because ovarian function is conserved. Women with severe and debilitating symptoms may request bilateral oophorectomy. This may be considered, but we recommend careful counselling of the woman to outline the drawbacks and consequences of a premature surgical menopause. It is important to replace oestrogen until the age of the natural menopause. Removing the uterus when oophorectomy is performed allows women to receive unopposed oestrogen replacement and avoid recurrent progestogen induced premenstrual symptoms. A trial of GnRH is advisable before deciding to perform bilateral oophorectomy and hysterectomy.

Women with severe premenstrual syndrome who are undergoing hysterectomy for another gynaecological indication may also elect to have their ovaries removed to avoid ongoing premenstrual symptoms.

Managing premenstrual disorders in general practice

The figure shows how different premenstrual disorders may be presented on the daily record of severity of problems chart. The diagnosis of a premenstrual disorder should be based on two months of recording using a paper or electronic based system of rating symptoms, and this is easily done in primary care. It is of course difficult to send away a severely affected patient without treatment but this initial process is essential. No woman should wait to be seen in secondary care only to be sent away for two months of chart recording because this can easily take place between referral and consultation. The prospective record of symptoms will give the clinician an idea of whether there is a positive diagnosis and how severely the woman is affected.

Women who have premenstrual symptoms that are debilitating but who are symptom free for at least one week after menstruation have core premenstrual disorder. Their symptoms may or may not fit the diagnostic criteria for premenstrual dysphoric disorder. Treat these women as outlined above according to their wishes after all information is presented. A hierarchical approach that takes into account the severity of symptoms, previous treatment, and background characteristics (table) is preferable.

Women with mild physiological premenstrual symptoms that have no substantial impact on their functioning may need no more than support and reassurance of normality. Advise good nutrition, exercise, and stress reduction, which are realistic and healthful, albeit unproved, non-medical approaches.

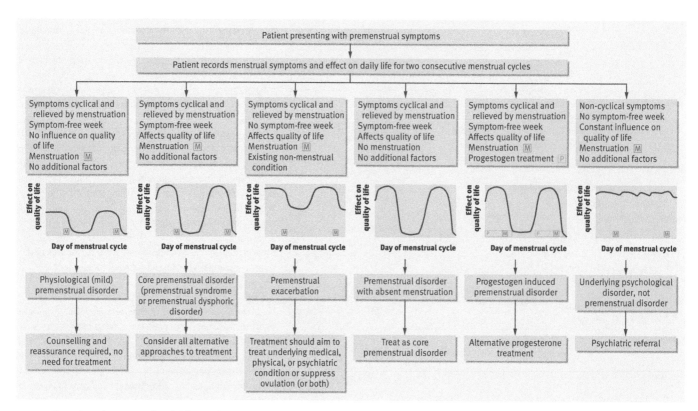

Fig 1 Schematic representation of daily record of severity of problems charts obtained on patients presenting with a presumed diagnosis of premenstrual disorder

---

A PATIENT'S PERSPECTIVE

I have always had severe mood swings, but over the past few years they got worse. They lasted for days and left me physically and emotionally exhausted. I was verbally aggressive and so nasty that when the mood had passed I would be devastated by my actions. This had a huge effect on my relationship with my son; I couldn't book holidays or outings because I would spoil them. I became a hermit for a couple of years.

I tried many prescription drugs including citalopram, over the counter remedies, and I trawled the internet but nothing came close to working. At this point I was desperate.

My general practitioner referred me to a consultant gynaecologist who gave me mood diaries to fill in. These showed that my symptoms occurred before menstruation and got better during my period—I had typical premenstrual syndrome. I received injections of a gonadotrophin releasing hormone agonist (Prostap) and later a levonorgestrel releasing intrauterine system and oestrogen patches. Initially, my moods were very up and down, then one day I suddenly realised that I hadn't had a symptom for a while. Now I can't remember when I had my last one.

Recently, I was talking to my son who gave me the biggest hug going and said "I've got my mum back."

AREAS FOR FUTURE RESEARCH

- To develop a simple one stop diagnostic test so that patients don't have to record symptoms for two months before they can start treatment
- To replace paper based rating techniques with electronic symptom recording using the internet from a computer, laptop, tablet, or mobile phone
- To develop a neuroimaging technique (such as functional magnetic resonance imaging) that can be conducted across menstrual cycles to distinguish patients with and without premenstrual disorders. This could provide the pathway to objective diagnosis and determination of the aetiology of premenstrual disorders
- To develop an agent that provides endometrial protection without regenerating premenstrual symptoms
- To validate a "GnRH test" that would enable us to identify the contributing component symptoms in patients with premenstrual exacerbation and predict the likely effect of removing the ovaries (GnRH would stop the menstrual cycle, removing all symptoms caused by it, so for premenstrual exacerbation it would show the level of the underlying condition and whether removing the ovaries during a hysterectomy would be beneficial)
- To develop a method of ovulation suppression that avoids hypo-oestrogenic side effects and does not reintroduce premenstrual symptoms

A patient who has debilitating symptoms but no symptom-free week may have an underlying psychological, psychiatric, or physical condition that is not related to the ovarian cycle and which is unlikely to be a premenstrual disorder. Explore alternative diagnoses and refer to psychiatric services if necessary. Symptoms of the perimenopause can be similar to the premenstrual syndrome but are also non-cyclical.

Women with a premenstrual syndrome-like cycle associated with progestogen treatment may be managed easily by changing type, dose, or duration of the treatment. Consider administration of progesterone via a levonorgestrel releasing intrauterine system. In women whose symptoms are caused by the oral contraceptive, consider changing the pill or changing to an intrauterine system.

Women who have substantial premenstrual impairment with only partial relief after menstruation could have an underlying psychological or physical condition with exacerbations related to ovarian function. In such cases consider one of the following approaches. Either treat the underlying condition adequately, in which case the premenstrual phase may become tolerable, or suppress ovulation to reduce luteal phase symptoms to the level of the follicular phase. Psychological interventions and psychotropic agents may achieve both aims simultaneously in these patients or in those with both a psychiatric disorder and premenstrual syndrome.

It is easy to overlook cyclical symptoms in the absence of a reference menstrual bleed. In women who do not menstruate (as a result of hysterectomy, endometrial ablation, or a levonorgestrel releasing intrauterine system) but report a regular pattern of symptoms, measuring progesterone blood concentrations and noting a peak of symptoms will help to show the association between symptoms and ovulation. Manage as for core premenstrual disorder. It will be more difficult to use luteal phase-only treatment without a menstrual cycle as a guide.

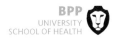

TIPS FOR NON-SPECIALISTS

- Diagnosis can be achieved only by the use of prospectively administered charts. The daily record of severity of problems is ideal for this. If a patient is referred to secondary care the charts must be completed while she is waiting for the appointment
- Careful diagnosis and classification of the disorder will limit the likelihood of treatment failure
- When patient led or non-drug based approaches fail, selective serotonin reuptake inhibitors or oral contraceptives may be considered. Identify a progestogen (oral or intrauterine) that does not reintroduce premenstrual symptoms—this may need to be done empirically on an individual basis
- Many patients will benefit from suppression of ovulation, which can be achieved in several ways; in primary care this is most easily achieved by use of transdermal estradiol and levonorgestrel releasing intrauterine systems

ADDITIONAL EDUCATIONAL RESOURCES

Resources for patients

- National Association for Premenstrual Syndrome (www.pms.org.uk)—Information and support for women with premenstrual syndrome
- Royal College of Obstetricians and Gynaecologists (www.rcog.org.uk/files/rcog-corp/ManagingPremenstrualSyndromePMSInformationForYou.pdf)—Patient information leaflet on managing premenstrual syndrome
- Medline Plus (www.nlm.nih.gov/medlineplus/premenstrualsyndrome.html)—Health information on premenstrual syndrome from the US National Library of Medicine
- American Congress of Obstetricians and Gynecologists (www.acog.org/publications/patient_education/bp057.cfm)—Patient education leaflet on premenstrual syndrome
- NHS choices (www.nhs.uk/conditions/premenstrual-syndrome)—Information on premenstrual syndrome

Resources for healthcare professionals

- Royal College of Obstetricians and Gynaecologists. Management of premenstrual syndrome. 2007. www.rcog.org.uk/files/rcog-corp/uploaded-files/GT48ManagementPremensturalSyndrome.pdf
- Map of medicine (http://eng.mapofmedicine.com/evidence/map/menstrual_cycle_irregularities_and_post_menopausal_bleeding_pmb_7.html)—Evidence-based, practice-informed care maps for the management of PMS
- Symptometrics (www.symptometrics.com/Information/MenstrualSymptometrics/PremenstrualDisorders.aspx)—Information about premenstrual disorders and prospective recording of data
- Medscape (http://emedicine.medscape.com/article/293257-overview)—Overview of premenstrual dysphoric disorder

Contributors: SO'B planned the article; the writing and research was carried out jointly by SO'B, TN, AR, and LD. SO'B is guarantor.

Competing interests: All authors have completed the Unified Competing Interest form at www.icmje.org/coi_disclosure.pdf (available on request from the corresponding author) and declare: no support from any organisation for the submitted work; SO'B and LD have been reimbursed by Bayer Schering (the manufacturer of Yaz) for attending several conferences, consulted to the company, been paid by for running educational programmes and speaking at symposiums, and received research grants from the company; SO'B has received fees for participating in an expert advisory group for the National Institute for Health and Clinical Excellence (NICE) and is editor in chief of obstetrics and gynaecology for Map of Medicine; SO'B has also been paid by AstraZeneca for attending a symposium and speaking; the International Society for Premenstrual Disorders (ISPMD), which is chaired by SO'B, received an unrestricted educational grant from Bayer Schering for the consensus meeting; Both SO'B and TN have received research funding for Symptometrics, the Keele University/University Hospital of North Staffordshire spin-out company, and for which they also have a contract as inventors of the innovation, which may generate income in the future. AR has no competing interests.

Provenance and peer review: Commissioned; externally peer reviewed.

Patient consent obtained.

1 Halbreich U, Borenstein J, Pearlstein T, Kahn LS The prevalence, impairment, impact, and burden of premenstrual dysphoric disorder (PMS/PMDD). Psychoneuroendocrinology 2003;28:1-23.
2 O'Brien PM, Bäckström T, Brown C, Dennerstein L, Endicott J, Epperson CN, et al. Towards a consensus on diagnostic criteria, measurement and trial design of the premenstrual disorders: the ISPMD Montreal consensus. Arch Womens Ment Health 2011;14:13-21.
3 O'Brien S, Ismail K. History of the premenstrual disorders. In: O'Brien PM, Rapkin AJ, Schmidt PJ. The premenstrual syndromes: PMS and PMDD. Informa Healthcare, 2007.
4 Wyatt K, Dimmock P, Jones P, Obhrai M, O'Brien S. Efficacy of progesterone and progestogens in management of premenstrual syndrome: systematic review. BMJ 2001;323:776.
5 Ford O, Lethaby A, Roberts H, Mol BW. Progesterone for premenstrual syndrome. Cochrane Database Syst Rev 2009;2:CD003415.
6 Rapkin AJ, Chang LC, Reading AE. Comparison of retrospective and prospective assessment of premenstrual symptoms. Psychol Rep 1988;62:55-60.
7 Royal College of Obstetricians and Gynaecologists. Premenstrual syndrome. Management. Green-top guideline 48. RCOG Press, 2007. www.rcog.org.uk/files/rcog-corp/uploaded-files/GT48ManagementPremensturalSyndrome.pdf.
8 Steiner M, Macdougall M, Brown E. The premenstrual symptoms screening tool (PSST) for clinicians. Arch Women's Ment Health 2003;6:203-9.
9 Dennerstein L, Lehert P, Keung LS, Pal SA, Choi D. A population-based survey of Asian women's experience of premenstrual symptoms. Menopause Int 2010;16:139-45.
10 Premenstrual dysphoric disorder. In: Diagnostic and statistical manual of mental disorders. 4th ed. American Psychiatric Press, 2000:771-4.
11 ACOG practice bulletin: premenstrual syndrome. Int J Gynecol Obstet 2001;73:183-91.
12 12Case AM, Reid RL. Effects of the menstrual cycle on medical disorders. Arch Intern Med 1998;158:1405-12.
13 Girman A, Lee R, Kligler B. An integrative medicine approach to premenstrual syndrome. Am J Obstet Gynecol 2003;188(suppl):S56-65.
14 Hunter MS, Ussher JM, Cariss M, Browne S, Jelley R, Katz M. Medical (fluoxetine) and psychological (cognitive-behavioural therapy) treatment for premenstrual dysphoric disorder. A study of treatment processes. J Psychosom Res 2002;53:811-7.
15 Wang M, Hammarbäck S, Lindhe BA, Bäckström T. Treatment of premenstrual syndrome by spironolactone: a double-blind, placebo-controlled study. Acta Obstet Gynecol Scand 1995;74:803-8.
16 Brown J, O'Brien PMS, Marjoribanks J, Wyatt K. Selective serotonin reuptake inhibitors for premenstrual syndrome. Cochrane Database Syst Rev 2009;2:CD001396.
17 Rapkin AJ, Winer SA. The pharmacologic management of premenstrual dysphoric disorder. Expert Opin Pharmacother 2008;9:1-17.
18 Steiner M, Pearlstein T, Cohen LS, Endicott J, Kornstein SG, Roberts C, et al. Expert guidelines for the treatment of severe PMS, PMDD, and co morbidities: the role of SSRIs. J Womens Health (Larchmt) 2006;15:57-69.
19 Tuccori M, Testi A, Antonioli L, Fornai M, Montagnani S, Ghisu N, et al. Safety concerns associated with the use of serotonin reuptake inhibitors and other serotonergic/noradrenergic antidepressants during pregnancy: a review. Clin Ther 2009;31:1426-53.
20 Freeman EW, Rickels K, Sondheimer SJ, Polansky M. A double blind trial of oral progesterone, alprazolam, and placebo in treatment of severe premenstrual syndrome. JAMA 1995;274:51-7.
21 Landen M, Eriksson O, Sundblad C, Andersch B, Naessén T, Eriksson E. Compounds with affinity for serotonergic receptors in the treatment of premenstrual dysphoria: a comparison of buspirone, nefazodone and placebo. Psychopharmacology 2001;155:292-8.
22 Lopez LM, Kaptein AA, Helmerhorst FM. Oral contraceptives containing drospirenone for premenstrual syndrome. Cochrane Database Syst Rev 2009;2:CD006586.
23 Yonkers KA, Brown C, Pearlstein TB, Foegh M, Sampson-Landers C, Rapkin A. Efficacy of a new low dose oral contraceptive with drospirenone in premenstrual dysphoric disorder. Obstet Gynecol 2005;106:492-501.
24 Pearlstein TB, Bachmann GA, Zacur HA, Yonkers KA. Treatment of premenstrual dysphoric disorder with a new drospirenone-containing oral contraceptive formulation. Contraception 2005;72:414-21.
25 Wyatt KM, Dimmock PW, Ismail KM, O'Brien PMS. The effectiveness of GnRHa with and without "add-back" therapy in treating premenstrual syndrome: a meta-analysis. Br J Obstet Gynaecol 2004;111:585-93.
26 Hahn PM, Van Vugt DA, Reid RL. A randomized, placebo-controlled, crossover trial of danazol for the treatment of premenstrual syndrome. Psychoneuroendocrinology 1995;20:193-209.
27 Watson NR, Studd JW, Savvas M, Garnett T, Baber RJ. Treatment of severe premenstrual syndrome with oestradiol patches and cyclical oral norethisterone. Lancet 1989;2:730-2.
28 Magos AL, Brincat M, Studd JWW. Treatment of the premenstrual syndrome by subcutaneous estradiol implants and cyclical oral norethisterone: placebo controlled study. BMJ 1986;292:1629-33.

Related links

bmj.com/archive
- The assessment and management of insomnia in primary care (2011;342:d2899)
- Diagnosis and management of schistosomiasis (2011;342:d2651)
- Advising on travel during pregnancy (2011;342:d2506)
- The management of tennis elbow (2011;342:d2687)

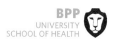

Contraception for women: an evidence based overview

Jean-Jacques Amy, editor in chief[1], Vrijesh Tripathi, lecturer[2]

[1]European Journal of Contraception and Reproductive Health Care, Opalfeneweg 3, B-1740 Ternat, Belgium

[2]Faculty of Science and Agriculture, University of West Indies, St Augustine, Trinidad and Tobago, West Indies

Correspondence to: J-J Amy, Florencestraat, 62, B-1050 Brussels, Belgium jeanjacques.amy@skynet.be

Cite this as: BMJ 2009;339:b2895

DOI: 10.1136/bmj.b2895

http://www.bmj.com/content/339/bmj.b2895

Contraception allows parents to choose the number and spacing of children. Each year, family planning programmes prevent an estimated 187 million unintended pregnancies, including 60 million unplanned births and 105 million abortions, and avert an estimated 2.7 million infant deaths and 215 000 pregnancy related deaths.[1]

The prevalence of contraceptive use differs across the world owing to differences in desired number of children, awareness, funding, and service delivery, with an overall prevalence of use worldwide of 63%. Female sterilisation and intrauterine devices account for nearly 40% in less developed regions, and pills, intrauterine devices, and condoms for the same proportion in more developed regions.[2] This article reviews evidence based information on contraceptive methods currently available for women.

The family planning consultation

Counselling

Counselling is thought to enable clients to make contraceptive choices that best fit their values and needs; it should lead to greater satisfaction and more correct and longer use of contraception, particularly when partners are involved. However, a Cochrane review of randomised controlled trials that acknowledged heterogeneity between studies found no conclusive evidence that counselling improves adherence to, and continuation of, the use of contraceptives.[3]

The World Health Organization identifies four types of clients according to their counselling needs: returning clients with no problems, returning clients with problems, new clients with a method in mind, and new clients with no method in mind.[4] Family planning providers must therefore be both knowledgeable and skilled in communicating information. Ideally, family planning counselling is holistic and encompasses sexual and reproductive health, but prevention of sexually transmitted infections is outside the scope of this review.

SOURCES AND SELECTION CRITERIA

We prepared this review by searching Cochrane reviews, PubMed, and our personal archives of references.

SUMMARY POINTS

- Combined oestrogen and progestogen contraceptives inhibit ovulation. Their biological effects and safety profiles are similar regardless of route of administration
- Progestogen-only methods act by various mechanisms and can be used by women in whom oestrogens are contraindicated
- Copper bearing intrauterine devices combine the highest efficacy with the lowest cost. The levonorgestrel releasing intrauterine system reduces menstrual blood loss
- When used correctly, the lactational amenorrhoea method prevents conception in more than 98% of women during the first six months after childbirth
- Levonorgestrel-only emergency contraceptive pills and copper bearing intrauterine devices are valuable methods of emergency contraception
- Emergency contraceptive pills prevent pregnancy; they should be taken as soon as possible, and not later than 72 hours after unprotected intercourse

Clinical aspects

According to WHO international guidelines, the minimum requirements before starting contraception with a combined oestrogen-progestogen product consists of asking for a personal and family history of deep vein thrombosis and measuring blood pressure at baseline and follow-up.[5] Combined agents are best avoided by women over 35 years who smoke.[5] Progestogens only can be started in healthy non-pregnant women without screening procedures.[5]

A recent Cochrane review found little evidence to support the idea that immediately starting hormonal contraception is associated with greater effectiveness, continuation, and acceptance than starting the contraception after the onset of the next menses.[6]

How do hormonal contraceptives work?

Combined oestrogen-progestogen products

Table 1 lists the currently available combined oestrogen-progestogen contraceptives. These products release an oestrogen (mostly ethinylestradiol) and a progestogen, which act systemically to inhibit ovulation. All, except the sequential pill, also increase the viscosity of cervical mucus—which inhibits migration of sperm to the uterine cavity—and suppress endometrial growth. Combined oral contraceptives, patches, and combined vaginal rings may be used cyclically, according to an extended regimen (with a medication-free interval), or continuously. According to WHO guidelines,[4] return to fertility on discontinuation of treatment is immediate, with the exception of monthly injectable preparations, which require five months on average after the last injection for fertility to return.

Progestogen-only products

Progestogen-only preparations (table 2) may be given to women in whom oestrogens are contraindicated. Progestogen-only pills are taken each day at the same time, with no pill-free interval. Progestogen-only pills and implants that release levonorgestrel act primarily by thickening the cervical mucus; ovulation is not always prevented. In addition to their effect on cervical mucus, desogestrel pills, depot medroxyprogesterone acetate, and etonogestrel releasing implants inhibit ovulation in most cycles. Fertility returns as soon as pills are discontinued, whereas it takes an average of 10 and six months to return after the last injection of depot medroxyprogesterone acetate and norethisterone enantate, respectively.[4]

How effective are hormonal contraceptives?

Effectiveness is related to the acceptability of the contraceptive method and to compliance. "Typical use" is considerably less effective than "perfect use" (correct and consistent use). A recent Cochrane review found that combined oral contraceptive pills, transdermal patches, and vaginal rings were equally efficacious[7]: they have a failure rate of 0.3 per 100 women per year with perfect use and 8 with typical use.[7] [8] Maintaining a regular schedule is more

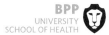
important for progestogen-only pills than for combined oral contraceptives—more than a three hour delay in taking the progestogen-only pill can cause failure of contraception. Implants, injectable preparations, and intrauterine contraceptives do not depend on daily compliance and have lower failure rates.[8] Implants (failure rate of 0.05 per 100 women per year with typical use) and injectable preparations (3) are among the most effective reversible contraceptives.[8] According to recently updated WHO recommendations, depot medroxyprogesterone acetate may be given up to four weeks late without pregnancy needing first to be ruled out.[5]

How is the effectiveness of hormonal contraceptives affected by drug interaction?

The efficacy of hormonal contraceptives may be reduced when liver enzyme inducing drugs are taken simultaneously.[5] Box 1 lists several drugs that interact with hormonal contraceptives. Certain antibiotics without liver enzyme inducing activity alter the enterohepatic recirculation of sex steroids and thereby reduce the efficacy of combined oral contraceptives. Additional contraceptive protection, such as a barrier method, should be used concurrently and for four weeks after discontinuing such drugs. Interactions of antiretrovirals with hormonal contraceptives are specific to the type of antiretroviral and hormonal contraceptive being used. HIV positive women should use a dual method of hormonal and barrier contraception.[9]

What are the non-contraceptive benefits of combined contraceptive pills?

Analysis of data from 45 observational studies from 21 countries showed that the overall relative risk of ovarian cancer decreased by 20% for each five years of use.[10] In women who had used combined oral contraceptives for 15 years the risk was halved. A protective effect with regard to both endometrial and ovarian malignancy can be detected in ex-users of contraceptives for up to 15 years.

Hormonal contraceptives may be used to treat dysfunctional uterine bleeding, dysmenorrhoea, and menorrhagia; their use is associated with a lower incidence of functional ovarian cysts, benign breast disease, and colorectal cancer.[w1] Their effect on bone mineral density depends on the dose of oestrogen and the age of the woman.

What are the adverse effects and complications of hormonal contraceptives?

The side effects and complications of combined oral contraceptives have been well investigated. A nationwide prospective study carried out in the United States showed that after six months of using an oral contraceptive 16% (switchers) to 32% (starters) of women had stopped taking their pill. Nearly half (46%) of the women who discontinued did so because of side effects, such as breakthrough bleeding and headache.[11]

Case-control studies have shown an increased relative risk of deep venous thrombosis and pulmonary embolism, ranging from 2.1 to 4.4.[12] This risk is related to the dose of oestrogen and the type of progestogen. Pills containing desogestrel or gestodene are associated with a twofold greater risk than those containing levonorgestel or norethisterone; those containing cyproterone acetate have a four times greater risk.[12] The data are insufficient to make conclusions about combined oral contraceptives containing other progestogens.[12] Women with thrombophilia are particularly at risk of thromboembolic events. A systematic review and meta-analysis of seven studies of women taking combined oral contraceptives found significant associations of the risk of thromboembolism with deficiencies of antithrombin, protein C, or protein S; raised concentrations of factor VIIIc; and the presence of factor V Leiden and prothrombin G20210A.[13]

Use of combined oral contraceptives is associated with an increased risk of myocardial infarction, stroke, gallbladder disease, hypertension, glycometabolic imbalance in people with diabetes, carcinoma of the cervix, hepatocellular carcinoma, and—to a lesser degree—breast cancer in current users. These risks are not modified when ethinylestradiol is given parenterally, or by the use of new progestogens not derived from 19-nortestosterone.[5] A Cochrane review found that transdermal patches cause more, and the vaginal ring causes fewer (except for vaginal discharge and vaginitis), side effects than combined oral contraceptives.[7] A cohort study found a more than twofold increase in deep venous thrombosis and pulmonary embolism in users of transdermal contraceptives compared with women taking a combined oral contraceptive containing 35 µg ethinylestradiol and norgestimate.[14] Box 2 lists contraindications to the use of combined hormonal contraceptives.

Table 1 Combined oestrogen-progestogen preparations

Type	Description
Combined oral contraceptives	Tablets that are taken daily, either cyclically, according to an extended regimen, or continuously
Monthly injectable preparations	Oily suspension of an oestrogen and a progestogen given monthly by deep intramuscular injection
Transdermal combined patch	Adhesive patch worn on the body that releases steroids via the skin into the bloodstream. The patch is changed weekly
Combined vaginal ring	Flexible ring placed in the vagina that releases steroids via the vaginal wall into the bloodstream. The ring is kept in place for 3 weeks, after which the ring is not worn for 1 week

---

Table 2 Progestogen-only preparations

Type	Description
Progestogen-only pills	Most contain a very low dose of progestogen. They are taken continuously and every day at the same time
Progestogen-only injectable preparations	Oily suspension of a progestogen given every 2 or 3 months by deep intramuscular injection
Implants	Small plastic rods which are surgically implanted under the skin medially in the upper arm. They are effective for either 3 or 5 years
Levonorgestrel intrauterine system	Intrauterine contraceptive which releases small quantities of levonorgestrel in the uterine cavity

---

BOX 1 DRUGS THAT INTERACT WITH HORMONAL CONTRACEPTIVES[5] [9]

Liver enzyme inducing drugs that reduce the efficacy of hormonal contraceptives

- Barbiturates
- Carbamazepine
- Oxcarbazepine
- Phenytoin
- Primidone
- Topiramate
- Modafinil
- Rifampicin
- Griseofulvin
- Certain antiretrovirals (such as ritonavir and nevirapine)

Other drugs

- Non-liver enzyme inducing antibiotics (various interactions)
- Lamotrigine (concentrations lowered by the contraceptive)
- Ciclosporin (concentrations raised by the contraceptive)
- Potassium sparing diuretics (risk of hyperkalaemia with pills containing drospirenone)

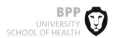

The use of a progestogen only is commonly associated with altered bleeding patterns.[w2 w3] Use of depot medroxyprogesterone acetate decreases bone mineral density, but this returns to baseline values after discontinuation of treatment.[w4]

How do intrauterine contraceptives work?

Copper bearing intrauterine devices act by immobilising sperm in the uterine cavity and preventing fertilisation. Of all contraceptive methods, these devices combine the highest efficacy with the lowest cost.[w5] The TCu-380A is approved for 10 years but could be effective for 12.

The levonorgestrel releasing intrauterine system causes marked (but reversible) atrophy of the endometrium. A Cochrane review of contraception trials found this system to be as effective as the TCu-380A.[15] It is approved for five years of use and is successful in treating menorrhagia and dysmenorrhoea. A systematic review of nine studies showed that menstrual bleeding over time is reduced by 74-97%.[16] A systematic overview of observational studies found limited evidence that this system benefits women with endometriosis, adenomyosis, fibroids, endometrial hyperplasia, and early stage endometrial cancer (in women unfit for surgery).[17] WHO guidelines state that fertility returns immediately after removal of all intrauterine contraceptives.[4]

What are the adverse effects and complications of intrauterine contraceptives?

Insertion of intrauterine devices can be painful. Rarely, uterine perforation occurs. Immediate postpartum or postabortum insertion has the advantages of high motivation, assurance that the woman is not pregnant, and convenience, but it is associated (particularly postpartum and after a second trimester abortion) with a higher expulsion rate than after interval insertion (box 3).[5]

Copper bearing intrauterine devices increase menstrual flow by 30% on average and may aggravate dysmenorrhoea. According to a recent Cochrane review, non-steroidal anti-inflammatory drugs reduce bleeding and pain associated with the use of intrauterine devices; tranexamic acid is a second line treatment for excessive bleeding.[18] A case-control study found that intrauterine devices do not raise the risk of tubal occlusion in nulligravid women,[19] and a meta-analysis of case-control studies showed that ectopic pregnancy is not more common in women who conceive with an intrauterine device in place.[20] According to observational evidence, intrauterine devices do not increase the risk of pelvic inflammatory disease unless inserted in women with pre-existing gonorrhoea or *Chlamydia* infection.[w6]

Women using a levonorgestrel releasing intrauterine system may have spotting and bleeding during the first months, acne (if already prone to it), mastalgia, or mood changes and they may develop functional ovarian cysts. The recurrence or persistence of side effects may require the removal of the device. Amenorrhoea occurs in about 20% of women one year after insertion of the levonorgestrel releasing intrauterine system. Women may consider it a reason for discontinuation if they were not counselled about the beneficial effect this may have on their health.

How useful are barrier methods?

All barrier methods offer the convenience of contraception "when needed," but their success rate depends on correct and consistent use. Typical use is associated with high failure rates (from 15 for the male condom to 32 per 100

BOX 2 CONTRAINDICATIONS TO COMBINED HORMONAL CONTRACEPTIVES[4 5]

Absolute contraindications (class 4 in the WHO classification)

- Pregnancy
- Undiagnosed genital bleeding
- Breast cancer
- Past or present circulatory disease (for example, arterial or venous thrombosis, ischaemic heart disease, and cerebral haemorrhage)
- Thrombophilia
- Pill induced hypertension
- Migraine with aura
- Active liver disease, cholestatic jaundice, Dubin-Johnson syndrome, acute porphyria
- Systemic lupus erythematosus
- Haemolytic-uraemic syndrome
- Thrombotic thrombocytopenic purpura

Relative contraindications (class 2 or 3 in the WHO classification)

- Smoker aged over 35 years
- Hypertension (blood pressure above 140/90 mm Hg)
- Diabetes
- Hyperprolactinaemia
- Gall bladder disease
- Migraine without aura
- Otosclerosis
- Sickle cell disease

---

women per year for the cervical cap used by multiparous women),[8] and all may cause allergy.

The female condom is a single-use polyurethane sheath, which is placed into the vagina. To insert the condom into the vagina, the movable and flexible inner ring at its closed end is compressed and introduced much like a diaphragm. The larger, fixed outer ring remains outside the vagina to cover part of the introitus. The penis should be manually placed (by either partner) into the sheath to prevent it from becoming wrongly positioned between the condom and the vaginal wall. The condom is removed immediately after intercourse.

The diaphragm is particularly suited for women over the age of 35, whose fertility is progressively decreasing and who show greater compliance. It should be inserted less than three hours before intercourse and left in situ for at least six hours afterwards. Its use increases the risk of urinary tract infections.

The cervical cap may be inserted up to 48 hours before coitus. Both the diaphragm and the cap must be coated with spermicide before insertion. Neither should be fitted within six to 12 weeks after childbirth or second trimester abortion, and neither protects against HIV. Women with a history of toxic shock syndrome should not use a diaphragm or a cap.

How useful are spermicides, used alone?

Spermicides are usually used with barrier devices, and they are not reliable if used alone, except in women whose natural fertility is reduced, particularly with increasing age. Their use many times a day (for example, by professional sex workers) may cause damage of the vaginal wall and facilitate HIV transmission.[w7]

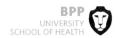

BOX 3 CONTRACEPTION FOR SPECIAL GROUPS

Adolescents

When accessible, adolescents mostly use pills (less often patches or rings) or male condoms. Dual protection with a condom and another contraceptive should be encouraged. Easy access to emergency contraception is a priority. Long acting reversible contraceptives protect more effectively against unwanted pregnancy; injectable preparations and implants are preferable to copper bearing intrauterine devices in this age group.

Post partum

Because of the higher risk of thrombosis during the first weeks after childbirth, combined oestrogen-progestogen preparations should not be used until 21 days after delivery. Progestogen-only pills may be started at once. Progestogen-only injectable preparations may cause heavy metrorrhagia if given before six weeks post partum. Intrauterine contraceptives may be inserted immediately after delivery or any time from six weeks post partum onwards (to lessen the risk of perforation). Diaphragms and cervical caps should not be fitted until six to 12 weeks post partum.

Lactating mothers

Breast feeding is a contraindication for the use of all hormonal methods except for progestogen-only pills, which have no known adverse effect on the infant or lactation.

Older (perimenopausal) women

Contraceptives (including 20 µg pills) that are well tolerated, effective, and not contraindicated should not be discontinued until menopause is confirmed or the age of 51. The levonorgestrel intrauterine system is particularly useful for premenopausal women with menorrhagia. Because of diminishing fertility, less effective methods (such as diaphragms and cervical caps) may provide sufficient protection in this age group.

Does evidence support the use of natural contraceptive methods?

Methods based on fertility awareness involve identifying "fertile days" of the cycle by observing changes in the basal body temperature or cervical secretions, or by monitoring cycle days, and abstaining from coitus or using a barrier contraceptive on those days. A Cochrane review, in which the authors searched five computerised databases for randomised controlled trials of these methods, concluded that—because of poor methodology and reporting—pregnancy rates could not be determined.[21] Although these methods may be the only ones deemed acceptable for personal or religious reasons, or the only ones available in resource poor settings, they are difficult to apply; couples who use them should be informed about the lack of evidence regarding their effectiveness and, where possible, counselled about other options they might consider.

Is the "lactational amenorrhoea method" reliable?

The lactational amenorrhoea method is an efficient physiological tool for spacing births. Suckling an infant reduces the release of gonadotrophins, which suppress ovulation and cause amenorrhoea. Reduced suckling leads to the return of ovulation.

For this method to be successful three conditions must be met: the baby must be exclusively or nearly exclusively breast fed on demand, day and night; the mother must be amenorrhoeic; and the method must not be relied on for more than six months. Another contraceptive method must be used as soon as these criteria are no longer fulfilled.

A Cochrane review established that the lactational amenorrhoea method, when correctly applied, is 98% effective.[22] The beneficial effects of exclusive breast feeding on the infant are important additional advantages.[w8]

When and how to use emergency contraception

Emergency contraception includes all methods that act after intercourse but before implantation. For maximal efficacy it should be used as soon as possible. Combined oral contraceptives, progestogen-only pills, mifepristone, and copper bearing intrauterine devices may be used. Hormonal emergency contraceptives can be offered at any time during the menstrual cycle, and even twice in a given cycle, if necessary.

Currently, the levonorgestrel-only emergency contraceptive is the most widely used. A recent Cochrane review found it to be more effective and better tolerated than the combined oral contraceptive, with no adverse effect on pregnancy.[23] A single 1500 µg dose regimen is simpler than 750 µg taken twice, 12 hours apart. When dedicated emergency contraceptive pills are not available, the Yuzpe method may be used: two tablets of a combined oral contraceptive, each containing 50 µg ethinylestradiol and 250 µg levonorgestrel, are taken twice at a 12 hour interval. The selective progesterone receptor modulator mifepristone (10 mg taken within five days of unprotected coitus) is also effective, but it may cause the next menstruation to be delayed,[24] which may increase anxiety.

A WHO multicentre randomised trial found that a single low dose of mifepristone vand both the single and the two dose regimens of levonorgestrel are equally efficacious.[25] A Cochrane review using information from eight randomised controlled trials found that advance provision of hormonal emergency contraceptives had no negative effect on sexual and reproductive health behaviours and outcomes.[26] Another systematic review showed that increased access to emergency contraceptive pills enhances use but does not reduce rates of unintended pregnancy.[27]

Postcoital (up to five days) insertion of a copper intrauterine device prevents implantation. The method is effective, even after multiple coital exposures during a short interval, and it has the advantage of providing ongoing contraception.

What are the drawbacks of sterilisation?

According to the guidelines of the International Planned Parenthood Federation, voluntary sterilisation should be available to all people who do not request it under duress, who are certain that they want no more children, and who understand the nature of the procedure after counselling. Verbal counselling must be backed by printed information to be read by the patient before the operation.[w9]

Female sterilisation is more risky than vasectomy. A large prospective multicentre cohort study showed that the cumulative probability of regret within 14 years after tubal sterilisation was considerably higher (20% v 6%) for women sterilised at the age of 30 or less than for those over 30.[28] Regret is more common after sterilisation immediately post partum or after an abortion than at a less emotional time. Unpredicted life events, like a change in marital status or the death of a child, are also sources of regret. Counsellors must mention that tubal occlusion is permanent and irreversible, and that it carries a low failure rate.

At what age can a woman stop using contraception?

Women who smoke and those with other cardiac risk factors should discontinue use of combined oral contraceptives at age 35 and switch to another method. In healthy non-smokers, any method that is well tolerated, including low dose (20 µg ethinylestradiol) combined oral contraceptives, can be used up to age 51, after which the risk of conceiving is negligible. Women who prefer to stop using hormonal or intrauterine contraceptives at an earlier age can use a barrier method until menopause is confirmed.

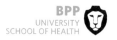

TIPS FOR NON-SPECIALISTS

- The best contraceptive method for a given woman is the one that is medically safe, that she uses consistently, and that she feels happy with
- Contraceptives containing an oestrogen (such as combined oral contraceptives) should not be used by women with hypertension or a history of deep vein thrombosis. Hormonal methods should not be used by women with breast cancer or serious liver disease
- For contraceptives that rely on compliance (such as pills and barrier methods), the failure rate with "typical use" is considerably higher than that associated with "perfect use"
- Long acting reversible contraceptives like intrauterine devices, injectable preparations, and implants depend least on the user and are as efficacious as sterilisation
- Return of fertility after use of contraceptive injectable preparations takes longer than after discontinuation of other methods
- After use of an emergency contraceptive a reliable method of contraception should be initiated

AREAS OF ONGOING AND FUTURE RESEARCH

- Replacing ethinylestradiol, which has many side effects, with natural oestrogens (such as oestradiol and estetrol) in certain circumstances
- Developing new progestogens that bind specifically to the progesterone receptor and will replace those currently used in certain applications
- Expanding the range of applications of progesterone receptor modulators such as mifepristone (for example, as oestrogen-free contraceptives given orally or by means of intrauterine systems or vaginal rings)
- Blocking the expression of newly identified genes implicated in gametogenesis, follicular rupture, development of the corpus luteum, sperm motility, or capacitation to create therapeutic modalities with few side effects
- Elucidating the mechanism of action of the levonorgestrel intrauterine system
- Investigating the effect of hormonal contraceptives on indicators of the progression of HIV infection and the mechanism whereby they increase genital shedding of virus in HIV positive women

ADDITIONAL EDUCATIONAL RESOURCES

Resources for healthcare professionals

- WHO (www.who.int/reproductive-health/)—*Medical eligibility criteria for contraceptive use*, 3rd ed. Geneva: Reproductive Health and Research, 2004 (type title into the search box)
- WHO (www.who.int/reproductive-health/publications/spr/spr_2008_update.pdf)—*Selected practice recommendations for contraceptive use: 2008 update* (click on "Family planning" first)
- Faculty of Sexual and Reproductive Healthcare (www.ffprhc.org.uk)—Provides method specific guidance (first click on "Good medical practice")
- International Planned Parenthood Federation. *Medical and service delivery guidelines.* (www.ippf.org/en/Resources/Guides-toolkits/)—These guidelines offer up to date evidence based guidance on various issues, including family planning
- Royal College of Obstetricians and Gynaecologists (www.rcog.org.uk/index.asp?PageID=699)—*Male and female sterilisation.* Evidence-based clinical guideline no 4. 2004 (type title in the search box)

Resources for patients

- Association of Reproductive Health Professionals (www.arhp.org/patienteducation/index.cfm)—Series of booklets on various reproductive health matters, including contraception
- Family Planning Council (www.familyplanning.org/)—Information on birth control methods
- Contraceptive.org.uk (www.contraceptive.org.uk/)—Refers to other sources of information
- Emergency Contraception Website (www.not-2-late.com)—Provides information on emergency contraception for "the morning after"
- Royal College of Obstetricians and Gynaecologists (www.rcog.org.uk/index.asp?PageID=703)—Patient information leaflet on sterilisation for women and men
- Society of Obstetricians and Gynaecologists of Canada (www.sexualityandu.ca)—Information adapted to different target groups, such as teenagers, adults, parents, teachers, and healthcare professionals

Contributors: J-JA wrote the first draft of the article and both authors helped review the evidence on which the paper is based. Both authors are guarantors.

Competing interests: J-JA has been paid by Bayer Schering Pharma and by Organon, part of Schering-Plough, for organising education.

Provenance and peer review: Commissioned; externally peer reviewed.

1. Singh S, Darroch JE, Vlassoff M, Nadeau J. *Adding it up: the benefits of investing in sexual and reproductive health care.* New York: Alan Guttmacher Institute, 2003. www.guttmacher.org/pubs/addingitup.pdf.
2. United Nations Department of Economics and Social Affairs Population Division. *World contraceptive use.* 2007. ww.un.org/esa/population/publications/contraceptive2007/contraceptive_2007_table.pdf .
3. Lopez LM, Steiner M, Grimes DA, Schulz KF. Strategies for communication effectiveness. *Cochrane Database Syst Rev* 2008;(4):CD006964.
4. WHO. *Selected practice recommendations for contraceptive use: 2008 update.* 2008. www.who.int/reproductive-health/publications/spr/spr_2008_update.pdf (click on "Family planning" first).
5. WHO. *Medical eligibility criteria for contraceptive use.* 3rd ed. 2004. www.who.int/reproductivehealth/publications/family_planning/9789290215080/en/index.html.
6. Lopez LM, Newmann SJ, Grimes DA, Nanda K, Schulz KF. Immediate start of hormonal contraceptives for contraception. *Cochrane Database Syst Rev* 2008;(2):CD006260.
7. Lopez LM, Grimes DA, Gallo MF, Schulz KF. Skin patch and vaginal ring versus combined oral contraceptives for contraception. *Cochrane Database Syst Rev* 2008;(1):CD003552.
8. Trussell J. Contraceptive efficacy. In: Hatcher RA, Trussell J, Stewart F, Nelson A, Cates W, Guest F, et al, eds. *Contraceptive technology.* 18th ed. New York: Ardent Media, 2004:355-63.
9. El-Ibiary SY, Cocohoba JM. Effects of HIV antiretrovirals on the pharmacokinetics of hormonal contraceptives. *Eur J Contracept Reprod Health Care* 2008;13:123-32.
10. Collaborative Group on Epidemiological Studies of Ovarian Cancer. Ovarian cancer and oral contraceptives: collaborative reanalysis of data from 45 epidemiological studies including 23 257 women with ovarian cancer and 87 303 controls. *Lancet* 2008;371:303-14.
11. Rosenberg MJ, Waugh MS. Oral contraceptive discontinuation: a prospective evaluation of frequency and reasons. *Am J Obstet Gynecol* 1998;179:577-82.
12. Martinez F, Avecilla A. Combined hormonal contraception and venous thromboembolism. *Eur J Contracept Reprod Health Care* 2007;12:97-106.
13. Wu O, Robertson L, Langhorne P, Twaddle S, Lowe GD, Clarke P, et al. Oral contraceptives, hormonal replacement therapy, thrombophilias and risk of venous thromboembolism: a systematic review. The Thrombosis: Risk and Economic Assessment of Thrombophilia Screening (TREATS) Study. *Thromb Haemost* 2005;94:17-25.
14. Cole JA, Norman H, Doherty M, Walker AM. Venous thromboembolism, myocardial infarction, and stroke among transdermal contraceptive system users. *Obstet Gynecol* 2007;109:339-46.
15. Grimes DA, Lopez LM, Manion C, Schulz KF. Cochrane systematic reviews of IUD trials: lessons learned. *Contraception* 2007;75(suppl):S55-9.
16. Hubacher D, Grimes DA. Noncontraceptive health benefits of intrauterine devices: a systematic review. *Obstet Gynecol Surv* 2002;57:120-8.
17. Varma R, Sinha D, Gupta JK. Non-contraceptive uses of levonorgestrel-releasing hormone system (LNG-IUS)—a systematic enquiry and overview. *Eur J Obstet Gynecol Reprod Biol* 2006;125:9-28.
18. Grimes DA, Hubacher D, Lopez LM, Schulz KF. Non-steroidal anti-inflammatory drugs for heavy bleeding or pain associated with intrauterine-device use. *Cochrane Database Syst Rev* 2006;(3):CD006034.
19. Hubacher D, Lara-Ricalde R, Taylor DJ, Guerra-Infante F, Guzman-Rodriguez R. Use of copper intrauterine devices and the risk of tubal infertility among nulligravid women. *N Engl J Med* 2001;345:561-7.
20. Xiong X, Buekens P, Wollast E. IUD use and the risk of ectopic pregnancy: a meta-analysis of case-control studies. *Contraception* 1995;52:23-34.
21. Grimes DA, Gallo MF, Halpern V, Nanda K, Schulz KF, Lopez LM. Fertility awareness-based methods for contraception. *Cochrane Database Syst Rev* 2007;(3):CD004860.
22. Van der Wijden C, Kleinen J. Lactational amenorrhea for family planning. *Cochrane Database Syst Rev* 2003;(4):CD001329.
23. Cheng L, Gülmezoglu AM, van Oel CJ, Piaggio G, Ezcurra E, van Look PF. Interventions for emergency contraception. *Cochrane Database Syst Rev* 2007;(4):CD001324.
24. Task Force on Postovulatory Methods of Fertility Regulation. Comparison of three single doses of mifepristone as emergency contraception: a randomised trial. *Lancet* 1999;353:697-702.
25. Von Hertzen H, Piaggio G, Ding J, Chen J, Song S, Bártfai G, et al. Low dose mifepristone and two regimens of levonorgestrel for emergency contraception: a WHO multicentre randomised trial. *Lancet* 2002;360:1803-10.
26. Polis CB, Schaffer K, Blanchard K, Glasier A, Harper C, Grimes DA. Advance provision of emergency contraception for pregnancy prevention. *Cochrane Database Syst Rev* 2007;(2):CD005497.
27. Raymond EG, Trussell J, Polis CB. Population effect of increased access to emergency contraceptive pills: a systematic review. *Obstet Gynecol* 2007;109:181-8.
28. Hillis SD, Marchbanks PA, Ratliff Tyler L, Peterson HB. Poststerilization regret: findings from the United States Collaborative Review of Sterilization. *Obstet Gynecol* 1999;93:889-95.

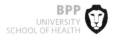

Recommendations for the administration of influenza vaccine in children allergic to egg

M Erlewyn-Lajeunesse, consultant in paediatric allergy [1], N Brathwaite, consultant in paediatric allergy[2], J S A Lucas, honorary consultant in allergy and respiratory paediatrics[1], senior lecturer in child health[3], J O Warner, professor of child health[4]

[1]Southampton University Hospitals NHS Trust, Southampton

[2]King's College Hospital, London

[3]Infection Inflammation and Immunology, School of Medicine, University of Southampton, Southampton

[4]Imperial College and Imperial College Healthcare NHS Trust, London

Correspondence to: M Lajeunesse, The Children's Allergy Clinic, Southampton University Hospitals NHS Trust, Southampton SO16 6YD mich.lajeunesse@soton.ac.uk

Cite this as: BMJ 2009;339:b3680

DOI: 10.1136/bmj.b3680

http://www.bmj.com/content/339/bmj.b3680

Egg allergy affects about 2.6% of preschool children by 3 years of age, and influenza immunisation using egg based vaccines has been classified as a "relative contraindication" (prescribe with extra caution) in this patient group.[1] Until now the numbers of children with egg allergy requiring immunisation has been low, but this may change with the potential for a mass immunisation campaign. This article reviews the literature on the safety of flu vaccines and provides guidelines for the administration of these vaccines to children with egg allergy. Although egg-free flu vaccines are expected to be available for this season, the provision of sufficient amounts of this vaccine cannot be guaranteed at the time of writing, and a pragmatic strategy for the safe immunisation of children with egg allergy is required.

Sources and selection criteria

We identified articles using PubMed and the search terms "influenza" and "egg allergy". We identified further references within relevant papers. We found two randomised clinical trials, but most evidence comes from small case series.

What vaccines are available?

This season two varieties of flu vaccine will be available: a pandemic A/H1N1 strain and the normal trivalent seasonal flu vaccine that will contain an A/H1N1 virus but will not protect against the pandemic strain. There is an egg-free flu vaccine for seasonal immunisation, and it is anticipated that there will be one available for the pandemic strain (table 1). These egg-free vaccines are produced using new viral culture techniques in a mammalian cell line.[2][3] Inactivated, split flu virus, split virion, subunit, or surface antigen flu vaccines are grown in hens' eggs and contain residual allergenic egg white proteins. Some but not all of last season's flu vaccines (2008) reported maximum egg protein content above the proposed safety cut-off of 1.2 µg/ml, with levels up to 2 µg/ml. Virosomal vaccines are highly purified, and although still grown in egg cultures, often have much less residual egg protein.[4]

What is the evidence for the current contraindications?

According to the Department of Health guidance on immunisation in the Green Book and manufacturer's product characteristics, flu immunisation is contraindicated by a confirmed anaphylaxis to a previous dose of the vaccine, to any component of the vaccine, or to egg products.[5] Despite the use of anaphylaxis as a severity cut-off, flu vaccines have been used cautiously in individuals with egg allergy. We will look at the evidence for each of these contraindications in turn.

Anaphylaxis as an adverse event after immunisation is a rare event at about one in a million doses.[6][7] There is a paucity of published data on the risk of allergic reaction to flu vaccine.[8] A large population based study in the United States in 1976 found 11 episodes of non-fatal anaphylaxis in 48 million doses.[9] None of the patients with an anaphylaxis to the flu vaccine reported a history of egg allergy.

Excipients in the vaccine can act as allergens in sensitised individuals, as seen with gelatin in the measles, mumps, and rubella vaccine (MMR vaccine) during the 1990s.[10] Common residues of production found in flu vaccines include the stabiliser polysorbate 80 and antibiotics such as gentamicin, neomycin, kanamycin, and polymyxin B. There are no reports of anaphylaxis to flu vaccine caused by sensitivity to these agents.

All reported cases of anaphylaxis after flu immunisation in individuals with egg allergy occurred over 20 years ago. At least one case of fatal anaphylaxis after influenza vaccine occurred in a child with egg allergy during the 1970s.[11] In 1946 Ratner and Untracht described two cases of adult anaphylaxis related to flu vaccine and egg intolerance from their literature review; they also documented two children who had immediate allergic reactions to full strength intradermal testing with flu vaccine.[12] The egg content of the vaccines causing these reactions was likely to have been much higher than those available today. The ovalbumin content of flu vaccines has been shown to change by manufacturer and by year.[13][14] More recently, manufacturers have published the maximum egg content of their vaccines in their "summary of product characteristics," which helps to make an assessment of their safety in egg allergy.

Can influenza vaccine be given safely in egg allergy?

Several reports have been published of the safe immunisation of individuals allergic to egg with flu vaccines containing egg (table 2). Initial case series excluded all who had a positive skin prick or intradermal testing to the flu vaccine.[11][15][16] Later case series showed that positive skin and intradermal tests to the vaccine did not predict reactivity, and that individuals with an anaphylaxis to egg have been immunised safely using a split dose protocol (six dose or two dose).[17][18][19]

SUMMARY POINTS

- Egg-free, mammalian culture based flu vaccines should be given preferentially to individuals allergic to egg
- If an egg-free vaccine is not available, only vaccines with a stated maximum egg content <1.2 µg/ml (0.6 µg per dose) should be used in individuals allergic to egg
- If egg based vaccine is administered to individuals with egg allergy, this should be done in a centre experienced in the management of anaphylaxis
- A single dose protocol is recommended for those with less severe egg allergy
- A two dose, split protocol can be used in those with anaphylaxis to egg or those with moderate or uncontrolled asthma

The most convincing evidence comes from a prospective multicentre controlled trial using a split dose protocol.[19] Flu vaccine was administered in two doses 30 minutes apart; the first dose was 1/10th (0.05 ml) and the second dose 9/10th (0.45 ml) of the recommended dose. The content of egg protein in the vaccines used in this trial was known to be less than 1.2 µg/ml (0.6 µg per 0.5 ml dose). Eighty three individuals with confirmed egg allergy were recruited, of whom 27 had a convincing history of anaphylaxis to egg. The 124 control participants without egg allergy received a standard single dose of the vaccine. All patients with egg allergy tolerated the split dose vaccination protocol without any significant allergic reaction. A controlled study also showed that a virosomal vaccine with a single dose protocol was safe in those with egg allergy.[20]

Although these studies have cautiously established the safety of flu vaccines in a small sample of individuals with egg allergy, the studies are too small to establish the risk of anaphylaxis; however, all subjects tolerated a cumulative full dose of vaccine.

What do current guidelines say?

The current guidance has interpreted these data in different ways.[14 21 22] The American Academy of Paediatrics' *Red Book* has recommended a graded, five injection protocol after an initial 0.05 ml of 1:10 vaccine dilution, in a setting with full resuscitation facilities.[22] Two variations of a two dose, split protocol have also been recommended: one using a 1:100 intradermal test before dosing, whereas the other forgoes diagnostics but excludes those with anaphylaxis to egg.[14] [21] Neither of these guidelines incorporates the evidence for the safe administration of vaccine either to those with anaphylaxis to egg or to those apparently sensitised to the vaccine (with a positive intradermal test) using a two dose split protocol.[19] The British Society of Allergy and Clinical Immunology has recently ratified guidelines based on our advice to members of the Paediatric Allergy Group for the 2008 flu season, which form the basis of our recommendations.[23]

What should we do?

Given the likelihood of mass immunisation to flu, including preschool children, a pragmatic approach is essential to ensure that individuals with egg allergy are protected, both from the disease and from the risks of immunisation.

Is the child allergic to egg?

Egg allergy is easily diagnosed from a clear history of immediate allergic reaction to egg or to a food containing egg. All children with immediate reactions to egg, including those with localised rashes on exposure, should have skin prick testing or estimation of specific IgE to confirm the diagnosis. Specialist advice may be needed if the diagnosis remains uncertain. We have outlined clinical decision steps in the algorithm (figure).

Anaphylaxis to chicken meat, feathers, and dander has been reported as a contraindication to flu vaccine by some manufacturers. Although such allergies are rare, no cases of anaphylaxis to flu immunisation in such individuals have been reported. These rare allergies remain a theoretical risk and in the absence of any firm clinical data should be treated in the same way as egg allergy.

Table 1   Brands of influenza vaccine available in the UK for the autumn 2009 immunisation campaign*

Influenza vaccine type	Pandemic A/H1N1	Seasonal 2009	Vaccine choice for individuals with egg allergy
Cell culture	Celvapan (Baxter)	Optaflu (Novartis)	First
Virosome	None available	Viroflu (Sanofi Pasteur MSD)	Second
Standard†‡	Pandemrix (GSK)	All other brands†	Third‡

*These brands will change between seasons, as will the egg content of standard vaccines.

†Standard vaccine types containing hens' egg protein are described as inactivated, split flu virus, split virion, subunit, or surface antigen.

‡Brands that contain hens' egg protein and are used in individuals with egg allergy should have a stated ovalbumin content preferably <1.2 µg/ml or 0.6 µg/dose to be in keeping with safety data (see text).

Table 2   Immunisation of individuals allergic to egg with influenza vaccine

	Influenza vaccine diagnostics	Positive vaccine diagnostics	Previous anaphylaxis to egg	Vaccine administration schedule	Immediate adverse events
Davies and Pepys[15]	SPT neat	7/22	Not stated	Not given	Nil*
Bierman et al[11]	SPT neat	0/142†	1/142	2 single doses, 4 weeks apart	Nil
	IDT 1:100	12/142	12/142 "severe"	Not given if IDT positive	Nil
Miller et al[16]	IDT 1:100	5/42	3/42 "severe"	Not given	Nil
Murphy and Strunk[17]	SPT 1:10, IDT 1:100	0/6 (SPT) 6/6 (IDT)	Not stated	Six doses, graded‡	All had asthma, 1 wheezed 20 min after second dose
Anolik et al[18]	IDT 1:100	8/8 (egg allergy group), 5/8 (controls)	Not stated	Six doses, graded‡	Nil
James et al[19]	SPT neat	4/83 (egg allergy group), 1/124 (controls)	27/83	Split dose§	Nil
Esposito et al[20]	SPT neat	0/44 (egg allergy group), 0/44 (controls)	11/44	Single dose of virosmal vaccine	Nil

ITD= intradermal dilutional testing.

SPT=skin prick testing.

*Two (of seven) reported adverse reactions to a previous dose of influenza vaccine.

†Two children allergic to eggs developed a positive IDT result before the second dose of vaccine, which was then withheld.

‡Six dose protocol of 0.05 ml (1:100 dilution); 0.05 ml (1:10); 0.05 ml neat vaccine; then 0.1 ml, 0.15 ml, and 0.2 ml (neat) at intervals of 15 minutes, with a further split dose four weeks later.

§Two dose, split protocol of 1/10th, followed by 9/10th 30 minutes later using a vaccine with <1.2 µg/ml ovalbumin content.

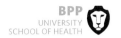

Many children outgrow their egg allergy in the first few years of life. If a child can eat lightly cooked egg (such as a spoonful of scrambled egg) without reaction then they are no longer allergic. We do not recommend testing children allergic to egg by a trial at home of food containing egg because of the risk of an unsupervised allergic reaction. A specialist should assess a child's current sensitivity. Children tolerating egg in baked products (such as cake) but not boiled or scrambled egg are still potentially at risk of severe reaction.

Which vaccine should be used?

We recommend that all individuals with egg allergy should be immunised with a mammalian culture based flu vaccine (table 1). If a mammalian cell culture vaccine is not available then we recommend using a virosomal vaccine for seasonal flu as this has the lowest egg content of any vaccine based on hens' egg and has clinical data to support its use.[20]

Table 3 Immunisation with an egg containing vaccine

	Worst previous reaction to egg	Vaccine protocol
Lower risk	Previous mild gastrointestinal or dermatological reaction to egg and positive diagnostics; or positive diagnostics but never knowingly exposed to egg	Single dose schedule 0.5 ml intramuscular dose of a virosomal vaccine or a vaccine with low egg content (<1.2 µg/ml) if virosomal not available
Higher risk	Previous respiratory or cardiovascular reaction to egg, and positive diagnostics; or "lower risk" individual with uncontrolled asthma treated at BTS/SIGN step 3 or higher	Two dose, split protocol of 0.05 ml intramuscularly, followed 30 minutes later by 0.45 ml of a virosomal vaccine or a vaccine with low egg content (<1.2 µg/ml) if virosomal not available

This table considers the approach if an egg-free vaccine is not available. Mild gastrointestinal and dermatological reactions include urticaria, angio-oedema, and vomiting. Anaphylaxis is characterised by symptoms involving the airway and respiratory tract, such as pharyngeal oedema, stridor, respiratory distress, and wheeze. Cardiovascular complications include circulatory shock, hypotension, severe abdominal pain, or collapse. Positive diagnostics are skin prick and specific IgE tests to egg protein.

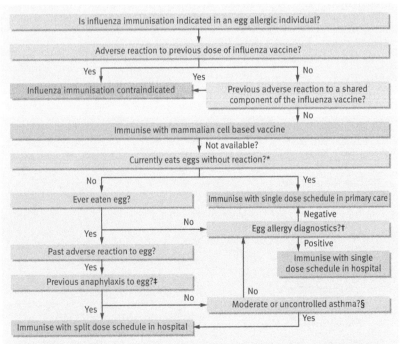

*Able to eat a portion of eggs (not just egg when baked in foods such as in cakes and biscuits) without immediate allergic reaction
†A positive skin prick test, specific IgE estimation, or food challenge
‡A history of a severe allergic reaction affecting at least one of the following areas: airway (throat tightness, sensation of closure, stridor, hoarseness); breathing (tachypnoea, respiratory distress, dyspnoea, wheeze, hypoxia); circulation (collapse, hypotension, shock with or without loss of consciousness, severe abdominal pain)
§Uncontrolled asthma or using preventer drugs at BTS/SIGN step 3 or higher

Algorithm for the immunisation of individuals allergic to egg with influenza vaccine

Flu vaccines that contain egg should be used with caution and only if other vaccines are not available. A careful assessment should weigh the risks of immunisation against risk of infection with the flu virus. The risk-benefit for each individual will depend on host factors such as underlying chronic illness and current or planned immunosuppression and on viral factors such as the local prevalence and virulence of the seasonal or pandemic virus. In keeping with available safety data, the vaccine should have a stated maximum egg content of <1.2 µg/ml (0.6 µg per dose).[19] The ovalbumin content of the pandemic vaccine Pandemrix (GSK) is not known. We recommend that the maximum egg concentration is added to the "summary of product characteristics" before its licensure.

Adverse events to any flu vaccine should be reported to the Medicines Healthcare Regulatory Agency's Yellow Card scheme (http://yellowcard.mhra.gov.uk).

Is all egg allergy the same?

Children with positive allergy diagnostics to egg by skin prick testing or specific IgE estimation have the potential for a generalised reaction when presented with allergen via the parenteral route of intramuscular immunisation, even if reactions on oral exposure have been mild. Until better safety data are available we recommend that these individuals are immunised in a facility with staff experienced in treating children with anaphylaxis, most likely secondary care.

We have divided individuals with egg allergy into two risk groups based on our opinion of their potential for anaphylaxis to the vaccine (table 3).[24] Most children with egg allergy have reactions involving the skin. For the easy application of our recommendations we have simplified the diagnosis of anaphylaxis.[25][26] If any uncertainty remains about the nature of the allergic reaction they should be considered to be in the higher risk group.

Asthma is a known risk factor for life threatening anaphylaxis, and so we have dealt with children with moderate to severe asthma differently, by including them in the higher risk group irrespective of the severity of their previous reactions to egg.[27]

As an arbitrary cut-off we have used step 3 of the British Thoracic Society/SIGN guidelines, where a long acting β2 agonist is added to inhaled corticosteroid therapy.[28] Children who have uncontrolled asthma should also be included in the higher risk group. We do not recommend that children with acute asthma are immunised; it should be deferred until they have recovered.

We recommend that high risk children should always be immunised in secondary care owing to the availability of advanced paediatric resuscitation facilities. Unlike normal immunisation advice to wait for 20 minutes after the procedure, we advise that higher risk patients should remain on the premises for 60 minutes after immunisation, in keeping with standard allergen immunotherapy practice (where allergic reaction is more commonly encountered) and to refrain from strenuous exercise for 24 hours.

The A/H1N1 vaccine

The A/H1N1 vaccine is expected to consist of two doses three weeks apart. Both doses should be provided in a centre experienced in the management of anaphylaxis. The second dose of the same vaccine can be given in a single 0.5 ml intramuscular injection provided that the first dose has been tolerated.

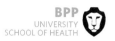

COMMON FALSE CONTRAINDICATIONS TO INFLUENZA IMMUNISATION

The following are not contraindications to immunisation with flu vaccine:

- A history of egg allergy but now able to eat eggs without reaction
- A family history of egg allergy—in a sibling or other family member
- A family history of reaction to flu or any other vaccine

ADDITIONAL EDUCATIONAL RESOURCES

For patients

- NHS Immunisation Information (www.immunisation.nhs.uk)—NHS website giving advice on vaccines, disease, and immunisation in the UK

For healthcare professionals

- *Immunisation against infectious disease—"the green book."* (www.dh.gov.uk/en/Publichealth/ Healthprotection/Immunisation/Greenbook/DH_4097254)—Department of Health publication providing advice on immunisation
- BSACI (www.bsaci.org/index.php?option=com_clinics&Itemid=26)—This website of the British Society for Allergy and Clinical Immunology provides information about where the UK NHS and Irish allergy clinics are located, and what services they operate

TIPS FOR NON-SPECIALISTS

- Celvapan (Baxter), a pandemic A/H1N1 vaccine, and Optiflu (Novartis), a seasonal influenza vaccine are grown in a mammalian cell culture system and are egg-free
- Other flu vaccines are prepared in hens' eggs and may contain small amounts of egg protein
- Individuals with severe egg allergy face a risk of anaphylaxis with flu vaccines that contain egg

Contributions: ME-L wrote the article based on previous documents written jointly by all authors. JSAL, NB, and JOW edited and reviewed the article.

Funding: No special funding.

Competing interests: ME-L has received reimbursement to attend scientific meetings from GSK and Wyeth and has an unrestricted educational grant for Sanofi Pasteur MSD.

Provenance and peer review: Not commissioned; externally peer reviewed.

1 Eggesbo M, Botten G, Halvorsen R, Magnus P. The prevalence of allergy to egg: a population-based study in young children. *Allergy* 2001;56:403-11.
2 Howard MK, Kistner O, Barrett PN. Pre-clinical development of cell culture (Vero)-derived H5N1 pandemic vaccines. *Biol Chem* 2008;389:569-77.
3 Barrett PN, Mundt W, Kistner O, Howard MK. Vero cell platform in vaccine production: moving towards cell culture-based viral vaccines. *Expert Rev Vaccines* 2009;8:607-18.
4 Kursteiner O, Moser C, Lazar H, Durrer P. Inflexal V—the influenza vaccine with the lowest ovalbumin content. *Vaccine* 2006;24:6632-5.
5 Salisbury D, Ramsay M, Noakes K. *Immunisation against infectious disease—the "green book ."* 4th ed. London: Stationery Office, 2006. www.dh.gov.uk/en/Publichealth/Healthprotection/Immunisation/Greenbook/DH_4097254
6 Bohlke K, Davis RL, Marcy SM, Braun MM, DeStefano F, Black SB, et al. Risk of anaphylaxis after vaccination of children and adolescents. *Pediatrics* 2003;112:815-20.
7 Peng MM, Jick H. A population-based study of the incidence, cause, and severity of anaphylaxis in the United Kingdom. *Arch Intern Med* 2004;164:317-9.
8 Coop CA, Balanon SK, White KM, Whisman BA, Rathkopf MM. Anaphylaxis from the influenza virus vaccine. *Int Arch Allergy Immunol* 2008;146(1):85-8.
9 Retailliau HF, Curtis AC, Storr G, Caesar G, Eddins DL, Hattwick MA. Illness after influenza vaccination reported through a nationwide surveillance system, 1976-1977. *Am J Epidemiol* 1980;111:270-8.
10 Pool V, Braun MM, Kelso JM, Mootrey G, Chen RT, Yunginger JW, et al. Prevalence of anti-gelatin IgE antibodies in people with anaphylaxis after measles-mumps rubella vaccine in the United States. *Pediatrics* 2002;110(6):e71.
11 Bierman CW, Shapiro GG, Pierson WE, Taylor JW, Foy HM, Fox JP. Safety of influenza vaccination in allergic children. *J Infect Dis* 1977;136(suppl):S652-5.
12 Ratner B, Untracht S. Allergy to virus and rickettsial vaccines. *JAMA* 1946;132:899-905.
13 Mark C. Large variations in the ovalbumin content in six European influenza vaccines. *Pharmeur Sci Notes* 2006;2006(1):27-9.
14 Zeiger RS. Current issues with influenza vaccination in egg allergy. *J Allergy Clin Immunol* 2002;110:834-40.
15 Davies R, Pepys J. Egg allergy, influenza vaccine, and immunoglobulin E antibody. *J Allergy Clin Immunol* 1976;57:373-83.
16 Miller JR, Orgel HA, Meltzer EO. The safety of egg-containing vaccines for egg-allergic patients. *J Allergy Clin Immunol* 1983;71:568-73.
17 Murphy KR, Strunk RC. Safe administration of influenza vaccine in asthmatic children hypersensitive to egg proteins. *J Pediatr* 1985;106:931-3.
18 Anolik R, Spiegel W, Posner M, Jakabovics E. Influenza vaccine testing in egg sensitive patients. *Ann Allergy* 1992;68(1):69.
19 James JM, Zeiger RS, Lester MR, Fasano MB, Gern JE, Mansfield LE, et al. Safe administration of influenza vaccine to patients with egg allergy. *J Pediatr* 1998;133:624-8.
20 Esposito S, Gasparini C, Martelli A, Zenga A, Tremolati E, Varin E, et al. Safe administration of an inactivated virosomal adjuvanted influenza vaccine in asthmatic children with egg allergy. *Vaccine* 2008;26:4664-8.
21 Piquer-Gibert M, Plaza-Martin A, Martorell-Aragones A, Ferre-Ybarz L, Echeverria-Zudaire L, Bone-Calvo J et al. Recommendations for administering the triple viral vaccine and antiinfluenza vaccine in patients with egg allergy. *Allergol Immunopathol (Madr)* 2007;35:209-12.
22 Committee on Infectious Diseases, American Academy of Pediatrics. Active immunization. In: Pickering LK, Baker CJ, Long SS, McMillan JA, eds. *Red book: report of the committee of infectious diseases .* 27th ed. Elk Grove Village, IL: American Academy of Pediatrics, 2006:9-54.
23 Nasser S, Brathwaite N. Swine flu vaccination in patients with egg allergy. *Clin Exp Allergy* 2009;39:1288-90.
24 Brown SG. Clinical features and severity grading of anaphylaxis. *J Allergy Clin Immunol* 2004;114:371-6.
25 Sampson HA, Munoz-Furlong A, Campbell RL, Adkinson NF Jr, Bock SA, Branum A, et al. Second symposium on the definition and management of anaphylaxis: summary report—second National Institute of Allergy and Infectious Disease/Food Allergy and Anaphylaxis Network symposium. *J Allergy Clin Immunol* 2006;117:391-7.
26 Ruggeberg JU, Gold MS, Bayas JM, Blum MD, Bonhoeffer J, Friedlander S, et al. Anaphylaxis: case definition and guidelines for data collection, analysis, and presentation of immunization safety data. *Vaccine* 2007;25:5675-84.
27 Colver AF, Nevantaus H, Macdougall CF, Cant AJ. Severe food-allergic reactions in children across the UK and Ireland, 1998-2000. *Acta Paediatr* 2005;94:689-95.
28 British Thoracic Society Scottish Intercollegiate Guidelines Network. British guideline on the management of asthma. *Thorax* 2008;63(suppl 4):1-121.

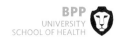

Childhood cough

Malcolm Brodlie, academic clinical lecturer in paediatrics[1][2],

Chris Graham, general practitioner registrar[3],

Michael C McKean, consultant respiratory paediatrician[2]

[1]Institute of Cellular Medicine, Newcastle University, Newcastle upon Tyne, UK

[2]Department of Paediatric Respiratory Medicine, Great North Children's Hospital, Newcastle upon Tyne, UK

[3]Northumbria Vocational Training Scheme, Postgraduate School of Primary Care, Northern Deanery, Newcastle upon Tyne, UK, UK

Correspondence to: M Brodlie, Old Children's Outpatients Department, Royal Victoria Infirmary, Newcastle upon Tyne NE1 4LP, UK malcolm.brodlie@ncl.ac.uk

Cite this as: BMJ 2012;344:e1177

DOI: 10.1136/bmj.e1177

http://www.bmj.com/content/344/bmj.e1177

Children often present with cough,[w1] and over the counter cough remedies are among the most common drugs given to children, despite lack of evidence to support their use.[1] Questionnaire based surveys of parents suggest that the prevalence of persistent cough in the absence of wheeze in children is high and ranges from 5% to 10% at any one time.[2] Cough is an important physiological protective reflex that clears airways of secretions or aspirated material. As a symptom it is non-specific, and many of the potential causes in children are different from those in adults.[3]

Chronic cough in a child may generate parental anxiety and disrupt other family members' sleep.[4] Lessons at school may also be disturbed. For children themselves persistent coughing may be distressing and may affect their ability to sleep, study, or exercise. Parents' reports of the frequency, duration, or intensity of coughing correlate poorly with objective observations,[w2] and reported severity seems to relate most closely to the impact of coughing on parents or teachers.[w3]

Acute cough is typically defined as being of less than three weeks' duration and chronic cough is variably defined as lasting from three to 12 weeks.[5] Most children with acute cough have a viral infection of the upper respiratory tract, which is self limiting.[6] Children with an atypical history, or with chronic cough, may be more challenging to assess and are commonly incorrectly diagnosed—with asthma for example—and inappropriately treated.[7][w4] Despite the wide differential diagnosis for a presenting symptom of cough in children, it is important to identify its cause and provide appropriate treatment.

We review evidence from systematic reviews and guidelines to present an overview of the causes of cough in childhood and approaches to its investigation and management, highlighting key factors that should prompt specialist referral.

SOURCES AND SELECTION CRITERIA

We based this review on British Thoracic Society guidelines published in 2008. We also consulted an evidence based review of the management of chronic non-specific cough in childhood, Cochrane reviews, and our personal archive of references. Clinical guidelines have also been published in America and Australia in recent years. All published guidelines agree on the current lack of good quality evidence on which to make evidence based statements for the diagnosis, investigation, and treatment of cough in children.

SUMMARY POINTS

- Acute cough usually resolves within three to four weeks, whereas chronic cough persists for longer than eight weeks
- Most cases of acute cough in otherwise normal children are associated with a self limiting viral infection of the upper respiratory tract
- Cough is a non-specific symptom, and in children the differential diagnosis is wide; however, careful systematic clinical evaluation will usually lead to an accurate diagnosis
- It is crucial to hear the cough because parents' reports of the nature, frequency, and duration of coughing are often unreliable
- Isolated cough without wheeze or breathlessness is rarely caused by asthma
- Adult cough algorithms are not useful when assessing children

What is the approach to assessing a child with acute cough?

Consider the potential causes of acute cough

By far the most common cause of acute cough in children is a viral infection of the upper respiratory tract that will need no specific clinical investigations.[6] Healthy children cough on a daily basis and experience upper respiratory tract infections several times a year.[8][w5] A systematic review of studies set in primary care found that 24% of preschool children continue to be symptomatic two weeks after the onset of an upper respiratory tract infection.[9] A child with an acute upper respiratory tract infection will characteristically have a runny nose and sneezing.[6] A prospective cohort study of non-asthmatic preschool children presenting to primary care with acute cough investigated factors that predict future complications—defined as any new symptom, sign, or diagnosis identified by a primary care clinician at a parent initiated reconsultation or hospital admission before resolution of the cough. With a 10% pretest probability, fever, tachypnoea, or chest signs were features most likely to predict future complications.[10]

However, acute cough may also be associated with a clinically important lower respiratory tract infection, allergy, or an inhaled foreign body, or it may rarely be the presenting symptom of a serious underlying disorder, such as cystic fibrosis or a primary immunodeficiency.

Take a careful history and perform a thorough clinical examination

The figure describes factors in the history and examination that point towards a specific diagnosis in a child with acute cough. Urgent referral for specialist assessment and rigid bronchoscopy is indicated if an inhaled foreign body is suspected.[5] Foreign body aspiration is not always accompanied by an obvious history; suggestive features include sudden onset of coughing or breathlessness.

Include in the clinical examination an initial rapid assessment to judge the child's general condition, incorporating objective measurements of respiratory rate, heart rate, oxygen saturations, and temperature. The National Institute for Health and Clinical Excellence has published guidance on the assessment of feverish illness in preschool children.[11] Promptly refer any child who is acutely unwell to specialist paediatric services.[w6] Examine for signs of an upper respiratory tract infection (for example, runny nose, inflamed tympanic membranes, and throat) or effects on the lower respiratory tract (for example, crackles, wheeze, or abnormal air entry). Systematic reviews have shown that the best single finding to rule out pneumonia is the absence of tachypnoea.[12][w7] Parental concern and the clinician's instinct that something is wrong remain important red flags for serious illness in settings with a low prevalence of serious infection.[12] Exclude the presence of any signs of a more chronic problem, such as poor growth or nutrition, finger clubbing, chest deformity, or atopy.

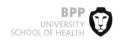

Pertussis is a cause of acute and chronic cough in children and is discussed further in the chronic cough section. In the acute setting be aware of the potential for severe disease in young and high risk infants, where it may be associated with apnoea and systemic illness.[w8]

When to consider specialist referral and further investigation

Table 1 summarises indications for performing chest radiography and considering specialist referral. Referral is especially appropriate when acute cough is progressive and severe beyond two to three weeks; if there are signs suggestive of a serious lower respiratory tract infection; if haemoptysis is present; or if the clinician suspects underlying pathology, such as cancer, tuberculosis, or an inhaled foreign body.[5]

How can acute cough be managed?

Supportive treatment only, including antipyretics as necessary and adequate intake of fluids, is indicated for viral infections of the upper respiratory tract. Antibiotics are not beneficial in the absence of signs of pneumonia, and bronchodilators are not effective for acute cough in children who do not have asthma.[13w9] A Cochrane review found no good evidence of effectiveness of over the counter drugs for acute cough, such as antihistamine or decongestant based preparations.[1w10] Young children have died from an overdose of over the counter drugs for cough, and in the United Kingdom such drugs have been withdrawn for children under 6 years.[14]

If pertussis is diagnosed, treatment with a macrolide antibiotic is indicated. Unless the diagnosis is established in the first two weeks of infection, which is clinically unlikely, the main role of these drugs is to reduce the period of infectivity.[15] There is currently no evidence to support the use of bronchodilators, steroids, or antihistamines in acute pertussis.[16]

Future unnecessary healthcare consultations may be reduced by explaining these points to parents, carefully exploring their worries, and providing them with information about what to expect.[w11] Precautionary advice about appropriate re-consultation if symptoms progress or do not improve is equally important.[12w11]

Acute cough associated with hay fever during the pollen season may be successfully treated with antihistamines or intranasal steroids.[17] Evidence based guidelines exist for the management of community acquired pneumonia,[18] bronchiolitis,[19] asthma,[20] and allergic rhinitis[17] in children.

What is the approach to assessing a child with chronic cough?

In the short to medium term most coughing in children relates to transient respiratory tract infections that will settle by three to four weeks.[9] British Thoracic Society guidelines define chronic cough as cough that lasts longer than eight weeks, with the stated caveat of a grey area of prolonged acute cough or subacute cough in children with pertussis or postviral cough that takes three to eight weeks to resolve.[5] A prospective cohort study of school aged children presenting to primary care with a cough lasting 14 days or more found that around a third had serological evidence of recent *Bordetella pertussis* infection, and nearly 90% of these children had been fully immunised.[21]

Consider the type of chronic cough

Children with chronic cough may be divided into three groups—normal children; children with specific cough and a clearly identifiable cause; and children with so called non-specific isolated cough, who are well with a persistent dry cough, no other respiratory symptoms or signs of an underlying disorder, and a normal chest radiograph.[5] Non-specific isolated cough is a label rather than a diagnosis, and such children need to be kept under careful review.[22] Children in this group have an increased frequency and severity of cough, although the specific cause has not been identified.[w12] If no specific cause can be found for the chronic cough, plan a follow-up visit to allow re-evaluation and assessment at a later date. Non-organic coughing includes habit cough and psychogenic cough. Recurrent cough refers to more than two protracted episodes of coughing a year that are not associated with a viral infection of the upper respiratory tract.[5]

BOX 1 IMPORTANT POINTS IN THE HISTORY OF A CHILD WITH CHRONIC COUGH[5]

- Nature of the cough:
- Severity
- Time course
- Diurnal variability
- Sputum production
- Associated wheeze
- Disappears during sleep?
- Any haemoptysis?
- Age of onset
- Relation to feeding and swallowing (is there a problem with aspiration?)
- Fever
- Contact with tuberculosis or HIV
- Chronic ear or nose symptoms (is there a problem with cilia function?)
- Foreign body aspiration
- Relieving factors, such as bronchodilators or antibiotics
- Exposure to cigarette smoke
- Possible allergies and triggers
- Immunisation status
- Use of drugs, such as angiotensin converting enzyme inhibitors
- Family history of atopy (is this asthma?) or chronic respiratory disorders
- General growth and development

BOX 2 RED FLAG FEATURES THAT SHOULD PROMPT SPECIALIST REFERRAL[5][22]

- Neonatal onset of the cough
- Chronic moist, wet, or productive cough
- Cough started and persisted after a choking episode
- Cough occurs during or after feeding
- Neurodevelopmental problems also present
- Auscultatory findings
- Chest wall deformity
- Haemoptysis
- Recurrent pneumonia
- Growth faltering
- Finger clubbing
- General ill health or comorbidities, such as cardiac disease or immunodeficiency

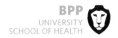
Table 1   British Thoracic Society guideline indications for performing a chest radiograph and considering specialist referral in a child with acute cough[5]

Indication	Features	Likely common diagnoses
Uncertainty about the diagnosis of pneumonia	Fever and rapid breathing in the absence of wheeze or stridor; localising signs in the chest; persistent high fever or unusual course in bronchiolitis; cough and fever persisting beyond 4-5 days	Pneumonia (chest radiograph not always indicated, see guidelines[18])
Possibility of an inhaled foreign body	Choking episode may not have been witnessed but cough of sudden onset or presence of asymmetrical wheeze or hyperinflation	Inhaled foreign body; expiratory film may be helpful but normal chest radiograph does not exclude diagnosis; bronchoscopy is the most important investigation
Pointers suggesting that this is a presentation of a chronic respiratory disorder	Growth faltering, finger clubbing, chest deformity	See chronic cough section in main text
Unusual clinical course	Cough is relentlessly progressive beyond 2-3 weeks*; recurrent fever after initial resolution	Pneumonia plus or minus associated pleural effusion or empyema; pertussis-like illness†; enlarging intrathoracic lesion; tuberculosis; inhaled foreign body; lobar collapse
Uncertainty about whether the child has true haemoptysis	To be differentiated from spitting out of blood from nose bleeds; cheek biting; or pharyngeal, oesophageal, or gastric bleeding	Acute pneumonia; underlying chronic lung disorder (such as cystic fibrosis); inhaled foreign body; tuberculosis; pulmonary haemosiderosis; tumour; arteriovenous malformation; vasculitis

*Becoming increasingly severe beyond 2-3 weeks, most acute coughs associated with infections of the upper respiratory tract should start abating in the second week.[5]
†See chronic cough section in main text.

Table 2   Characteristic cough qualities in children[22]

Quality	Possible causes
Barking or "brassy" cough	Croup, bronchomalacia, tracheomalacia, "TOF cough" after repair of a tracheo-oesophageal fistula, habit cough
Honking cough	Psychogenic
Paroxysmal cough (with or without whoop)	Pertussis
Chronic wet "fruity" cough	Suppurative lung disease

Table 3   Basic investigations in a child with chronic cough[5]

Investigation*	Rationale
Chest radiograph	Overview of the lungs (normal radiograph does not exclude serious pathology, however—for example, in bronchiectasis)
Spirometry with or without bronchodilator responsiveness or bronchial hyper-reactivity	Overview of lung volumes and airway calibre (only possible in school aged children); bronchial hyper-reactivity may not correlate with responsiveness to asthma treatment in children with chronic cough
Sputum sample	Microbiology (bacteria and viruses); differential cytology (may be difficult to obtain in young children)
Allergy testing	Skin prick or specific IgE testing

*This is not an exhaustive list of investigations and suspicion of serious underlying disease should prompt rapid referral to a paediatric respiratory specialist.

Table 4   Potentially serious disorders that are associated with chronic coughing in children[5 22]

Condition	Investigations*
Cystic fibrosis	Sweat test, genotyping
Immunodeficiency	Differential white cell count, lymphocyte subsets, immunoglobulin concentrations and subsets, functional antibody responses, neutrophil function
Primary ciliary disorders	Ex vivo studies of cilial ultrastructure and function, nasal nitric oxide, genotyping
Persistent bacterial bronchitis	Chest radiography, sputum culture, response to prolonged antibiotics and physiotherapy; high resolution computed tomography to rule out bronchiectasis
Bronchiectasis	Chest radiograph, high resolution computed tomography
Recurrent aspiration, laryngeal cleft, H-type tracheoesophageal fistula, swallowing incoordination with or without neurodevelopmental or neuromuscular disorder, gastro-oesophageal reflux	Barium swallow, video fluorosocopy, milk isotope scan, bronchoscopy, pH and impedance studies, upper gastrointestinal endoscopy, fistulography
Retained inhaled foreign body	Rigid bronchoscopy, chest radiography; high resolution computed tomography may show focal disease
Tuberculosis	Chest radiography, sputum culture, Mantoux testing, early morning gastric aspirates, bronchoscopy, interferon γ release assays
Anatomical abnormality, tracheomalacia, bronchomalacia, congenital lung malformation—for example, congenital cystic adenomatoid malformaltion	Bronchoscopy, high resolution computed tomography
Interstitial lung disease or obliterative bronchiolitis	Spirometry, chest radiography, high resolution computed tomography, lung biopsy
Cardiac disease	Chest radiography, echocardiography

*This is not an exhaustive list of investigations and suspicion of any of the above problems should prompt rapid referral to a paediatric respiratory specialist.

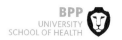

History and examination

A careful history and examination will enable the clinician to identify features that may be suggestive of an important underlying disease process that requires specialist opinion or targeted intervention.

Box 1 lists points to consider when taking a history. It is vital to clarify what the child or parent means by cough. Some causes produce a characteristic cough, and it is important to hear the cough because parents' reports of respiratory symptoms such as wheeze, stridor, and nocturnal cough may not be accurate.[w3] Table 2 presents specific types of cough. Most young children do not expectorate sputum so it is important to determine the nature of the cough—wet or dry. Ask parents if they have observed phlegm in the child's vomitus. If the cough is episodic and cannot be heard at the time of consultation ask the parent to try to bring the child in during an episode. Ask about environmental factors that may contribute to cough, particularly exposure to tobacco smoke or allergens. Consider and carefully ask about psychological problems, and explore parents' concerns and expectations.

Table 5 Aspects of the management of chronic cough in children[5]

Aspect of management	Explanation
Watchful waiting in an otherwise well child	Limit to 6-8 weeks and follow by a thorough review to check that the cough has resolved and no specific features have developed
Non-specific isolated cough in an otherwise well child	Evidence is sparse and no treatments are particularly effective; parents will need to be reassured; the cough usually gradually subsides with time; careful review is needed
Removal of exposure to aeroirritants, such as tobacco smoke	Although there is limited evidence that removal of aeroirritants is helpful, there is considerable evidence that environmental exposure is associated with increased coughing, so it is sensible to remove such exposure
Trial of anti-asthma treatment	Treatment should be effectively delivered in adequate doses with clearly defined outcomes recorded over a set time period—for example, 8-12 weeks—followed by cessation of treatment
Trial of allergen avoidance and rhinosinusitis treatment	Little evidence to support in terms of respiratory symptoms, but a trial of allergen avoidance, antihistamines, and intranasal corticosteroids may be beneficial
Empirical trial of gastro-oesophageal reflux treatment	Not recommended owing to the lack of evidence in non-specific cough in children without specific diagnosis of gastro-oesophageal reflux disease
Treatment of specific cause, such as cystic fibrosis, immunodeficiency, asthma, primary ciliary dyskinesia, and tuberculosis	See condition specific evidence based guidelines
Antibiotics for persistent bacterial bronchitis	Once other conditions have been excluded, and a positive sputum culture has been obtained, persistent bacterial bronchitis may benefit from early access to prolonged courses of antibiotics and physiotherapy to prevent development of bronchiectasis in later life[23]
Behavioural approaches to psychogenic cough	Behaviour modification regimens may be helpful[w15]

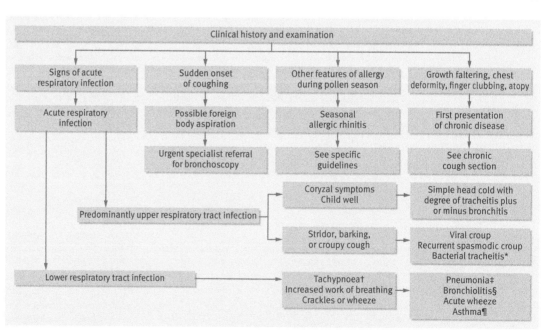

Factors that point towards a specific diagnosis in a child with acute cough. *Bacterial tracheitis is a rare but life threatening condition (croupy cough helps distinguish it from epiglottitis) that is associated with a high fever and progressive upper airway obstruction; it requires prompt specialist care—normally securing of the airway and intravenous antibiotics against *Staphylococcus aureus*, *Haemophilus influenzae* B, and streptococci. †Respiratory rate varies with age in children; tachypnoea is usually defined as >60 breaths/min in those under 2 months, >50 breaths/min at age 2-12 months, and >40 breaths/min in those over 1 year. ‡In the absence of stridor or wheeze, cough, fever, and signs of respiratory distress are suggestive of pneumonia. §Bronchiolitis is suggested in an infant with cough associated with crackles, with or without audible wheeze, during the winter respiratory syncytial virus season. ¶Asthma is suggested if cough is associated with wheezing plus or minus other atopic features and family history

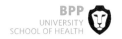

A thorough general examination should look for signs of atopy and clubbing of the fingers. Plot a growth chart and check whether the child's growth rate has recently slowed. When the child coughs feel the chest for palpable vibration owing to partial airway obstruction by retained secretions. Note any chest deformity suggestive of a chronic problem, such as increased anteroposterior diameter, sternal bowing, pectus carinatum, or Harrison's sulcus above the costal margins. Auscultate the chest listening for the quality, nature, and symmetry of air entry along with any added crackles, wheeze, or rubs. Listen for upper airway sounds and perform an ear, nose, and throat examination, particularly looking for signs of allergic rhinitis, including nasal polyps.

When should further investigation and referral be considered? Systematic reviews and guidelines point to several red flags that should prompt swift referral to specialist care for investigation (box 2).[5][22] In particular, the presence of a chronic wet cough is abnormal and should trigger referral for investigation of chronic suppurative lung disease.

In 2007 screening was introduced for cystic fibrosis in the UK as part of the newborn bloodspot programme. This programme will not detect every child with cystic fibrosis and some will still present clinically with chronic respiratory symptoms, malabsorption, or growth faltering.[W13]

TIPS FOR NON-SPECIALISTS

- Most episodes of acute cough in children are related to self limiting viral upper respiratory tract infections
- In most cases, a diagnosis can be made by taking a careful history, exploring parental concerns and expectations, and conducting a systematic examination
- In a child with acute cough, signs of respiratory compromise, suggestion of foreign body aspiration or serious underlying disease should prompt swift referral to a specialist
- In children with chronic cough, quickly refer those with faltering growth, neurodevelopmental abnormalities, wet productive cough, or other signs of underlying disease
- Most children with a non-specific isolated cough will improve with time

ADDITIONAL EDUCATIONAL RESOURCES

Resources for healthcare professionals
- Shields MD, Bush A, Everard ML, McKenzie S, Primhak R. BTS guidelines: recommendations for the assessment and management of cough in children. *Thorax* 2008;63(suppl 3):iii1-15
- Harnden A. Whooping cough. *BMJ* 2009;338:b1772
- National Institute for Health and Clinical Excellence. Feverish illness in children—assessment and initial management in children younger than 5 years. 2007. www.nice.org.uk/CG047
- British Thoracic Society and Scottish Intercollegiate Guidelines Network. British guideline on the management of asthma. A national clinical guideline. 2011. www.sign.ac.uk/pdf/sign101.pdf
- Harris M, Clark J, Coote N, Fletcher P, Harnden A, McKean M, et al. British Thoracic Society guidelines for the management of community acquired pneumonia in children: update 2011. *Thorax* 2011;66(suppl 2):ii1-23
- Vance G, Lloyd K, Scadding G, Walker S, Jewkes F, Williams L, et al. The "unified airway": the RCPCH care pathway for children with asthma and/or rhinitis. *Arch Dis Child* 2011;96(suppl 2):i10-4

Resources for patients
- NHS Choices. Cough (www.nhs.uk/conditions/Cough/Pages/Introduction.aspx)—Provides a basic explanation and advice about cough
- NHS Choices. Vaccinations for kids (www.nhs.uk/Planners/vaccinations/Pages/Vaccinesforkidshub.aspx)—A useful guide to childhood vaccinations

UNANSWERED QUESTIONS AND AREAS FOR FUTURE RESEARCH

- Acute and chronic cough are common conditions in childhood; what is the real impact of cough on children, families, and society?
- Evidence from good quality research studies is needed to inform the management of cough in children
- What factors accurately predict the causes and natural course of acute and chronic cough in children?

Table 3 outlines basic investigations to be considered in a child with a chronic cough. Table 4 briefly outlines some of the potentially serious lung conditions associated with chronic coughing and the investigations performed in secondary or tertiary care that may uncover them. Persistent bacterial bronchitis in children is increasingly recognised.[23] Such children have a chronic productive wet cough but the diagnosis can be made only after underlying causes (table 4) have been excluded and a positive sputum culture result.

Do children with isolated chronic cough have asthma?
Subsequent prospective studies have supported the opinion expressed in 1994 by McKenzie that—in the absence of wheeze or dyspnoea—very few children with non-specific isolated cough have asthma.[7][24] Only a small proportion of children with non-specific isolated cough have eosinophilic airway inflammation.[25] Bronchial hyper-reactivity is associated with wheeze but not with isolated dry or nocturnal cough.[26] Children with a recurrent dry cough may, however, have genuinely increased cough sensitivity.[27]

If clinical features—such as wheeze, atopy, or a strong family history—suggest that the child has asthma, consider a trial of an inhaled corticosteroid as anti-asthma treatment.[5] Ensure the effective delivery of appropriate doses of drug, as advised by evidence based asthma management guidelines—for example, in a 6 year old child 100 µg of beclometasone dipropionate delivered twice daily via a spacer device.[20] Clearly define outcomes that will be recorded over a set period, such as a symptom and peak flow diary recorded over 8-12 weeks. After the trial stop the treatment to allow assessment of its effect.[5] If the child can perform spirometry or peak flow measurements, BTS asthma guidelines recommend an assessment of the reversibility of airway obstruction in response to an inhaled bronchodilator.[20] Asthma is unusual in children under 2 years of age. The clinical diagnosis of asthma in children is often challenging, and specialist referral is appropriate if there is uncertainty or symptoms are difficult to control.[20]

Is gastro-oesophageal reflux a cause of chronic cough in children?
The association between gastro-oesophageal reflux and non-specific isolated cough in children has not been fully elucidated.[28] In otherwise healthy children there is little evidence to suggest that gastro-oesophageal reflux alone is a cause of cough. Gastro-oesophageal reflux is common in infancy and is only sometimes associated with cough. An empirical trial of drugs for reflux in children with non-specific isolated cough is not currently recommended because evidence of their efficacy is lacking.[5][28]

How can psychogenic cough be recognised?
Many clinicians will be familiar with the phenomenon of a dry repetitive habit cough that persists for some time after an upper respiratory tract infection has cleared.[5] Psychogenic cough may be disruptive, bizarre, and honking, with no organic cause in an otherwise well child. Characteristically, psychogenic cough is less prominent at night or when the child is distracted and more prominent in the presence of carers or teachers. The habit may be reinforced by secondary gain derived, such as time off school. Consider Tourette's syndrome or other tic disorders, particularly if features other than an isolated cough are present.[W14]

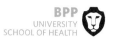

An approach to managing a child with chronic cough

Appropriate management of chronic cough in children depends on reaching an accurate diagnosis that allows targeted treatment. Treatment algorithms used for chronic cough in adults are not useful in children because the three main causes of chronic cough in adults—cough variant asthma, gastro-oesophageal reflux, and postnasal drip—are rarely relevant in children.[3] Table 5 outlines specific considerations in the management of chronic cough in children as recommended by BTS guidelines.[5]

Contributors: MB wrote the original draft of the review and collated the final version. CG and MCMcK commented on the first draft and contributed to subsequent versions. MCMcK is guarantor.

Funding: None received.

Competing interests: All authors have completed the ICMJE uniform disclosure form at www.icmje.org/coi_disclosure.pdf (available on request from the corresponding author) and declare: no support from any organisation for the submitted work; no financial relationships with any organisations that might have an interest in the submitted work in the previous three years; no other relationships or activities that could appear to have influenced the submitted work.

Provenance and peer review: Not commissioned; externally peer reviewed.

1   Smith SM, Schroeder K, Fahey T. Over-the-counter medications for acute cough in children and adults in ambulatory settings. *Cochrane Database Syst Rev* 2008;1:CD001831.
2   Faniran AO, Peat JK, Woolcock AJ. Measuring persistent cough in children in epidemiological studies: development of a questionnaire and assessment of prevalence in two countries. *Chest* 1999;115:434-9.
3   Chang AB. Pediatric cough: children are not miniature adults. *Lung* 2010;188(suppl 1):S33-40.
4   Marchant JM, Newcombe PA, Juniper EF, Sheffield JK, Stathis SL, Chang AB. What is the burden of chronic cough for families? *Chest* 2008;134:303-9.
5   Shields MD, Bush A, Everard ML, McKenzie S, Primhak R. BTS guidelines: recommendations for the assessment and management of cough in children. *Thorax* 2008;63(suppl 3):iii1-15.
6   Pappas DE, Hendley JO, Hayden FG, Winther B. Symptom profile of common colds in school-aged children. *Pediatr Infect Dis J* 2008;27:8-11.
7   McKenzie S. Cough—but is it asthma? *Arch Dis Child* 1994;70:1-2.
8   Munyard P, Bush A. How much coughing is normal? *Arch Dis Child* 1996;74:531-4.
9   Hay AD, Wilson AD. The natural history of acute cough in children aged 0 to 4 years in primary care: a systematic review. *Br J Gen Pract* 2002;52:401-9.
10 Hay AD, Fahey T, Peters TJ, Wilson A. Predicting complications from acute cough in pre-school children in primary care: a prospective cohort study. *Br J Gen Pract* 2004;54:9-14.
11 National Institute for Health and Clinical Excellence. Feverish illness in children—assessment and initial management in children younger than 5 years. 2007. www.nice.org.uk/CG047
12 Van den Bruel A, Haj-Hassan T, Thompson M, Buntinx F, Mant D. Diagnostic value of clinical features at presentation to identify serious infection in children in developed countries: a systematic review. *Lancet* 2010;375:834-45.
13 Arroll B, Kenealy T. Antibiotics for the common cold. *Cochrane Database Syst Rev* 2002;3:CD000247.
14 Medicines and Healthcare Products Regulatory Agency. Children's over-the-counter cough and cold medicines: New advice, 2010. www.mhra.gov.uk/Safetyinformation/Safetywarningsalertsandrecalls/Safetywarningsandmessagesformedicines/CON038908.
15 Health Protection Agency. Guidelines for the public health managment of pertussis. 2011. www.hpa.org.uk/webc/HPAwebFile/HPAweb_C/1287142671506
16 Bettiol S, Thompson MJ, Roberts NW, Perera R, Heneghan CJ, Harnden A. Symptomatic treatment of the cough in whooping cough. *Cochrane Database Syst Rev* 2010;1:CD003257.
17 Vance G, Lloyd K, Scadding G, Walker S, Jewkes F, Williams L, et al. The "unified airway": the RCPCH care pathway for children with asthma and/or rhinitis. *Arch Dis Child* 2011;96(suppl 2):i10-14.
18 Harris M, Clark J, Coote N, Fletcher P, Harnden A, McKean M, et al. British Thoracic Society guidelines for the management of community acquired pneumonia in children: update 2011. *Thorax* 2011;66(suppl 2):ii1-23.
19 Scottish Intercollegiate Guidelines Network. Bronchiolitis in children. A national clinical guideline. 2006. www.sign.ac.uk/pdf/sign91.pdf
20 British Thoracic Society and Scottish Intercollegiate Guidelines Network. British guideline on the management of asthma. A national clinical guideline. 2011. www.sign.ac.uk/pdf/sign101.pdf.
21 Harnden A, Grant C, Harrison T, Perera R, Brueggemann AB, Mayon-White R, et al. Whooping cough in school age children with persistent cough: prospective cohort study in primary care. *BMJ* 2006;333:174-7.
22 Gupta A, McKean M, Chang AB. Management of chronic non-specific cough in childhood: an evidence-based review. *Arch Dis Child Educ Pract Ed* 2007;92:33-9.
23 Donnelly D, Critchlow A, Everard ML. Outcomes in children treated for persistent bacterial bronchitis. *Thorax* 2007;62:80-4.
24 Wright AL, Holberg CJ, Morgan WJ, Taussig LM, Halonen M, Martinez FD. Recurrent cough in childhood and its relation to asthma. *Am J Respir Crit Care Med* 1996;153:1259-65.
25 Gibson PG, Simpson JL, Chalmers AC, Toneguzzi RC, Wark PA, Wilson AJ, et al. Airway eosinophilia is associated with wheeze but is uncommon in children with persistent cough and frequent chest colds. *Am J Respir Crit Care Med* 2001;164:977-81.
26 Chang AB. Cough, cough receptors, and asthma in children. *Pediatr Pulmonol* 1999;28:59-70.
27 Chang AB, Phelan PD, Sawyer SM, Del Brocco S, Robertson CF. Cough sensitivity in children with asthma, recurrent cough, and cystic fibrosis. *Arch Dis Child* 1997;77:331-4.
28 Chang AB, Lasserson TJ, Gaffney J, Connor FL, Garske LA. Gastro-oesophageal reflux treatment for prolonged non-specific cough in children and adults. *Cochrane Database Syst Rev* 2011;1:CD004823.

Related links

bmj.com/archive

Previous articles in this series
- Managing retinal vein occlusion (2012;344:e499)
- New recreational drugs and the primary care approach to patients who use them (2012;344:e288)
- Diagnosis and management of Raynaud's phenomenon (2012;344:e289)
- Improving healthcare access for people with visual impairment and blindness (2012;344:e542)

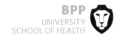

Management of atrial fibrillation

Carmelo Lafuente-Lafuente, consultant, internal medicine[1],
Isabelle Mahé, professor of therapeutics[2],
Fabrice Extramiana, associate professor of cardiology[3]

[1]Service de Médecine A, Hôpital Lariboisière, Université Paris 7, Paris

[2]Service de Médecine Interne 5, Hôpital Louis Mourier, Université Paris 7, Paris

[3]Service de Cardiologie, Hôpital Lariboisière, Université Paris 7, Paris

Correspondence to: Dr C Lafuente-Lafuente, Service de Médecine A, Clinique Thérapeutique, Hôpital Lariboisière, Assistance Publique–Hôpitaux de Paris, Université Paris 7 Diderot, 2, rue Ambroise Paré, 75010 Paris, France c.lafuente@nodo3.net

Cite this as: BMJ 2009;339:b5216

DOI: 10.1136/bmj.b5216

http://www.bmj.com/content/339/bmj.b5216

Atrial fibrillation is the commonest sustained arrhythmia encountered in clinical practice. Its prevalence increases with age, rising from 0.7% in people aged 55-59 years to 18% in those older than 85 years.[1] Consequently, the public health burden associated with atrial fibrillation is increasing.[w1] The therapeutics of atrial fibrillation is evolving. In recent years, publication of several randomised controlled trials and meta-analyses have improved our understanding of the advantages and inconveniences of rate and rhythm control strategies, and effective, new non-pharmacological treatments have been introduced. New antiarrhythmic and anticoagulant drugs are expected in the near future.

Clinical manifestations of atrial fibrillation: what is important to know?

Atrial fibrillation is characterised by a chaotic electrical activity in the atria that induces an irregular and usually rapid contraction of the ventricles (figure 1). Patients may be asymptomatic; may have mild symptoms, such as palpitations, weariness, and reduced effort capacity; or may present with syncope, heart failure, or angina. Many of the presenting symptoms, as well as their intensity, are related to the degree of associated tachycardia. Aside from tachycardia, the major complication of atrial fibrillation is systemic embolism, usually cerebral.

Atrial fibrillation may be self limiting (paroxysmal, which may recur) or sustained (termed "persistent" if lasting more than seven days). "Permanent" atrial fibrillation refers to persistent atrial fibrillation in which cardioversion has failed or restoration of sinus rhythm is no longer considered possible (table 1). An individual can have different types of atrial fibrillation over time—for example, it can evolve from paroxysmal to persistent.

In most cases, atrial fibrillation is associated with hypertension, coronary disease, heart failure, valvular diseases, or cardiomyopathies that result in a dysfunctional heart muscle. Correct recognition and treatment of underlying conditions is essential.

SUMMARY POINTS

- Atrial fibrillation is common and highly variable in its clinical presentation and evolution; it causes substantial morbidity and mortality, including impaired quality of life, heart failure, systemic emboli, and stroke

- The first priority is to control heart rate (if tachycardia is present) and provide adequate antithrombotic treatment for preventing complications of embolism

- Patients with moderate to high risk of stroke require warfarin long term for preventing emboli; aspirin is adequate in patients with low risk of stroke

- When a patient should but cannot take warfarin, aspirin plus clopidogrel can be an intermediate option

- For long term treatment of atrial fibrillation, rate control matches rhythm control in terms of mortality and major cardiovascular events but has fewer adverse events related to the treatment and fewer hospital admissions

- Consider referring for rhythm control younger patients with lone atrial fibrillation, patients with symptomatic atrial fibrillation, and patients with atrial fibrillation secondary to a corrected precipitant

- If antiarrhythmic drugs fail to maintain sinus rhythm, percutaneous catheter ablation is an alternative for rhythm control

SOURCES AND SELECTION CRITERIA

We searched the Cochrane database of systematic reviews, Clinical Evidence, and the US National Guideline Clearinghouse up to 20 September 2009. We also used personal databases (www.nodo3.net/) and reference collections. We selected well conducted systematic reviews, meta-analyses, and large randomised controlled trials. When no study of those types was available, we considered small randomised controlled trials and cohort studies

How should we investigate a patient presenting with atrial fibrillation?

Diagnosis of atrial fibrillation requires electrocardiographic documentation. In patients with suspected symptoms but in sinus rhythm at the time of consultation, ambulatory electrocardiography (a 24 hour monitor or an event recorder) may be needed. History taking and physical examination are important for defining whether the atrial fibrillation is paroxysmal or persistent and which symptoms it produces, and for enabling detection of possible causes and precipitating factors, as well as any underlying heart disease (table 2).

US and UK guidelines recommend transthoracic echocardiography in all patients with atrial fibrillation to identify underlying heart disease and to assess signs associated with increased risk of recurrence and embolism (dilated atria, presence of thrombus).[2][3] The US guidelines also recommend measurement of serum electrolytes, blood count, and renal, hepatic, and thyroid function in all patients at least once. Sometimes referral will be needed for specialised investigations, such as transoesophageal echocardiography in patients in whom a cardioversion without previous anticoagulation is being considered, electrophysiological study in patients with wide QRS complex tachycardia, or exercise testing when ischaemia is suspected (table 2).

What are the general principles of the treatment?

Managing acutely unwell patients

Current guidelines for atrial fibrillation agree in several aspects.[2][3][w2] Patients presenting with rapid atrial fibrillation and acute symptoms (hypotension, syncope, chest pain, dyspnoea, heart failure, or neurological symptoms) require urgent control of their heart rate and possibly emergency cardioversion, in a hospital setting.

It is usual to admit to hospital any patient with symptomatic atrial fibrillation of recent onset, even if stable, to expedite investigation and treatment. Some experts advocate trying early restoration of sinus rhythm in these patients to prevent further atrial remodelling and reduce the risk of persistence and recurrence of the arrhythmia.[w3] However, this approach has not been tested in randomised trials.

Managing patients who are stable at presentation

For patients who are haemodynamically stable and have few or tolerable symptoms the initial management is to slow down the heart rate to the normal range and provide adequate treatment to prevent emboli. Subsequent long

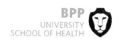
term management will focus on rate control or rhythm control. Additionally, adequate treatment of cardiovascular risk factors, especially of hypertension, and avoiding hypokalaemia when using diuretics, can contribute to reduce recurrences of atrial fibrillation.

Which drugs should be used to control heart rate?

Table 3 lists the most common drugs used for controlling heart rate. A systematic review of randomised trials found that first generation calcium channel blockers, β blockers, digoxin, or a combination of these drugs are more effective than placebo in slowing tachycardia associated with atrial fibrillation.[4] Digoxin seemed less effective at controlling heart rate during exercise than β blockers or diltiazem (mean difference 15 to 30 beats/min higher with digoxin). In the AFFIRM trial,[5] a large randomised trial that studied rate versus rhythm control, β blockers were the most effective drugs for slowing heart rate, but frequent treatment changes or combination with other drugs were often needed to achieve adequate rate control.

A randomised trial found that intravenous diltiazem was better than intravenous digoxin (90% versus 74% of patients were well controlled at 24 hours) for rapid rate control of acute, symptomatic, uncomplicated atrial fibrillation.[w4] In patients with decompensated heart failure, current US guidelines recommend intravenous administration of digoxin or amiodarone to slow heart rate, and avoidance of acute use of calcium channel blockers or acute large doses of β blockers as both are negative inotropes.[2]

How do we choose an antithrombotic treatment?

Full anticoagulation is warranted whenever pharmacological or electrical cardioversion is considered, for at least three weeks before and four weeks after the procedure, except when atrial fibrillation has existed for less than 48 hours.[2] If pharmacological or electrical cardioversion is not considered, then a systematic assessment of embolic and haemorrhagic risk in each patient with atrial fibrillation should guide the choice of antithrombotic treatment.[2] [w5] Several scores have been developed to help in this assessment. A large cohort study found that the CHADS-2 tool was the best of three schemes for estimating the risk of stroke in patients with atrial fibrillation not associated with valvular disease (box 1).[6] Echographic demonstration of intra-auricular thrombus or an enlarged left atrium also indicate increased risk of emboli.[7] A score for predicting the risk of bleeding in outpatients treated with warfarin has also been developed (box 2).[8]

Which patients should receive aspirin?

Systematic reviews of randomised trials show that aspirin reduces the risk of stroke by about 22-36%.[9] [10] According to guidelines, aspirin is adequate for (a) patients at low risk of stroke (those aged under 75 years with no prior thromboembolism and no additional risk factor such as hypertension, diabetes, or heart failure) and (b) when warfarin is contraindicated.[2] [3] [11]

Which patients should receive warfarin?

In well conducted systematic reviews warfarin reduced rate of stroke by 65-68% compared with placebo and 32-47% compared with aspirin, at the expense of increasing haemorrhages (2.5 to 5 major bleedings per 100 patient years, compared with one to two major bleedings in aspirin treated patients).[9] [10] [12] Guidelines strongly recommend

warfarin for patients with atrial fibrillation and moderate to high risk of stroke, such as those with (a) mitral stenosis or prosthetic heart valve, (b) a history of prior ischaemic stroke or systemic embolism, or (c) two or more thromboembolic risk factors (box 2).[2] [3] [11]

In patients with an intermediate to low risk of stroke (no previous stroke and only one risk factor), either aspirin or warfarin is reasonable. A patient's individual characteristics and preferences should be considered. It is important to (a) explain clearly to patients that their disease carries a risk of embolism and stroke and that they need to take a treatment continuously to reduce this risk and (b) describe the relative advantages and inconveniences of aspirin and warfarin (especially the needs of regular monitoring and dose adaptations). A semiquantitative ("low, moderate, or high") or quantitative ("x cases in every 100 persons every year") estimate of patients' individual risks may be given. A large randomised trial[13] and a cohort study[w5] have found that elderly patients obtain greater net benefit from warfarin despite their higher haemorrhagic risk.

What about paroxysmal atrial fibrillation?

Cohort studies have found that thromboembolic risk in recurrent paroxysmal atrial fibrillation is closely similar to persistent or permanent atrial fibrillation.[w6] Current guidelines recommend using the same criteria to select antithrombotic treatment irrespective of the pattern of atrial fibrillation.[2] [3] Anticoagulation is commonly stopped some weeks after cardioversion, but in a retrospective analysis of data from a large randomised trial this approach was associated with increased incidence of stroke.[w7]

Are there alternatives to aspirin or warfarin for preventing thromboembolic events?

Two large randomised trials, the ACTIVE trials, have studied outcomes in patients treated with aspirin plus clopidogrel. In one of them, aspirin plus clopidogrel proved inferior to warfarin in preventing embolism.[w8] The other found that in patients with atrial fibrillation who were considered unsuitable for warfarin, aspirin and clopidogrel combined reduced stroke and major cardiovascular events further than aspirin alone (relative risk 0.89).[14] However, the combination increased major bleeding by a similar magnitude.

Which long term treatment strategy: rate or rhythm control?

In rate control, in which the aim of treatment is to slow the heart rate and prevent emboli, atrial fibrillation is tolerated. In rhythm control, the objective is to restore and maintain sinus rhythm. To restore sinus rhythm, pharmacological or electrical cardioversion can be used, always after adequate anticoagulation. Pharmacological cardioversion can be tried with antiarrhythmic drugs, administered intravenously or orally; patients receive the treatment usually as inpatients but sometimes as outpatients. In electrical cardioversion, a low voltage electric current, synchronised with the R wave, is delivered through pads placed appropriately on the chest and back. The shock is painful, so it requires sedation or anaesthesia. After cardioversion, atrial fibrillation often recurs (70-85% of patients at one year[15]), so most patients need treatment with antiarrhythmic drugs to stay in sinus rhythm.

Several good quality randomised trials,[16] [17] [w9] pooled in meta-analysis,[18] [19] have compared rate and rhythm control in a variety of patients with atrial fibrillation. No study found

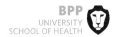

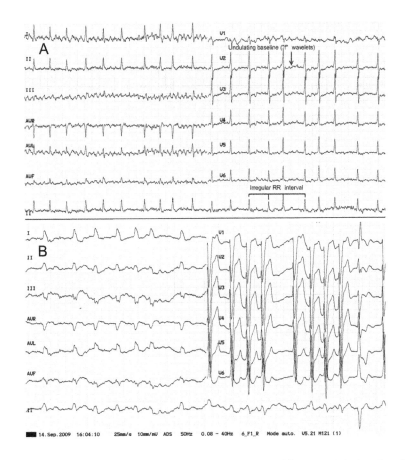

Fig 1 Top panel (A): Typical electrocardiogram of patient with atrial fibrillation. Bottom panel (B): Atrial fibrillation in patient with concomitant left bundle branch block causing enlarged and abnormal QRS complexes

Table 1   Classification of atrial fibrillation*

Type	Definition	Recurrence
Recent onset or first detected	First diagnosed episode (sometimes an incidental diagnosis and precise duration is not known)	May or may not recur
Paroxysmal	Terminates spontaneously in <7 days	Tends to recur
Persistent	Sustained beyond 7 days; rarely terminates spontaneously	Often recurs
Permanent	Cardioversion has failed or restoration of sinus rhythm is no longer considered possible	Established

*Adapted from joint guidelines from the American College of Cardiology, American Heart Association, and European Society of Cardiology.[2]

any difference between the strategies in terms of mortality, major cardiovascular events, or stroke. Rate control was better for some secondary outcomes: it produced fewer side effects and fewer admissions to hospital. Regardless of whether patients received rate control or rhythm control, those who were in sinus rhythm reported better scores for quality of life. However, when the results were analysed on the basis of intention to treat, quality of life scores did not differ for rate control and rhythm control.[w10 w11]

On the basis of these findings, many specialists consider rate control to be the default strategy for most patients with atrial fibrillation.[w2] However, these result are averaged over a wide range of patients, and many patients in the studies had persistent atrial fibrillation and were aged over 65 years. Other specialists believe that rhythm control might provide better outcomes or quality of life in some subgroups of patients.

Which patients should be referred for rhythm control?

Current guidelines recommend considering rhythm control in patients with (a) lone atrial fibrillation, especially younger patients; (b) symptomatic atrial fibrillation, such as frequent symptomatic paroxysmal atrial fibrillation or symptoms despite rate control; or (c) atrial fibrillation secondary to a corrected precipitant.[3] In addition, patients who should but cannot take warfarin might reduce their risk of stroke if sinus rhythm is restored. Nevertheless, rhythm control in those subgroups has not yet been proved in controlled trials to be better than rate control.

Rhythm control has also been recommended for patients with heart failure. However, a recent large randomised trial in patients with systolic heart failure found no difference between rate and rhythm control for any outcome, including worsening heart failure.[17]

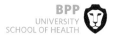

Table 2 Investigations in patients with atrial fibrillation

Investigation	Purpose
Basic evaluation (history)	
Presence of symptoms, type, intensity	To assess clinical impact
Date of onset or discovery, frequency, duration	To characterise as paroxysmal or persistent
Antecedents, cardiac and non-cardiac diseases, cardiovascular risk factors, alcohol and drugs intake	To look for possible causes, precipitating factors, and possible underlying heart disease
Any previous treatment and response	To plan future treatment
Basic evaluation (physical examination)	
Blood pressure	To rule out hypertension
Heart rate	To establish degree of tachycardia
Heart murmurs, signs of heart failure	To consider probability of heart disease
Enlarged or nodular thyroid	To consider lung and thyroid diseases (possible causes of atrial fibrillation)
Signs of respiratory disease	**Basic evaluation (other)**
	Transthoracic echocardiography
To identify heart disease: valvular disease, left ventricle size, hypertrophy, and function	To establish precise risk of recurrence and of embolism: atrial size, presence of thrombus in left atria (low sensibility)
Blood tests: electrolytes, thyroid function	To identify possible causes or precipitating factors
Blood tests: blood count, renal and hepatic function	To adequately establish dose of drugs and follow side effects
Additional testing	
24 hour electrocardiographic monitoring or event recorder	To diagnose the type of arrhythmia if unknown, and to assess adequacy of rate control
Six-minute walk test	To assess adequacy of rate control
Exercise testing	To evaluate ischaemia if suspected, reproduce exercise induced atrial fibrillation, assess adequacy of rate control
Transoesophageal echocardiography	To identify thrombus in left atrium (high sensibility) and guide cardioversion accordingly
Electrophysiological study	To clarify the mechanism of wide QRS complex tachycardia (accessory pathway?) and to study further any patient considered for ablation of atrial fibrillation, of atrioventricular node, or of other supraventricular arrhythmias
Chest radiography	To identify lung diseases if suggested by clinical findings

*Adapted from joint guidelines from the American College of Cardiology, American Heart Association, and European Society of Cardiology.[2]

Table 3 Drugs commonly used to control heart rate in atrial fibrillation

Drug	Dose range	Use in heart failure	Major and common side effects
β blockers			
Atenolol	25-100 mg daily	Negative inotropes. Avoid in acute decompensated heart failure. Recommended in chronic, stable systolic heart failure	Hypotension, bradycardia, atrioventricular block, heart failure, bronchospasm, impotence, asthenia, depression
Bisoprolol	2.5-10 mg daily		
Metoprolol	Intravenously 2.5-5 mg (up to three doses) or orally 25-200 mg every 12 hours		
Any other β blocker at appropriate doses			
Calcium channel blockers			
Diltiazem	Intravenously 0.25 mg/kg ororally 120-360 mg daily, in two to three doses	Negative inotropes. Use caution in decompensated heart failure	Hypotension, bradycardia, atrioventricular block, heart failure
Verapamil	120-360 mg daily in two to three doses		
Digoxin	Intravenously 0.25 mg every two hours, up to 1-1.5 mg, or orally 0.125-0.5 mg daily	Positive inotrope. Improves symptoms of heart failure	Bradycardia; intoxication (nausea, abdominal pain, vision changes, confusion, various arrhythmias)

Which antiarrhythmic drugs are used to maintain sinus rhythm?

Two meta-analyses and a systematic review[15 20 21] have found that several class I and III antiarrhythmics (table 4) are effective in reducing recurrences of atrial fibrillation, but all of them cause adverse effects, many have a proarrhythmic activity (that is, they may induce or aggravate arrhythmias), and none improve survival. Furthermore, class IA drugs were associated with increased mortality.

Amiodarone does not increase mortality, can be given to patients with heart failure, and seems to be more effective than other drugs in maintaining sinus rhythm. Unfortunately,

amiodarone causes frequent and varied adverse effects, which can be severe.[22 w12] Overall, the benefit to risk ratio of antiarrhythmic drugs is low and they should be prescribed by experienced specialists.

Are there other alternatives for rhythm control?

Patients with infrequent paroxysmal atrial fibrillation may receive no treatment between episodes. If their atrial fibrillation recurs they may have repeated electrical or pharmacological cardioversion, sometimes following a "pill in the pocket" approach (that is, patients who have been given flecainide or propafenone in hospital to reduce paroxysmal

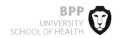

atrial fibrillation, and tolerate them well, can be prescribed a single, oral loading dose of flecainide or propafenone for them to take outside hospital if they experience sudden and persistent heart palpitations). A prospective non-controlled trial found that this approach was effective and safe in patients with no underlying heart disease.[23]

Which non-pharmacological treatments can be used for atrial fibrillation?

Atrioventricular nodal catheter ablation with permanent ventricular pacing is used as a palliative approach for controlling ventricular rate in patients with symptomatic atrial fibrillation refractory to medical treatment. A meta-analysis of randomised and non-randomised studies showed that this technique is highly effective and significantly improves quality of life.[24] The main limitations are a small risk of sudden death during the few months after ablation and lifelong dependency on a pacemaker.

Non-pharmacological interventions aiming to "cure" atrial fibrillation have been tried, initially using open surgery.[w13] A more successful approach has been the development of closed chest endocardial ablation, after the discovery that in many patients atrial fibrillation is triggered and/or perpetuated by extrasystoles originating in the pulmonary veins.[25] Briefly, catheters are introduced into the left atrium after a transeptal puncture, and atrial tissue is selectively destroyed (by radiofrequency or cryoenergy) to electrically isolate pulmonary veins. In experienced centres, the success rates are above 70% at one year for paroxysmal atrial fibrillation. In persistent atrial fibrillation, pulmonary vein isolation alone is not sufficient to achieve acceptable success rates, and atrial substrate modification (discrete ablation and/or linear ablations) is usually necessary. Redoing procedures is required in 9-20% of patients. The rate of related major complications of ablation is below 5%.[w14] The advances obtained with endocardial catheter ablation have also led to the development of off-pump, epicardial surgical ablation, following the same principles.

BOX 1 SCORING SYSTEM FOR ESTIMATING RISK OF STROKE PATIENTS WITH ATRIAL FIBRILLATION NOT ASSOCIATED WITH VALVULAR DISEASE*

Risk factors
- Age >75 years—1 point
- Hypertension—1 point
- Diabetes mellitus—1 point
- Congestive heart failure—1 point
- History of stroke or transient ischaemic attack—2 points

Annual risk of stroke (based on points accrued)
- 0 points—1.9%
- 1 point—2.8%
- 2 points—4.0%
- 3 points—5.9%
- 4 points—8.5%
- 5 points—12.5%
- 6 points—18.2%

Using the CHADS-2 tool[6]

BOX 2 SCORING SYSTEM FOR ESTIMATING RISK OF MAJOR BLEEDING RELATED TO WARFARIN*

Risk factors
- Age >65 years—1 point
- History of stroke—1 point
- History of gastrointestinal bleeding—1 point
- Any, or several combined, of the following—1 point:
- -Diabetes mellitus
- -Recent myocardial infarction
- -Packed cell volume <30%
- -Creatinine >1.5 mg/l

Annual risk of stroke (based on points accrued)
- Low risk (0 points)—0.8%
- Intermediate risk (1 to 2 points)—2.5%
- High risk (3 to 4 points)—10.6%

Using the bleeding risk index[8]

Table 4 Antiarrhythmic drugs commonly used to maintain sinus rhythm*

Drug	Maintenance dose	Use in heart failure	Major and common side effects
Class IA			
Quinidine, disopyramide	Not applicable	Avoid (owing to increased mortality)	Avoid (owing to increased mortality)
Class IC			
Flecainide	50-200 mg every 12 hours	No (negative inotropes); risk of increasing mortality in patients with structural heart disease	Heart failure, gastrointestinal and neurological side effects, blurred vision, proarrhythmia
Propafenone	150-300 mg every 8 hours		Gastrointestinal, dizziness, proarrhythmia
Class III			
Sotalol	80-160 mg every 12 hours	No (negative inotrope)	Hypotension, bradycardia, heart failure, neurological side effects, proarrhythmia
Dofetilide†	125-500 micrograms every 12 hours; monitor QTc interval; start in inpatient setting	Possible	Headache, dizziness, nausea, bradycardia, proarrhythmia
Amiodarone‡	100-200 mg daily	Yes	Bradycardia, atrioventricular block. Thyroid, dermatological, pulmonary, corneal, and liver toxicities

*Antiarrhythmic drugs should be withdrawn in any patients presenting with a long QT interval, new or increasing QRS widening, pronounced bradycardia, or unexplained syncope. β blockers might have a modest effect in preventing recurrences of atrial fibrillation, according to some randomised controlled trials.[w27] [w28]
†Not available in Europe.
‡Not approved by the US Food and Drug Administration for this indication.

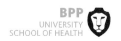

Which patients should be referred for catheter ablation?
Catheter ablation for patients with atrial fibrillation has become widely used only recently and has not yet been tested in large randomised studies with a mortality end point. However, several well conducted randomised trials and systematic reviews have shown that, in both paroxysmal and persistent atrial fibrillation, catheter ablation is better than antiarrhythmic drugs at preventing recurrences of atrial fibrillation.[26] [27] [W14-W17] According to recent guidelines, prevention of recurrence of atrial fibrillation by ablation is justified only when atrial fibrillation is associated with disabling symptoms, and its use depends on the type of atrial fibrillation.[2]

In patients with paroxysmal symptomatic atrial fibrillation, catheter ablation may be considered after failure of a first line antiarrhythmic drug. Hence, in patients with a structurally normal heart, ablation is an alternative to amiodarone if a class IC antiarrhythmic fails. When amiodarone is the first line treatment because class IC drugs are contraindicated, ablation can be considered if amiodarone fails.

The guidelines are less clear for patients with persistent atrial fibrillation. In such patients, catheter ablation can be considered for "severely symptomatic recurrent atrial fibrillation after failure of greater than or equal to one antiarrhythmic drug plus rate control."[2] This recommendation is not based on strong evidence but is supported by small case series and randomised studies showing that restoration of sinus rhythm by catheter ablation may be associated with a significant improvement in left ventricular ejection fraction in patients with either heart failure induced by tachycardia or pre-existing heart failure.[28] [W18]

Can we expect any new treatments for atrial fibrillation?

New antiarrhythmic drugs are being developed. In a randomised trial, vernakalant, a new atrial selective agent, was effective for rapid cardioversion of recent onset atrial fibrillation.[W19] In several randomised trials, dronedarone, a derivative of amiodarone, was more effective than placebo in maintaining sinus rhythm and reducing admission to hospital[29] [W20] but increased mortality in patients with heart failure.[W21] The results from a study comparing dronedarone with amiodarone are expected soon.

New oral anticoagulant drugs not requiring blood tests for monitoring are being developed. In a recent large randomised trial, dabigatran, a direct thrombin inhibitor, was as good as warfarin for the primary end point of stroke or systemic embolism and was associated with comparable or lower rates of major haemorrhage.[30]

A randomised trial has shown that percutaneous occlusion of left atrial appendage is as good as warfarin in preventing stroke in patients with atrial fibrillation.[W22] The best indications for such devices remain to be determined.

Contributors: CL-L coordinated the review and wrote the introduction and the sections on rate control, rhythm control, and antiarrhythmic drugs. IM wrote about anticoagulants and the choice of antithrombotic treatment. FE wrote about non-pharmacological treatments, ablation, and percutaneous procedures. All the authors revised the draft and approved the complete final version. CL-L is the guarantor.

Competing interests: None declared.

Provenance and peer review: Commissioned; externally peer reviewed.

TOPICS FOR FUTURE RESEARCH

- Understand the mechanism of atrial remodelling (the changes in atrial substrate that usually precede the development of atrial fibrillation and are accentuated by its persistence) and find effective treatments for preventing or reducing it
- Clarify the utility of angiotensin converting enzyme inhibitors and angiotensin II receptor blockers to prevent atrial fibrillation or reduce recurrences. Results of randomised trials and one meta-analysis have been contradictory[W23-W26]
- Compare new oral anticoagulants (dabigatran, rivaroxaban, factor VIIa/tissue factor inhibitors, tecarfarin) with warfarin, the current treatment of choice
- Establish the indications of percutaneous occlusion of left atrial appendage for preventing emboli
- Define the role of new antiarrhythmic drugs (dronedarone, vernakalant) in the management of atrial fibrillation
- Determine the best treatment for elderly patients
- Evaluate the effect of percutaneous catheter ablation of atrial fibrillation on mortality

TIPS FOR NON-SPECIALISTS

- Patients with tachycardia plus syncope, chest pain, dyspnoea, or acute neurological symptoms should be sent immediately to hospital for urgent treatment
- Use β blockers, diltiazem, or digoxin (if heart failure is present), or a combination of these drugs at standard doses to slow heart rate in atrial fibrillation if tachycardia is present

ADDITIONAL EDUCATIONAL RESOURCES

For healthcare professionals

- National Institute for Health and Clinical Excellence. Atrial fibrillation. Clinical guideline CG36. www.nice.org.uk/Guidance/CG36
- ACC/AHA/ESC 2006 guidelines for the management of patients with atrial fibrillation. (Executive summary: http://circ.ahajournals.org/cgi/content/full/114/7/700; full guidelines: http://content. onlinejacc.org/cgi/reprint/48/4/e149.pdf; pocket guidelines: www.acc.org/qualityandscience/ clinical/pdfs/AF_PocketGuide.pdf)
- NHS Clinical Knowledge Summaries—source of evidence based information and practical "know how" about common conditions managed in primary care; provides answers to questions that arise in the consultation, with links to answers outlining the evidence (www.cks.nhs.uk/ atrial_fibrillation)

For patients

- Shea JB, Sears SF. A patient's guide to living with atrial fibrillation. *Circulation.* 2008;117:e340-43. http://circ.ahajournals.org/cgi/content/full/117/20/e340
- Medline Plus. www.nlm.nih.gov/medlineplus/atrialfibrillation.html
- NHS Clinical Knowledge Summaries (patient information leaflet, atrial fibrillation). www.cks.nhs. uk/patient_information_leaflet/Atrial_fibrillation (Free access)
- Wikipedia. http://en.wikipedia.org/wiki/Atrial_fibrillation

1   Heeringa J, van der Kuip DA, Hofman A, Kors JA, van Herpen G, Stricker BH, et al. Prevalence, incidence and lifetime risk of atrial fibrillation: the Rotterdam study. *Eur Heart J* 2006;27:949-53.
2   Fuster V, Ryden LE, Cannom DS, Crijns HJ, Curtis AB, Ellenbogen KA, et al. ACC/AHA/ESC 2006 guidelines for the management of patients with atrial fibrillation. *Circulation* 2006;114:e257-354.
3   National Institute for Health and Clinical Excellence (NICE). Atrial fibrillation. (Clinical guideline CG36.) 2006. www.nice.org.uk/Guidance/ CG36.
4   Segal JB, McNamara RL, Miller MR, Kim N, Goodman SN, Powe NR, et al. The evidence regarding the drugs used for ventricular rate control. *J Fam Pract* 2000;49(1):47-59.
5   AFFIRM Investigators. The atrial fibrillation follow-up investigation of rhythm management (AFFIRM) study: approaches to control rate in atrial fibrillation. *J Am Coll Cardiol* 2004;43:1201-8.
6   Gage BF, Waterman AD, Shannon W, Boechler M, Rich MW, Radford MJ. Validation of clinical classification schemes for predicting stroke: results from the National Registry of Atrial Fibrillation. *JAMA* 2001;285:2864-70.
7   Atrial Fibrillation Investigators. Echographic predictors of stroke in patients with atrial fibrillation: a prospective study of 1066 patients from three clinical trials. *Arch Intern Med* 1998;158:1316-20.
8   Aspinall SL, DeSanzo BE, Trilli LE, Good CB. Bleeding risk index in an anticoagulation clinic assessment by indication and implications for care. *J Gen Intern Med* 2005;20:1008-13.
9   Cooper NJ, Sutton AJ, Lu G, Khunti K. Mixed comparison of stroke prevention treatments in individuals with nonrheumatic atrial fibrillation. *Arch Intern Med* 2006;166:1269-75.
10   Hart RG, Pearce LA, Aguilar MI. Meta-analysis: antithrombotic therapy to prevent stroke in patients who have nonvalvular atrial fibrillation. *Ann Intern Med* 2007;146:857-67.
11   Singer DE, Dalen JE, Fang MC, Go AS, Halperin JL, Lip GJH, et al. Antithrombotic therapy in atrial fibrillation: American College of Chest Physicians evidence-based clinical practice guidelines (8th edition). *Chest* 2008;133:S546-92.

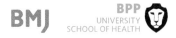

12 Aguilar MI, Hart R, Pearce LA. Oral anticoagulants versus antiplatelet therapy for preventing stroke in patients with non-valvular atrial fibrillation and no history of stroke or transient ischemic attacks. *Cochrane Database Syst Rev* 2007;(3):CD006186.

13 BAFTA investigators, Midland Research Practices Network (MidReC); Mant J, Hobbs FD, Fletcher K, Roalfe A, et al. Warfarin versus aspirin for stroke prevention in an elderly community population with atrial fibrillation (the Birmingham atrial fibrillation treatment of the aged study, BAFTA): a randomised controlled trial. *Lancet* 2007;370:493-503.

14 ACTIVE Investigators; Connolly SJ, Pogue J, Hart RG, Hohnloser SH, Pfeffer M, et al. Effect of clopidogrel added to aspirin in patients with atrial fibrillation. *N Engl J Med* 2009;360:2066-78.

15 Lafuente-Lafuente C, Mouly S, Longas-Tejero MA, Bergmann JF. Antiarrhythmics for maintaining sinus rhythm after cardioversion of atrial fibrillation. *Cochrane Database Syst Rev* 2007;(4):CD005049.

16 Atrial Fibrillation Follow-up Investigation of Rhythm Management (AFFIRM) Investigators; Wyse DG, Waldo AL, DiMarco JP, Domanski MJ, Rosenberg Y, et al. A comparison of rate control and rhythm control in patients with atrial fibrillation (the AFFIRM STUDY). *N Engl J Med* 2002;347:1825-33.

17 Atrial Fibrillation and Congestive Heart Failure (AF-CHF) Investigators; Roy D, Talajic M, Nattel S, Wyse DG, Dorian P, et al. Rhythm control versus rate control for atrial fibrillation and heart failure. *N Engl J Med* 2008;358:2667-77.

18 De Denus S, Sanoski CA, Carlsson J, Opolski G, Spinler SA. Rate vs rhythm control in patients with atrial fibrillation: a meta-analysis. *Arch Intern Med* 2005;165:258-62.

19 Testa L, Biondi-Zoccai GG, Russo AD, Bellocci F, Andreotti F, Crea F. Rate-control vs rhythm-control in patients with atrial fibrillation: a meta-analysis. *Eur Heart J* 2005;26:2000-6.

20 Miller MR, McNamara RL, Segal JB, Kim N, Robinson KA, Goodman SN, et al. Efficacy of agents for pharmacologic conversion of atrial fibrillation and subsequent maintenance of sinus rhythm: a meta-analysis of clinical trials. *J Fam Pract* 2000;49:1033-46.

21 Nichol G, McAlister F, Pham B, Laupacis A, Shea B, Green M, et al. Meta-analysis of randomised controlled trials of the effectiveness of antiarrhythmic agents at promoting sinus rhythm in patients with atrial fibrillation. *Heart* 2002;87:535-43.

22 Doyle JF, Ho KM. Benefits and risks of long-term amiodarone therapy for persistent atrial fibrillation: a meta-analysis. *Mayo Clin Proc* 2009;84:234-42.

23 Alboni P, Botto GL, Baldi N, Luzi M, Russo V, Gianfranchi L, et al. Outpatient treatment of recent-onset atrial fibrillation with the "pill-in-the-pocket" approach. *N Engl J Med* 2004;351:2384-91.

24 Wood MA, Brown-Mahoney C, Kay GN, Ellenbogen KA. Clinical outcomes after ablation and pacing therapy for atrial fibrillation: a meta-analysis. *Circulation* 2000;101:1138-44.

25 Haïssaguerre M, Jaïs P, Shah DC, Takahashi A, Hocini M, Quiniou G, et al. Spontaneous initiation of atrial fibrillation by ectopic beats originating in the pulmonary veins. *N Engl J Med* 1998;339:659-66.

26 Noheria A, Kumar A, Wylie Jr, Josephson ME. Catheter ablation vs antiarrhythmic drug therapy for atrial fibrillation: a systematic review. *Arch Intern Med* 2008;168:581-6.

27 Jaïs P, Cauchemez B, Macle L, Daoud E, Khairy P, Subbiah R, et al. Catheter ablation versus antiarrhythmic drugs for atrial fibrillation: the A4 study. *Circulation* 2008;118:2498-505.

28 PABA-CHF Investigators; Khan MN, Jaïs P, Cummings J, di Biase L, Sanders P, et al. Pulmonary-vein isolation for atrial fibrillation in patients with heart failure. *N Engl J Med* 2008;359:1778-85.

29 ATHENA Investigators; Hohnloser SH, Crijns HJ, van Eickels M, Gaudin C, Page RL, et al. Effect of dronedarone on cardiovascular events in atrial fibrillation. *N Engl J Med* 2009;360:668-78.

30 RE-LY Steering Committee and Investigators; Connolly SJ, Ezekowitz MD, Yusuf S, Eikelboom J, Oldgren J, et al. Dabigatran versus warfarin in patients with atrial fibrillation. *N Engl J Med* 2009;361:1139-51.

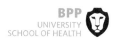

Preventing exacerbations in chronic obstructive pulmonary disease

Drug and Therapeutics Bulletin

[1]Drug and Therapeutics Bulletin
Editorial Office, London WC1H
9JR, UK

dtb@bmjgroup.com

Cite this as: *BMJ* 2011;342:c7207

DOI: 10.1136/bmj.c7207

http://www.bmj.com/content/342/
bmj.c7207

Acute exacerbations of chronic obstructive pulmonary disease (COPD) are associated with significant morbidity and mortality. Patients with frequent exacerbations have high levels of anxiety and depression, significantly impaired health status and faster disease progression.[1][2] Exacerbations are also the most common cause of emergency respiratory admissions to UK hospitals[3] and are costly to health services.[2] Here we assess whether and how drug and non-drug interventions can help in preventing exacerbations.

Background

COPD is defined by the Global Initiative for Chronic Lung Disease (GOLD) as "a preventable and treatable disease ... characterised by airflow limitation that is not fully reversible. It is a progressive systemic disease that results in debility over time."[4] Cigarette smoking is the most important causal factor for the development of the disease and smoking cessation is a crucial intervention that can both reduce the rate of decline in lung function and improve survival.[5][6] The severity of COPD is defined in terms of the reduction in forced expiratory volume in 1 second (FEV1) relative to that predicted for age, height, and sex. This measure is considered the most significant (but not only) predictor of prognosis in the disease.[7] Mild COPD is defined as an FEV1 of 80% of predicted, moderate as 50-79%, severe as 30-49%. and very severe <30%.[8]

There is no standard definition for an exacerbation. GOLD describes it as "an event in the natural course of the disease characterised by a change in the patient's baseline dyspnoea, cough, and/or sputum production that is beyond normal day-to-day variation, is acute in onset, and may warrant a change in regular medication."[4] COPD exacerbations develop because of complex interactions between respiratory viruses, airway bacteria, ambient air pollution, and host factors, which then result in an inflammatory cascade. Consequences of the inflammatory processes in the airway include increased sputum production, bronchospasm, and airway oedema and these in turn result in worsening airflow limitation and breathlessness.[9] The frequency of episodes increases with disease severity.[2] On average, people with moderate to severe COPD have around three exacerbations per year compared with an average of around two for patients with mild disease.[2]

In trials of interventions in COPD, exacerbations are sometimes defined according to severity. For example, a moderate exacerbation might be defined as a worsening of respiratory symptoms requiring treatment with an antibacterial and/or oral corticosteroid, while a severe episode is often described as one requiring hospitalisation.

Preventive measures
Single drugs
Long-acting antimuscarinic drugs
A Cochrane systematic review of nine randomised controlled trials (involving a total of 6584 patients with moderately severe COPD) found that, compared with placebo or ipratropium (a shorter-acting antimuscarinic), tiotropium reduced the likelihood of exacerbations (defined as a complex of respiratory symptoms lasting at least three days and usually associated with a therapeutic intervention; odds ratio 0.74, 95% CI 0.66 to 0.83) and related hospitalisations (0.64, 95% CI 0.51 to 0.82).[10] In a more recently published four-year placebo-controlled trial in 5993 patients with moderate to severe COPD (the "Understanding Potential Long-term Impacts on Function with Tiotropium" [UPLIFT] study), tiotropium did not reduce the rate of decline in FEV1 (the primary outcome measure).[11] However, it did increase the time to the next exacerbation (16.7 months, 95% CI 14.9 to 17.9 v 12.5 months, 11.5 to 13.8) and reduced the mean number of exacerbations by 14% (P<0.001; all secondary outcome measures). Exacerbations were defined as an increase in, or the new onset of, more than one respiratory symptom lasting three days or more and requiring treatment with an antibacterial or systemic corticosteroid.

Antimuscarinics can cause unwanted effects such as visual disorders, dry mouth, constipation, micturition difficulties and arrhythmias. A meta-analysis of 17 randomised controlled trials (involving a total of 14 783 patients) assessing tiotropium or ipratropium found that such treatment slightly increased the likelihood of cardiovascular death, myocardial infarction, or stroke in patients with COPD (1.9% v 1.2% for control, relative risk 1.60, 95% CI 1.22 to 2.10).[12] However, the UPLIFT study (which did not exclude patients with cardiac disease) showed a lower likelihood of unwanted cardiac events with tiotropium compared with placebo at four years (relative risk of cardiac events 0.84, 95% CI 0.73 to 0.98).[11]

Long-acting beta2 agonists (LABAs)
A Cochrane systematic review of double-blind randomised controlled trials evaluating LABAs in patients who had COPD with poor reversibility to short-acting bronchodilators (and an FEV1 of 75% or less of predicted) found that the chances of experiencing an exacerbation (undefined in the report) were reduced with salmeterol 50 µg compared with placebo (odds ratio 0.72, 95% CI 0.57 to 0.90; data from six trials involving a total of 1741 patients).[13] The authors calculated a number needed to treat (NNT) of 24 (95% CI 14 to 98) to prevent one exacerbation in the short term. This review found insufficient evidence to draw a conclusion about other LABAs or other doses of salmeterol. Subsequently, a large double-blind randomised controlled trial (known as "Towards a Revolution in COPD Health" [TORCH]) evaluated salmeterol in poorly reversible COPD. The trial included 6112 patients with COPD and an FEV1 below 60% of predicted.[14] There was no difference in the time to death with salmeterol plus fluticasone compared with each of the components alone (the primary outcome measure). However, compared with placebo, salmeterol 50 µg twice daily reduced the annual rate of moderate or severe exacerbations (a secondary outcome measure, defined as a symptomatic deterioration requiring antibacterial or oral corticosteroid

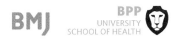

therapy or hospitalisation or a combination of these) by 15% (95% CI 7% to 22%, P<0.001). According to the authors, this corresponded to a NNT of 4 to prevent one exacerbation in one year.

LABAs can cause tremor, nervous tension, headache, muscle cramps, and palpitations. There is a theoretical risk of LABA therapy causing tachyarrhythmias in COPD due to beta-adrenergic stimulation. However, a meta-analysis of individual patient data from seven trials (involving a total of 1410 patients who had received salmeterol 50 μg twice daily for up to one year) found no significant increase in the risk of adverse cardiovascular events.[15]

Inhaled corticosteroids

A Cochrane systematic review included 47 randomised placebo-controlled trials (involving a total of 13 139 patients) of inhaled corticosteroids in the treatment of patients with COPD (FEV1 36–87% of predicted).[16] Long-term (more than six months) use of inhaled corticosteroids slightly reduced the rate of exacerbations (undefined in the report) (weighted mean difference −0.26 exacerbations per patient per year, P<0.0001).

A more recent meta-analysis of data from 11 published randomised placebo-controlled trials of inhaled corticosteroids (involving a total of 8164 patients with COPD and each lasting at least one year) also showed a moderate reduction in exacerbations (undefined) (0.82, 95% CI 0.73 to 0.92), with a subgroup analysis suggesting that such benefit occurred only in patients with an FEV1 below 50% of predicted.[17]

Associated unwanted effects of inhaled corticosteroids include oropharyngeal candidiasis and hoarseness. The drugs also increase the likelihood of pneumonia in patients with COPD (relative risk 1.60, 95% CI 1.33 to 1.92).[18] Such evidence led the Medicines and Healthcare products Regulatory Agency (MHRA) to advise that doctors should remain vigilant for pneumonia and other infections of the lower respiratory tract in patients with COPD treated with inhaled products that contain corticosteroids.[19] Inhaled corticosteroid-only preparations are not licensed for use in COPD. The MHRA also advises that they should not be used alone in COPD and should be introduced only when COPD progresses to severe disease.[20]

Drug combinations
LABA plus inhaled corticosteroid

A Cochrane systematic review identified seven double-blind randomised controlled trials (involving a total of 5708 patients with moderate to severe COPD).[21] Adding a LABA to an inhaled corticosteroid was found to reduce the rate of exacerbations relative to control by only 9% (95% CI 3% to 15%). Also, one of the trials (TORCH) showed a reduction in hospital admissions (a secondary outcome measure) with combination therapy compared with placebo, but not compared with either salmeterol or fluticasone alone.[14]

A systematic review of randomised controlled trials assessing the combination of a LABA plus an inhaled corticosteroid (involving 18 studies in a total of 12 446 patients) found such a combination to be no better than a LABA alone at preventing severe exacerbations (that is, requiring hospitalisation or withdrawal), but marginally better at preventing moderate exacerbations (needing antibacterials or systemic corticosteroids) (exacerbation rate 17.5% v 20.1% of patients, P=0.008; NNT 31, 95% CI 20 to 93).[22]

A Cochrane systematic review of randomised controlled trials comparing the combination of an inhaled corticosteroid plus a LABA with inhaled tiotropium found three trials (involving a total of 1507 patients).[23] Owing partly to differences in trial durations, no meta-analysis was performed. In the largest trial ("Investigating New Standards for Prophylaxis in Reducing Exacerbations" [INSPIRE], which included 1323 patients with a mean FEV1 of 39%), the rate of exacerbations (the primary outcome measure, defined as those requiring treatment with oral corticosteroids and/or antibacterials or requiring hospitalisation) were similar with the two treatments.[24]

Antimuscarinic plus corticosteroid plus LABA

A recently published Canadian Health Technology Assessment evaluated the efficacy of triple therapy for moderate to severe COPD through a systematic review of the evidence.[25] It found four randomised trials evaluating triple therapy (either tiotropium together with fluticasone plus salmeterol, or tiotropium with budesonide plus formoterol). The trials were found to have heterogeneous populations and varying methodological problems. Overall, the authors concluded there was insufficient evidence to show whether triple therapy was superior to a combination of a corticosteroid plus a bronchodilator or combination of a LABA plus an antimuscarinic.

Other drugs and vaccinations

A meta-analysis of data from 28 randomised controlled trials (involving a total of 7042 patients with COPD) found that mucolytic therapy reduced the mean number of exacerbations per patient by 0.04 per month; some of the evidence suggests that this benefit may only be seen in patients who are not already using an inhaled corticosteroid.[26]

There is insufficient clinical trial evidence to support the use of prophylactic antibacterial therapy to prevent exacerbations.

A Cochrane systematic review identified two randomised controlled trials (involving a total of 187 patients with COPD) assessing the effect of influenza vaccination on exacerbations.[27] Vaccination reduced the exacerbation rate relative to placebo (weighted mean difference in number of exacerbations −0.37, 95% CI −0.64 to −0.11, P=0.006). Another Cochrane review, which included four randomised controlled trials (involving a total of 937 patients with COPD), found no overall evidence of benefit for anti-pneumococcal vaccines on morbidity or mortality.[28]

Oxygen therapy and non-invasive ventilation

Long term oxygen therapy (usually given over a minimum of 15 hours a day) increases survival duration in patients who are severely hypoxaemic due to COPD (odds ratio for five-year survival versus no oxygen therapy 0.42, 95% CI 0.18 to 0.98).[29] However, there is no proven effect of long term oxygen therapy in preventing COPD exacerbations, although hypoxaemic patients who do not receive long term oxygen therapy are more likely to be admitted to hospital.[30] Similarly, there is no robust evidence to suggest that domiciliary non-invasive positive pressure ventilation for patients with COPD reduces exacerbation frequency.

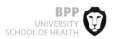

Other interventions
Pulmonary rehabilitation

Pulmonary rehabilitation programmes, which comprise graded exercise training, education and psychological/behavioural interventions (including smoking reduction strategies), have several benefits in COPD, including reduction of symptoms and improvement of quality of life.[31] However, such programmes are not universally available to UK patients. A Cochrane systematic review of randomised controlled trials comparing pulmonary rehabilitation of any duration after exacerbation of COPD with conventional care identified six trials (involving a total of 219 patients).[32] The authors concluded that the evidence (small studies of moderate methodological quality) suggested that pulmonary rehabilitation was a highly effective and safe intervention for reducing hospital admissions (NNT 3, 95% CI 2 to 4) and mortality (NNT 6, 95% CI 5 to 30) and improving health related quality of life. In a subsequently published trial involving 60 patients with COPD who had been admitted to hospital because of an exacerbation, fewer of those randomised to outpatient acute pulmonary rehabilitation (within a week of hospital discharge) were readmitted to receive treatment for an exacerbation within the following 3 months (7% v 33% of those given usual care, P=0.02).[33]

Patient education

Several controlled trials have examined the effects of education programmes aimed to teach self-medication, guide health behaviour change, and provide emotional support for patients with COPD. Data from these studies suggest that such programmes reduce the likelihood of hospital admission but there is insufficient evidence to formulate clear recommendations about the form and content of self-management education programmes.[34] [35] [36]

Disease management programmes

A systematic review of nine randomised controlled trials (total number of patients not included in the report) failed to find any consistent benefits of nurse led disease management for patients with stable COPD.[37] In a subsequently published trial, 155 patients who had been admitted to hospital for a COPD exacerbation were randomised to either integrated care (consisting of a comprehensive assessment, self-management support, an individual care plan and enhanced accessibility to healthcare professionals through a call centre and video conferencing) or usual care.[38] Patients receiving integrated care had fewer hospital admissions during one year (1.5 v 2.1, P=0.033) and more avoided re-admissions (49% v 31%, P=0.03).

In a randomised controlled study, 122 patients with moderate to severe COPD admitted to hospital with an acute exacerbation received a nurse led care package incorporating initial pulmonary rehabilitation and self-management education, a written COPD action plan, monthly telephone calls and three-monthly home visits over 24 months of follow-up.[39] Compared to patients receiving usual care, those receiving the nurse led intervention were more likely to start self-medication with antibacterials or corticosteroids during exacerbations and required fewer unscheduled primary care consultations than those receiving usual care. There were also significantly fewer COPD related deaths in the intervention group (one v eight), although rates of hospitalisation were similar. This was the first study to demonstrate a mortality benefit resulting from an integrated care intervention in COPD. As with other studies, it is unclear which element(s) of the programme were the most important, but it is likely that prompt self-medication mitigated the severity of exacerbations and accounted for the fewer COPD related deaths.

NICE advice

The updated National Institute for Health and Clinical Excellence (NICE) guideline on managing COPD[8] makes the following recommendations.

- All patients with COPD still smoking, regardless of age, should be encouraged to stop, and offered help to do so, at every opportunity
- People with stable COPD who remain breathless or have exacerbations despite using short-acting bronchodilators as required should be offered (if FEV1 is 50% or more of predicted) either a long-acting beta-2 agonist (LABA) or long-acting antimuscarinic as maintenance therapy; or (if FEV1 is below 50% of predicted) either a LABA plus an inhaled corticosteroid in a combination inhaler or a LABA plus a long-acting antimuscarinic;
- People with COPD who remain breathless or have exacerbations despite taking a LABA plus inhaled corticosteroid, should be offered a long-acting antimuscarinic in addition, irrespective of their FEV1
- Pulmonary rehabilitation should be available to all appropriate patients with COPD, including those who have had a recent hospitalisation for an acute exacerbation.

Conclusion

Exacerbations of chronic obstructive pulmonary disease (COPD) cause significant morbidity and mortality, and have a huge impact on healthcare services in terms of activity and costs.

The most effective intervention for patients with COPD is stopping smoking, which can reduce the decline in lung function and improve survival rate. Drugs can help to reduce the frequency of exacerbations, although their overall effect is modest. In general, the stepwise approach to using medicines recommended in the updated guideline from NICE on COPD seems reasonable on current evidence. However, there is insufficient evidence to show that any further benefit is gained from triple therapy, one of NICE's recommendations (a long-acting beta agonist plus a long-acting antimuscarinic plus an inhaled corticosteroid). Decisions about drug treatment should take into consideration the frequency of exacerbations in the particular patient and the possibility of unwanted effects of treatment (including a risk of pneumonia with inhaled corticosteroids). Pulmonary rehabilitation appears highly effective in reducing hospital admissions and mortality and should be available to all patients with moderate to severe COPD, which is currently not the case in all areas of the UK.

- This article was originally published with the title *Preventing exacerbations in COPD* in *Drug and Therapeutics Bulletin* (*DTB* 2010;48:74-7).
- *DTB* is a highly regarded source of unbiased, evidence based information and practical advice for healthcare professionals. It is independent of the pharmaceutical industry, government, and regulatory authorities, and is free of advertising.
- *DTB* is available online at http://dtb.bmj.com.

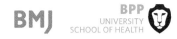

1   Donaldson GC Seemungal TAR, Bhowmik A, Wedzicha JA. Relationship between exacerbation frequency and lung function decline in chronic obstructive pulmonary disease. *Thorax* 2002;57:847-52.

2   O'Reilly JF, Williams AE, Holt K, Rice L. Defining COPD exacerbations: impact on estimation of incidence and burden in primary care. *Prim Care Respir J* 2006;15:346-53.

3   British Thoracic Society. Burden of lung disease report, 2nd ed. 2006. www.brit-thoracic.org.uk/Portals/0/Library/BTS%20Publications/burdeon_of_lung_disease2007.pdf.

4   Global Initiative for Chronic Obstructive Lung Disease. Global strategy for the diagnosis, management, and prevention of chronic obstructive pulmonary disease. 2009. www.goldcopd.com/Guidelineitem.asp?l1=2&l2=1&intId=2003.

5   Anthonisen NR, Connett JE, Kiley JP, Murray D, Altose MD, Bailey WC, et al. Effects of smoking intervention and the use of an inhaled anticholinergic bronchodilator on the rate of decline of FEV1. The Lung Health Study. *JAMA* 1994;272:1497-505.

6   Anthonisen NR, Skeans MA, Wise RA, Manfreda J, Kanner RE, Connett JE, et al. The effects of a smoking cessation intervention on 5-year mortality. *Ann Intern Med* 2005;142:233-9.

7   Thomason MJ, Strachan DP. Which spirometric indices best predict subsequent death from chronic obstructive pulmonary disease? *Thorax* 2000;55:785-8.

8   National Clinical Guideline Centre. Chronic obstructive pulmonary disease: management of chronic obstructive pulmonary disease in adults in primary and secondary care. 2010. http://guidance.nice.org.uk/CG101/Guidance/pdf/English.

9   O'Donnell DE, Parker CM. COPD exacerbations. 3: Pathophysiology. *Thorax* 2006;61:354-61.

10 Barr RG, Bourbeau J, Camargo CA, Ram FS. Inhaled tiotropium for stable chronic obstructive pulmonary disease. *Cochrane Database Syst Rev* 2005,2:CD002876.

11 Tashkin DP, Celli B, Senn S, Burkhart D, Kesten S, Menjoge S, et al. A 4-year trial of tiotropium in chronic obstructive pulmonary disease. *N Engl J Med* 2008;359:1543-54.

12 Singh S, Loke YK, Furberg CD. Inhaled anticholinergics and risk of major adverse cardiovascular events in patients with chronic obstructive pulmonary disease: a systematic review and meta-analysis. *JAMA* 2008;300:1439-50.

13 Appleton S, Poole P, Smith B, Veale A, Lasserson TJ, Chan MM. Long-acting beta2-agonists for poorly reversible chronic obstructive pulmonary disease. *Cochrane Database Syst Rev* 2006;3:CD001104.

14 Calverley PM, Anderson JA, Celli B, Ferguson GT, Jenkins C, Jones PW, et al. Salmeterol and fluticasone propionate and survival in chronic obstructive pulmonary disease. *N Engl J Med* 2007;356:775-89.

15 Ferguson GT, Funck-Brentano C, Fischer T, Darken P, Reisner C. Cardiovascular safety of salmeterol in COPD. *Chest* 2003;123:1817-24.

16 Yang IA, Fong KM, Sim EH, Black PN, Lasserson TJ. Inhaled corticosteroids for stable chronic obstructive pulmonary disease. *Cochrane Database Syst Rev* 2007;2:CD002991.

17 Agarwal R, Aggarwal AN, Gupta D, Jindal SK. Inhaled corticosteroids vs placebo for preventing COPD exacerbations: a systematic review and metaregression of randomized controlled trials. *Chest* 2010;137:318-25.

18 Singh S, Amin AV, Loke YK. Long-term use of inhaled corticosteroids and the risk of pneumonia in chronic obstructive pulmonary disease: a meta-analysis. *Arch Intern Med* 2009;169:219-29.

19 Medicines and Healthcare products Regulatory Agency. Inhaled corticosteroid: pneumonia. *Drug Safety Update* 2007;1:5-6.

20 Medicines and Healthcare products Regulatory Agency. Use of long-acting   -agonists in chronic obstructive pulmonary disease. *Drug Safety Update* 2009;2:7-8.

21 Nannini LJ et al. Combined corticosteroid and long-acting beta-agonist in one inhaler versus inhaled steroids for chronic obstructive pulmonary disease. *Cochrane Database Syst Rev* 2007;4:CD006826.

22 Rodrigo GJ, Cates CJ, Lasserson TJ, Poole P. Safety and efficacy of combined long-acting beta-agonists and inhaled corticosteroids vs long-acting beta-agonists monotherapy for stable COPD: a systematic review. *Chest* 2009;136:1029-38.

23 Welsh EJ et al. Combination inhaled steroid and long-acting beta2-agonist versus tiotropium for chronic obstructive pulmonary disease. *Cochrane Database Syst Rev* 2010;5:CD007891.

24 Wedzicha JA, Calverley PM, Seemungal TA, Hagan G, Ansari Z, Stockley RA; INSPIRE Investigators. The prevention of chronic obstructive pulmonary disease exacerbations by salmeterol/fluticasone propionate or tiotropium bromide. *Am J Respir Crit Care Med* 2008;177:19-26.

25 Canadian Agency for Drugs and Technologies in Health. Triple therapy for moderate-to-severe chronic obstructive pulmonary disease. 2006. www.cadth.ca/index.php/en/hta/reports-publications/search/publication/1690.

26 Poole PJ, Black PN. Mucolytic agents for chronic bronchitis or chronic obstructive pulmonary disease. *Cochrane Database Syst Rev* 2010;2:CD001287.

27 Poole P, Chacko E, Wood-Baker RW, Cates CJ. Influenza vaccine for patients with chronic obstructive pulmonary disease. *Cochrane Database Syst Rev* 2006;1:CD002733.

28 Granger R, Walters J, Poole PJ, Lasserson TJ, Mangtani P, Cates CJ, et al. Injectable vaccines for preventing pneumococcal infection in patients with chronic obstructive pulmonary disease. *Cochrane Database Syst Rev* 2006;4:CD001390.

29 Cranston JM. Domiciliary oxygen for chronic obstructive pulmonary disease. *Cochrane Database Syst Rev* 2005;4:CD001744.

30 Ringbaek TJ, Viskum K, Lange P. Does long-term oxygen therapy reduce hospitalisation in hypoxaemic chronic obstructive pulmonary disease? *Eur Respir J* 2002;20:38-42.

31 Drug and Therapeutics Bulletin. Managing stable chronic obstructive pulmonary disease. *DTB* 2001;39:81-5.

32 Puhan M, Scharplatz M, Troosters T, Walters EH, Steurer J. Pulmonary rehabilitation following exacerbations of chronic obstructive pulmonary disease. *Cochrane Database Syst Rev* 2009;1:CD005305.

33 Seymour JM, Moore L, Jolley CJ, Ward K, Creasey J, Steier JS, et al. Outpatient pulmonary rehabilitation following acute exacerbations of COPD. *Thorax* 2010;65:423-8.

34 Bourbeau J, Julien M, Maltais F, Rouleau M, Beaupré A, Bégin R, et al. Reduction of hospital utilization in patients with chronic obstructive pulmonary disease: a disease-specific self-management intervention. *Arch Intern Med* 2003;163:585-91.

35 Blackstock F, Webster K. Disease-specific health education for COPD: a systematic review of changes in health outcomes. *Health Educ Res* 2007;22:703-17.

36 Effing T, Monninkhof EM, van der Valk PD, van der Palen J, van Herwaarden CL, Partidge MR, et al. Self-management education for patients with chronic obstructive pulmonary disease. *Cochrane Database Syst Rev* 2007;4:CD002990.

37 Taylor SJ, Candy B, Bryar RM, Ramsay J, Vrijhoef HJ, Esmond G, et al. Effectiveness of innovations in nurse led chronic disease management for patients with chronic obstructive pulmonary disease:systematic review of evidence. *BMJ* 2005;331:485.

38 Casas A, Troosters T, Garcia-Aymerich J, Roca J, Hernández C, Alonso A, et al. Integrated care prevents hospitalisations for exacerbations in COPD patients. *Eur Respir J* 2006;28:123-30.

39 Sridhar M, Taylor R, Dawson S, Roberts NJ, Partridge MR. A nurse led intermediate care package in patients who have been hospitalised with an acute exacerbation of chronic obstructive pulmonary disease. *Thorax* 2008;63:194-200.

Related links

bmj.com/archive

Pervious articles in this series

- Islet transplantation in type 1 diabetes (2011;342:d217)
- Diagnosis and management of hereditary haemochromatosis (2011;342:c7251)
- Diagnosis and management of soft tissue sarcoma (2010;341:c7170)
- Recent advances in the management of rheumatoid arthritis (2010;341:b6942)

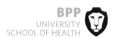
Dyspepsia

Alexander C Ford, senior lecturer and honorary consultant gastroenterologist[12],
Paul Moayyedi, chief of gastroenterology[3]

[1]Leeds Gastroenterology Institute, St James's University Hospital, Leeds, UK

[2]Leeds Institute of Biomedical and Clinical Sciences, Leeds University, Leeds, UK

[3]Gastroenterology Division, McMaster University, Health Sciences Center, Hamilton, ON, Canada

Correspondence to: AC Ford
alexf12399@yahoo.com

Cite this as: BMJ 2013;347:f5059

DOI: 10.1136/bmj.f5059

http://www.bmj.com/content/347/bmj.f5059

Definitions of the term dyspepsia vary but generally describe pain or discomfort in the epigastric region. People with dyspepsia have a normal life expectancy,[1] but symptoms impair quality of life,[2][3] and affect productivity.[4] Dyspepsia is estimated to cost the United Kingdom more than £1bn (€1.16bn; $1.55bn) annually,[5] so it is important to manage the condition appropriately. We summarise recent systematic reviews, meta-analyses, and randomised controlled trials to provide the general reader with an update on how to deal with this disorder effectively.

What is dyspepsia and who gets it?

Dyspepsia is a symptomatic diagnosis. A variety of definitions have been proposed, but a reasonable working definition for the primary care doctor is epigastric pain or discomfort for at least three months, in a patient who does not report predominant heartburn or regurgitation (although these symptoms can be part of the overall symptom complex). Gastro-oesophageal reflux disease (GORD) becomes the more likely diagnosis if symptoms of heartburn or regurgitation predominate, although this is one of the main areas of contention surrounding the definition of dyspepsia. The condition is common worldwide, with 20-40% of the world's population affected,[6] depending on the definition used. Epidemiological surveys show no consistent association with sex, age, socioeconomic status, smoking, or alcohol use.[3][7]

Dyspepsia is more common in people who take non-steroidal anti-inflammatory drugs (NSAIDs) and drugs such as calcium antagonists, bisphosphonates, nitrates, and theophyllines. It is also more common in people infected with Helicobacter pylori.[7] A population based study also found an association between anxiety and dyspepsia symptoms,[8] and certain genetic polymorphisms are more prevalent in those with the condition.[9] There is a strong overlap between irritable bowel syndrome, gastro-oesophageal reflux symptoms, and dyspepsia,[10][11] suggesting that common genetic or environmental factors are involved in the development of these disorders.

SOURCES AND SELECTION CRITERIA

We searched Medline, Embase, the Cochrane Database of Systematic Reviews, and Clinical Evidence online using the search term "dyspepsia", as well as recent conference proceedings. We limited studies to those conducted in adults and focused on systematic reviews, meta-analyses, and high quality randomised controlled trials published during the past five years whenever possible.

SUMMARY POINTS

- Dyspepsia is common—about a fifth of people are affected at some point in their lives
- The condition is chronic, with a relapsing and remitting nature
- There is no evidence that dyspepsia adversely affects survival
- In most patients, no cause for dyspepsia is detected at endoscopy
- Gastro-oesophageal cancer is extremely rare in patients with dyspepsia who have no alarm symptoms
- Most treatments are safe and well tolerated, but there is little evidence that they have any long term effect on the natural course of the disorder

What causes dyspepsia?

Several diseases can cause symptoms of dyspepsia. A systematic review identified nine studies (5389 participants) that performed endoscopy in a general population sample with dyspepsia.[12] Overall, there was a 13% prevalence of erosive oesophagitis and 8% prevalence of peptic ulcer disease, with gastric or oesophageal cancer occurring in less than 0.3% of endoscopies. Oesophagitis was more prevalent in Western populations than in Asian ones (25% v 3%), whereas the opposite was true for peptic ulcer disease (3% v 11%). Overall, 70-80% of people with dyspepsia had no clinically significant findings at endoscopy. Such patients are classed as having functional dyspepsia. The Rome III criteria for functional dyspepsia divide it into two separate syndromes. In epigastric pain syndrome, patients report intermittent pain or burning localised to the epigastric region. Patients with postprandial distress syndrome have bothersome postprandial fullness after an ordinary sized meal or early satiation that prevents a meal being finished.[13]

The pathophysiology of dyspepsia depends on the underlying disease. Peptic ulcer disease is usually caused by H pylori infection, with a few cases being associated with NSAIDs. GORD is caused by a combination of failure of the gastro-oesophageal junction to prevent acid reflux and impaired clearance of acid from the oesophagus. Although technically distinct from dyspepsia, it may present with dyspeptic-type symptoms, rather than heartburn or regurgitation.[14] Acid reflux may be severe enough to damage the oesophageal mucosa, in which case erosive oesophagitis will be visible at endoscopy.

Around 70-80% of patients with epigastric pain will have functional dyspepsia, and the causes of this disorder are poorly understood. Gastroduodenal dysmotility, and sensitivity to both distension and acid,[15] have all been proposed as possible causes. As well as peripheral mechanisms, there are changes in brain activity,[16][17] suggesting that central processing is also abnormal. Functional dyspepsia has therefore been described as multifactorial, which is probably why any individual treatment is effective only in a small proportion of patients.

The causes of the central nervous system abnormalities, dysmotility, and hypersensitivity seen in functional dyspepsia are poorly understood. Several hypotheses have been proposed, including a subtle increase in inflammatory mediators in the upper gastrointestinal tract.[18] An observation that has garnered the most attention recently is the presence of eosinophils in the duodenum.[19] This has led to the hypothesis that the resulting increase in immune activation and inflammation may cause neuromodulation that gives rise to dysmotility, hypersensitivity, and central nervous system changes. The cause of this immune activation is uncertain, but it is most likely to be an infective process. The obvious candidate would be H pylori infection, but other infections can give rise to immune activation of the upper gastrointestinal tract. In support of this, it has been observed that dyspepsia is more common after an episode of acute gastroenteritis.[20]

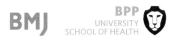

UPPER GASTROINTESTINAL ALARM SYMPTOMS (TAKEN FROM NATIONAL INSTITUTE FOR HEALTH AND CARE (FORMERLY CLINICAL) EXCELLENCE REFERRAL GUIDELINES FOR SUSPECTED CANCER[23])

- Age .55 years with new onset dyspepsia
- Chronic gastrointestinal bleeding
- Dysphagia
- Progressive unintentional weight loss
- Persistent vomiting
- Iron deficiency anaemia
- Epigastric mass
- Suspicious barium meal result

How can the cause of dyspepsia be established?

Symptoms do not reliably distinguish between organic and functional disease,[21] and even alarm features (box), such as weight loss, are not particularly helpful.[22] Despite this, in the UK the presence of any of these alarm features is an indication for urgent specialist referral for endoscopy, to exclude upper gastrointestinal cancer.[23] Otherwise, endoscopy is not mandated in the management of dyspepsia, although it is the only way to accurately establish the underlying cause, including functional dyspepsia, which is a diagnosis of exclusion made in the absence of organic findings. However, no country can afford to perform endoscopy in all patients, and most guidelines recommend managing people under the age of 55 years with dyspepsia but no alarm features by testing for H pylori non-invasively with the urea breath test or stool antigen. Patients with positive results should be treated with eradication therapy and those with negative results given acid suppression therapy.[24] Gastric scintigraphy may help confirm delayed gastric emptying, particularly in patients with postprandial distress-type symptoms, to direct treatment, although the correlation between gastric emptying rates and symptoms is poor.[25]

What are the treatment options?

Uninvestigated dyspepsia in primary care or the community
An individual patient data meta-analysis of randomised controlled trials found that—although prompt endoscopy was superior to testing patients with uninvestigated dyspepsia for H pylori, and treating with eradication therapy if positive, in terms of symptom control at 12 months—it was not cost effective.[26] However, it is unclear whether a test and treat approach is preferable to empirical acid suppression first line, because a second individual patient data meta-analysis found no significant difference in symptoms or costs between the two.[27] Current guidelines state that either option can be used.[28] If the prevalence of H pylori in the population is known, it makes sense to use an acid suppression strategy first if prevalence is low (<10%) and an H pylori test and treat strategy if the prevalence is higher.[24] If these strategies are unsuccessful, other options (discussed below) can be considered, or the patient can be referred to secondary care for advice and further investigation if appropriate.

A six month primary care based Dutch trial compared two management strategies for uninvestigated dyspepsia based around empirical acid suppression.[29] One strategy used a step-up approach, starting with antacids, with treatment escalated to H2 antihistamines and then proton pump inhibitors (PPIs) if symptoms remained uncontrolled. The second used a step-down approach, with the drugs given in the reverse order and de-escalated if symptoms improved.

Treatment success (adequate relief of symptoms) was similar at six months (72% with step-up v 70% with step-down), but costs were significantly lower with the step-up approach. This, together with the small treatment effect in favour of step-up, meant that it came out top in a cost effectiveness analysis.

Another group of primary care patients who may benefit from H pylori test and treat are those who do not consult with dyspepsia very often but who require PPIs long term. A trial screened long term PPI users for H pylori and randomised those who were positive to eradication therapy or placebo.[30] Eradication therapy significantly reduced symptom scores, PPI prescriptions, consultations for dyspepsia, and dyspepsia related costs. The costs of detection and treatment were less than the money saved after two years of follow-up. Sensitivity analysis showed that the prevalence of H pylori would need to be less than 12% before this was no longer cost saving.

It has been estimated that 5% of dyspepsia in the community is attributable to H pylori,[7] so population screening and treatment for this organism could theoretically reduce dyspepsia related costs. Results from follow-up studies of people recruited to two large randomised controlled trials of population based screening (and eradication therapy or placebo if H pylori positive) in the UK suggest this might be the case, with significantly lower costs and fewer consultations after seven to 10 years.[31 32] However, these studies did not follow up all recruited people successfully, so currently there is insufficient evidence to institute population screening and treatment in the UK.

Peptic ulcer disease

The causal role of H pylori in peptic ulcer disease is well established, and patients with H pylori positive disease should receive eradication therapy. A Cochrane review found that the number needed to treat (NNT) with eradication therapy to prevent one duodenal ulcer relapse (26 placebo controlled trials) was 2 and for gastric ulcer (nine trials) the number was 3.[33] Although there was significant heterogeneity between studies in both analyses, all but one trial showed a significant benefit with eradication therapy. PPI triple therapy (a PPI plus two antibiotics (clarithromycin with amoxicillin or metronidazole)) should be used in areas like the UK where clarithromycin resistance is less than 10%, with bismuth quadruple therapy (bismuth plus a PPI and two antibiotics) being given where resistance is higher.[34] Most cases of H pylori negative peptic ulcer disease are caused by NSAIDs, and trials show that PPIs are superior to H2 antihistamines for ulcer healing in this situation.[35 36] H pylori negative, NSAID negative peptic ulcer disease is rare and probably requires long term PPI treatment.

Functional dyspepsia

Diet and lifestyle

Food diaries from a small study of 29 patients suggest that people with functional dyspepsia eat fewer meals and consume less energy and fat than healthy controls,[37] but whether this is a cause or a consequence of symptoms is unclear. Although the prevalence of undiagnosed coeliac disease is higher in people with symptoms of irritable bowel syndrome,[38] this is not the case in dyspepsia.[39] It is also unclear whether non-coeliac gluten sensitivity is involved in symptom generation in some patients with functional dyspepsia. Doctors often advise people with dyspepsia to lose weight, avoid fatty food and alcohol, or stop smoking, but there is little evidence that these measures improve symptoms.[40] As a result, drugs are the mainstay of treatment.

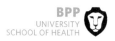

Acid suppression therapy

Antacids neutralise gastric acid, the production of which is controlled by gastrin, histamine, and acetylcholine receptors. Once stimulated, these receptors activate proton pumps in the parietal cell. H2 antihistamines and PPIs reduce acid production by blocking H2 receptors or the proton pump, respectively. Because PPIs act on the proton pump itself, these drugs lead to more profound acid suppression than H2 antihistamines or antacids.

A Cochrane review has studied the efficacy of acid suppressants in functional dyspepsia.[41] One placebo controlled trial of antacids showed no benefit. Twelve randomised controlled trials of H2 antihistamines versus placebo found that these drugs were effective for the treatment of functional dyspepsia (NNT=7). However, there was significant heterogeneity between studies, which was not explained by sensitivity analysis, and evidence of funnel plot asymmetry, suggesting publication bias or other small study effects. Their efficacy may therefore have been overestimated. Ten trials studied PPIs. Again, there was a significant benefit over placebo, although this was modest (NNT=10). There was significant heterogeneity between studies, with no obvious explanation, but no funnel plot asymmetry. A subgroup analysis conducted according to predominant symptom showed that PPIs were most beneficial in patients with reflux-type symptoms and more effective than placebo in patients with epigastric pain. However, they were no more effective than placebo in those with dysmotility-like functional dyspepsia.[42]

Most trials used PPIs for four to eight weeks. This seems a reasonable duration, especially as concerns have been raised recently about the safety of long term PPI use. Observational studies suggest that hip fracture, community acquired pneumonia, and *Clostridium difficile* infection are more common in PPI users,[43] [44] although all these associations were extremely modest, and direct causation cannot be assumed from studies such as these.

H pylori eradication therapy

The benefit of eradication therapy is less pronounced in functional dyspepsia than in peptic ulcer disease, but treatment is still more effective than placebo. In a Cochrane review of 21 placebo controlled trials the NNT for improvement in symptoms after eradicating *H pylori* was 14, with no heterogeneity between studies and no evidence of funnel plot asymmetry.[45]

Prokinetic drugs

Prokinetics enhance gastrointestinal motility. Examples include 5-hydroxytryptamine-4 (5-HT4) receptor agonists, such as cispride and mosapride, and the dopamine antagonists metoclopramide and domperidone. A Cochrane review identified 24 placebo controlled trials of prokinetics in functional dyspepsia.[41] Most used cisapride, which has been withdrawn owing to concerns over cardiac safety, with only one trial studying mosapride or domperidone, and no randomised controlled trials of metoclopramide. Overall, these drugs seemed to be highly effective (NNT=6). However, there was significant heterogeneity between studies, which was not explained by sensitivity analysis, and funnel plot asymmetry, which suggests that their apparent efficacy may be due to publication bias. In addition, when only high quality trials were included in the analysis the benefit was no longer apparent.[46]

Antidepressants and psychological therapies

Patients with functional dyspepsia, as with most other functional gastrointestinal disorders, have higher rates of anxiety, depression, and other psychological conditions than healthy people.[47] Antidepressants seem to be of benefit in irritable bowel syndrome,[48] and three trials have recently been conducted in functional dyspepsia. In a Chinese study, a low dose of the tricyclic antidepressant imipramine was significantly more effective than placebo (response rate 64% v 44%).[49] In another Chinese trial the selective serotonin reuptake inhibitor sertraline was not superior to placebo (28% experienced complete symptom resolution in both treatment arms).[50] Finally, in a placebo controlled trial of the tricyclic antidepressant amitriptyline or the selective serotonin reuptake inhibitor escitalopram, only amitriptyline showed a significant benefit over placebo.[51] Withdrawal owing to adverse events was more common with antidepressants in all three trials. These findings suggest that, if an antidepressant is used, a tricyclic is preferable.

A Cochrane review of the efficacy of psychological interventions in functional dyspepsia identified four trials.[52] Formal meta-analysis was not possible because of incomplete data reporting. The authors concluded that insufficient evidence existed for any benefit. Little has been published since this systematic review. A small randomised controlled trial of patients in whom conventional treatments had failed compared cognitive behavioural therapy (CBT) as an adjunct to intensive medical treatment (including testing for and targeting motor and sensory abnormalities) with intensive medical treatment alone or standard medical treatment.[53] A response was significantly more likely with intensive medical therapy combined with CBT compared with standard treatment (54% v 17%), but response rates were similar with intensive medical treatment alone (46%), suggesting that CBT may have no additive benefit. Despite the lack of evidence for any benefit, it seems reasonable to consider psychological treatments in patients with troublesome symptoms who have coexistent anxiety or depression.

Alternative therapies

In a randomised controlled trial that compared acupuncture with a sham procedure in functional dyspepsia, response rates were significantly higher with true acupuncture (71% v 35%).[54] A smaller sham controlled trial,[55] which included neurological imaging studies, found that acupuncture led to deactivation of the anterior cingulate cortex, insula, thalamus, and hypothalamus, which are all involved in processing painful visceral stimuli, perhaps explaining its therapeutic mechanism.

The herbal preparation iberogast, also known as STW5, which is a combination of plant extracts, has been tested in several trials of functional dyspepsia. Iberogast significantly improved symptom scores compared with placebo in one trial,[56] and in another 43% of patients randomised to iberogast reported resolution of symptoms at eight weeks compared with only 3% with placebo.[57] A single placebo controlled trial also found that peppermint oil, combined with caraway oil, was beneficial in functional dyspepsia.[58] At the time of writing, no randomised controlled trials have investigated probiotics in dyspepsia.

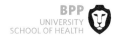

TIPS FOR NON-SPECIALISTS

- Treat peptic ulcer disease with eradication therapy if *Helicobacter pylori* is present or proton pump inhibitors if non-steroidal anti-inflammatory drugs are implicated
- Eradication therapy may be beneficial in *H pylori* positive functional dyspepsia, although the effect is modest
- Proton pump inhibitors, H2 antihistamines, and prokinetics may be beneficial in *H pylori* negative functional dyspepsia or in patients who do not benefit from eradication therapy
- Proton pump inhibitors are beneficial in patients with functional dyspepsia who mainly have reflux symptoms or epigastric pain, but not in those with dysmotility-like symptoms
- Increasing evidence suggests that tricyclic antidepressants, but not selective serotonin reuptake inhibitors, are beneficial in functional dyspepsia
- There is no evidence that psychological treatments are of benefit in functional dyspepsia
- Alternative therapies should be reserved for patients with functional dyspepsia whose symptoms are not relieved by conventional treatments

ADDITIONAL EDUCATIONAL RESOURCES BOX

Resources for healthcare professionals

- Leontiadis GI, Moayyedi P, Ford AC. Helicobacter pylori infection. *Clin Evid (Online)* 2009;pii:0406. An up-to-date summary of the evidence for the eradication of *Helicobacter pylori* in various situations
- National Institute for Clinical Excellence. Dyspepsia. Managing dyspepsia in adults in primary care. www.nice.org.uk/nicemedia/live/10950/29460/29460.pdf . NICE clinical guideline

Resources for patients

- Patient.co.uk (www.patient.co.uk/health/dyspepsia-indigestion)—Patient information on dyspepsia (indigestion)
- NHS Choices (www.nhs.uk/Conditions/Indigestion/Pages/Introduction.aspx)—Information from the NHS on indigestion

QUESTIONS FOR FUTURE RESEARCH

- Are psychological treatments of benefit in functional dyspepsia?
- Does dietary manipulation have a role to play in the management of functional dyspepsia?
- Is non-coeliac gluten sensitivity implicated in symptom generation in a proportion of patients with presumed functional dyspepsia?

Contributors: Both authors conceived and designed the article, drafted the manuscript, and approved the final version. ACF is guarantor.

Competing interests: We have read and understood the BMJ Group policy on declaration of interests and declare the following interests: ACF has received speaker's fees from Shire Pharmaceuticals; PM has received speakers fees from Shire Pharmaceuticals, Forest Canada, and AstraZeneca; his chair is funded in part by an unrestricted donation from AstraZeneca to McMaster University.

Provenance and peer review: Commissioned; externally peer reviewed.

1 Ford AC, Forman D, Bailey AG, Axon ATR, Moayyedi P. Effect of dyspepsia on survival: a longitudinal 10-year follow-up study. *Am J Gastroenterol* 2012;107:912-21.
2 Ford AC, Forman D, Bailey AG, Axon ATR, Moayyedi P. Initial poor quality of life and new onset of dyspepsia: Results from a longitudinal 10-year follow-up study. *Gut* 2007;56:321-7.
3 Mahadeva S, Yadav H, Rampal S, Everett SM, Goh K-L. Ethnic variation, epidemiological factors and quality of life impairment associated with dyspepsia in urban Malaysia. *Aliment Pharmacol Ther* 2010;31:1141-51.
4 Brook RA, Kleinman NL, Choung RS, Melkonian AK, Smeeding JE, Talley NJ. Functional dyspepsia impacts absenteeism and direct and indirect costs. *Clin Gastroenterol Hepatol* 2010;8:498-503.
5 Moayyedi P, Mason J. Clinical and economic consequences of dyspepsia in the community. *Gut* 2002;50(suppl 4):10-2.
6 Marwaha A, Ford AC, Lim A, Moayyedi P. Worldwide prevalence of dyspepsia: Systematic review and meta-analysis. *Gastroenterology* 2009;136(suppl 1):A182.
7 Moayyedi P, Forman D, Braunholtz D, Feltbower R, Crocombe W, Liptrott M, et al. The proportion of upper gastrointestinal symptoms in the community associated with Helicobacter pylori, lifestyle factors, and nonsteroidal anti-inflammatory drugs. *Am J Gastroenterol* 2000;95:1448-55.
8 Aro P, Talley NJ, Ronkainen J, Storskrubb T, Vieth M, Johansson SE, et al. Anxiety is associated with uninvestigated and functional dyspepsia (Rome III criteria) in a Swedish population-based study. *Gastroenterology* 2009;137:94-100.
9 Mujakovic S, ter Linde JJ, de Wit NJ, van Marrewijk CJ, Fransen GA, Onland-Moret NC, et al. Serotonin receptor 3A polymorphism c.-42C › T is associated with severe dyspepsia. *BMC Med Genet* 2011;12:140.
10 Ford AC, Marwaha A, Lim A, Moayyedi P. Systematic review and meta-analysis of the prevalence of irritable bowel syndrome in individuals with dyspepsia. *Clin Gastroenterol Hepatol* 2010;8:401-9.
11 Choung RS, Locke III GR, Schleck CD, Zinsmeister AR, Talley NJ. Overlap of dyspepsia and gastroesophageal reflux in the general population: one disease or distinct entities? *Neurogastroenterol Motil* 2012;24:229-34.
12 Ford AC, Marwaha A, Lim A, Moayyedi P. What is the prevalence of clinically significant endoscopic findings in subjects with dyspepsia? Systematic review and meta-analysis. *Clin Gastroenterol Hepatol* 2010;8:830-7.
13 Tack J, Talley NJ, Camilleri M, Holtmann G, Hu P, Malagelada JR, et al. Functional gastroduodenal disorders. *Gastroenterology* 2006;130:1466-79.
14 Moayyedi P, Talley NJ. Gastro-oesophageal reflux disease. *Lancet* 2006;367:2086-100.
15 Moayyedi P. Dyspepsia. *Curr Opin Gastroenterol* 2012;28:602-7.
16 Zhou G, Qin W, Zeng F, Liu P, Yang X, von Deneem KM, et al. White-matter microstructural changes in functional dyspepsia: a diffusion tensor imaging study. *Am J Gastroenterol* 2013;108:260-9.
17 Zeng F, Qin W, Liang F, Liu J, Tang Y, Liu X, et al. Abnormal resting brain activity in patients with functional dyspepsia is related to symptom severity. *Gastroenterology* 2011;141:499-506.
18 Liebregts T, Adam B, Bredack C, Gururatsakul M, Pilkington KR, Brierley SM, et al. Small bowel homing T cells are associated with symptoms and delayed gastric emptying in functional dyspepsia. *Am J Gastroenterol* 2011;106:1089-98.
19 Talley NJ, Walker MM, Aro P, Ronkainen J, Storskrubb T, Hindley LA, et al. Non-ulcer dyspepsia and duodenal eosinophilia: an adult endoscopic population-based case-control study. *Clin Gastroenterol Hepatol* 2007;5:1175-83.
20 Ford AC, Thabane M, Collins SM, Moayyedi P, Garg AX, Clark WF, et al. Prevalence of uninvestigated dyspepsia 8 years after a large waterborne outbreak of bacterial dysentery: a cohort study. *Gastroenterology* 2010;138:1727-36.
21 Moayyedi P, Talley NJ, Fennerty MB, Vakil N. Can the clinical history distinguish between organic and functional dyspepsia? *JAMA* 2006;295:1566-76.
22 Vakil N, Moayyedi P, Fennerty MB, Talley NJ. Limited value of alarm features in the diagnosis of upper gastrointestinal malignancy: systematic review and meta-analysis. *Gastroenterology* 2006;131:390-401.
23 National Institute for Health and Clinical Excellence. Referral guidelines for suspected cancer. 2005. www.nice.org.uk/nicemedia/live/10968/29814/29814.pdf.
24 American Gastroenterological Association. American Gastroenterological Association technical review on the evaluation of dyspepsia. *Gastroenterology* 2005;129:1756-80.
25 Talley NJ, Locke GR III, Lahr BD, Zinsmeister AR, Tougas G, Ligozio G,, et al. Functional dyspepsia, delayed gastric emptying, and impaired quality of life. *Gut* 2006;55:933-9.
26 Ford AC, Qume M, Moayyedi P, Arents NLA, Lassen AT, Logan RFA, et al. Helicobacter pylori "test and treat" or endoscopy for managing dyspepsia? An individual patient data meta-analysis. *Gastroenterology* 2005;128:1838-44.
27 Ford AC, Moayyedi P, Jarbol DE, Logan RFA, Delaney BC. Meta-analysis: Helicobacter pylori "test and treat" compared with empirical acid suppression for managing dyspepsia. *Aliment Pharmacol Ther* 2008;28:534-44.
28 National Institute for Clinical Excellence. Dyspepsia. Managing dyspepsia in adults in primary care. 2004. www.nice.org.uk/nicemedia/pdf/CG017fullguideline.pdf.
29 Van Marrewijk CJ, Mujakovic S, Fransen GAJ, Numans ME, de Wit NJ, Muris JWM, et al. Effect and cost-effectiveness of step-up versus step-down treatment with antacids, H2-receptor antagonists, and proton pump inhibitors in patients with new onset dyspepsia (DIAMOND study): a primary-care-based randomised controlled trial. *Lancet* 2009;373:215-25.
30 Raghunath AS, Hungin AP, Mason J, Jackson W. Helicobacter pylori eradication in long-term proton pump inhibitor users in primary care: A randomized controlled trial. *Aliment Pharmacol Ther* 2007;25:585-92.
31 Ford AC, Forman D, Bailey AG, Axon ATR, Moayyedi P. A community screening program for Helicobacter pylori saves money: ten-year follow-up of a randomised controlled trial. *Gastroenterology* 2005;129:1910-7.
32 Harvey RF, Lane JA, Nair P, Egger M, Harvey I, Donovan J, et al. Clinical trial: prolonged beneficial effect of Helicobacter pylori eradication on dyspepsia consultations—the Bristol helicobacter project. *Aliment Pharmacol Ther* 2010;32:394-400.
33 Ford AC, Delaney BC, Forman D, Moayyedi P. Eradication therapy in Helicobacter pylori positive peptic ulcer disease: systematic review and economic analysis. *Am J Gastroenterol* 2004;99:1833-55.
34 Malfertheiner P, Megraud F, O'Morain CA, Atherton J, Axon AT, Bazzoli F, et al; European Helicobacter Study Group. Management of Helicobacter pylori infection: the Maastricht IV Florence consensus report. *Gut* 2012;61:646-64.

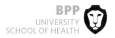

35 Yeomans ND, Tulassay Z, Juhasz L, Racz I, van Rensburg CJ, Swannell AJ, et al. A comparison of omeprazole with ranitidine for ulcers associated with nonsteroidal antiinflammatory drugs. Acid Suppression Trial: Ranitidine versus Omeprazole for NSAID-associated Ulcer Treatment (ASTRONAUT) study group. *N Engl J Med* 1998;338:719-26.

36 Agrawal NM, Campbell DR, Safdi MA, Lukasik NL, Huang B, Haber MM. Superiority of lansoprazole vs ranitidine in healing nonsteroidal anti-inflammatory drug-associated gastric ulcers: results of a double-blind, randomized, multicenter study. NSAID-Associated Gastric Ulcer Study Group. *Ann Intern Med* 2000;160:1455-61.

37 Pilichiewicz AN, Horowitz M, Holtmann G, Talley NJ, Feinle-Bisset C. Relationship between symptoms and dietary patterns in patients with functional dyspepsia. *Clin Gastroenterol Hepatol* 2009;7:317-22.

38 Ford AC, Chey WD, Talley NJ, Malhotra A, Spiegel BMR, Moayyedi P. Yield of diagnostic tests for celiac disease in subjects with symptoms suggestive of irritable bowel syndrome: Systematic review and meta-analysis. *Arch Intern Med* 2009;169:651-8.

39 Ford AC, Ching E, Moayyedi P. Meta-analysis: yield of diagnostic tests for coeliac disease in dyspepsia. *Aliment Pharmacol Ther* 2009;30:28-36.

40 Feinle-Bisset C, Azpiroz F. Dietary and lifestyle factors in functional dyspepsia. *Nat Rev Gastroenterol Hepatol* 2013;10:150-7.

41 Moayyedi P, Soo S, Deeks J, Delaney B, Innes M, Forman D. Pharmacological interventions for non-ulcer dyspepsia. *Cochrane Database Syst Rev* 2006;4:CD001960.

42 Moayyedi P, Delaney BC, Vakil N, Forman D, Talley NJ. The efficacy of proton pump inhibitors in non-ulcer dyspepsia: a systematic review and economic analysis. *Gastroenterology* 2004;127:1329-37.

43 Moayyedi P, Leontiadis GI. The risks of PPI therapy. *Nat Rev Gastroenterol Hepatol* 2012;9:132-9.

44 Ngamruengphong S, Leontiadis GI, Radhi S, Dentino A, Nugent K. Proton pump inhibitors and risk of fracture: a systematic review and meta-analysis of observational studies. *Am J Gastroenterol* 2011;106:1209-18.

45 Moayyedi P, Soo S, Deeks J, Delaney B, Harris A, Innes M, et al. Eradication of Helicobacter pylori for non-ulcer dyspepsia. *Cochrane Database Syst Rev* 2006;2:CD002096.

46 Abraham NS, Moayyedi P, Daniels B, Veldhuyzen Van Zanten SJO. The methodological quality of trials affects estimates of treatment efficacy in functional (non-ulcer) dyspepsia. *Aliment Pharmacol Ther* 2004;19:631-41.

47 Koloski NA, Jones M, Kalantar J, Weltman M, Zaguirre J, Talley NJ. The brain-gut pathway in functional gastrointestinal disorders is bidirectional: a 12-year prospective population-based study. *Gut* 2012;61:1284-90.

48 Ford AC, Talley NJ, Schoenfeld PS, Quigley EMM, Moayyedi P. Efficacy of antidepressants and psychological therapies in irritable bowel syndrome: systematic review and meta-analysis. *Gut* 2009;58:367-378.

49 Wu JC, Cheong PK, Chan Y, Lai LH, Ching J, Chan A, et al. A randomized, double-blind, placebo-controlled trial of low dose imipramine for treatment of refractory functional dyspepsia. *Gastroenterology* 2011;140(suppl 1):S50.

50 Tan VP, Cheung TK, Wong WM, Pang R, Wong BC. Treatment of functional dyspepsia with sertraline: a double-blind randomized placebo-controlled pilot study. *World J Gastroenterol* 2012;18:6127-33.

51 Locke GR, Bouras EP, Howden CW, Brenner DM, Lacy BE, Dibaise JK, et al. The functional dyspepsia treatment trial (FDTT) key results. *Gastroenterology* 2013;144(suppl 1):S140.

52 Soo S, Moayyedi P, Deeks JJ, Delaney B, Lewis M, Forman D. Psychological interventions for non-ulcer dyspepsia. *Cochrane Database Syst Rev* 2005;2:CD002301.

53 Haag S, Senf W, Tagay S, Langkafel M, Braun-Lang U, Pietsch A, et al. Is there a benefit from intensified medical and psychological interventions in patients with functional dyspepsia not responding to conventional therapy? *Aliment Pharmacol Ther* 2007;25:973-86.

54 Ma TT, Yu SY, Li Y, Liang FR, Tian XP, Zheng H, et al. Randomised clinical trial: an assessment of acupuncture on specific meridian or specific acupoint vs sham acupuncture for treating functional dyspepsia. *Aliment Pharmacol Ther* 2012;35:552-61.

55 Zeng F, Qin W, Ma T, Sun J, Tang Y, Yuan K, et al. Influence of acupuncture treatment on cerebral activity in functional dyspepsia patients and its relationship with efficacy. *Am J Gastroenterol* 2012;107:1236-47.

56 Von Arnim U, Peitz U, Vinson B, Gundermann KJ, Malfertheiner P. STW 5, a phytopharmacon for patients with functional dyspepsia: results of a multicenter, placebo-controlled double-blind study. *Am J Gastroenterol* 2007;102:1268-75.

57 Madisch A, Holtmann G, Mayr G, Vinson B, Hotz J. Treatment of functional dyspepsia with a herbal preparation. A double-blind, randomized, placebo-controlled, multicenter trial. *Digestion* 2004;69:45-52.

58 May B, Kohler S, Schneider B. Efficacy and tolerability of a fixed combination of peppermint oil and caraway oil in patients suffering from functional dyspepsia. *Aliment Pharmacol Ther* 2000;14:1671-7.

Related links

bmj.com
- Get CME credits with this article

bmj.com/archive
Previous articles in this series
- Tourette's syndrome (2013;347:f4964)
- Developing role of HPV in cervical cancer prevention (2013;347:f4781)
- Frontotemporal dementia (2013;347:f4827)
- Strongyloides stercoralis infection (2013;347:f4610)
- An introduction to patient decision aids (2013;347:f4147)

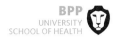

Irritable bowel syndrome

Alexander C Ford, senior lecturer and honorary consultant gastroenterologist[12],
Nicholas J Talley, professor of medicine[3]

[1]Leeds Gastroenterology Institute, St James's University Hospital, Leeds, UK

[2]Leeds Institute of Molecular Medicine, Leeds University, Leeds, UK

[3]Faculty of Health, University of Newcastle, New South Wales, Australia

Correspondence to: A Ford, Leeds Gastroenterology Institute, St James's University Hospital, Leeds LS9 7TF, UK alexf12399@yahoo.com

Cite this as: BMJ 2012;345:e5836

DOI: 10.1136/bmj.e5836

http://www.bmj.com/content/345/bmj.e5836

Irritable bowel syndrome (IBS) is one of the commonest gastrointestinal conditions encountered in primary or secondary care. The disorder is more common in younger people, and women. The diagnosis should be reached using symptom based clinical criteria, rather than excluding underlying organic disease by exhaustive investigation. There is no single known unifying cause, but biological markers have been identified. Treatment should be directed towards relief of the predominant symptom (or symptoms) reported, although these may change over time. Since there is no medical therapy established to alter the natural history of IBS in the longer term, the disorder represents a considerable financial burden to the health service, owing to medical consultations and the consumption of other valuable resources. Since the publication of management guidelines from the National Institute for Health and Clinical Excellence in 2008,[w1] there have been some significant developments in terms of synthesis of existing evidence, as well as emerging therapies. We therefore summarise recent systematic reviews, meta-analyses, and randomised controlled trials in order to provide a general update as to how to effectively identify and manage this disorder.

What is IBS and who gets it?

IBS is a chronic functional disorder of the lower gastrointestinal tract. Characteristic symptoms are abdominal pain or discomfort in association with the onset of either an alteration in stool form or frequency. Other symptoms such as the relief of pain or discomfort by defecation, or abdominal bloating are considered supportive of the diagnosis. The current classification system for the functional gastrointestinal disorders, the Rome criteria,[w2] further subdivides patients with IBS according to the predominant stool type produced. Thus, patients are classed as diarrhoea predominant (IBS-D), constipation predominant (IBS-C), or mixed (IBS-M), where stool type fluctuates between diarrhoea and constipation. Some patients cannot be classified, and the predominant stool type often changes with time.[w3]

Population based studies have shown that the prevalence of symptoms compatible with IBS in the community varies from around 5% to more than 20%. A recent systematic review of 80 cross sectional surveys in the community confirmed that prevalence varied considerably with geography, with a pooled prevalence of 7% in South East Asia, 12% in northern Europe and North America, and 21% in South America.[1] According to predominant stool form, IBS-D was the commonest subtype, with a pooled prevalence of 40%, and IBS-M the least common, with a pooled prevalence of 23%. The odds of IBS were significantly lower in people aged 50 years or more than in those under 50 years. Few studies provided data concerning the effect of socioeconomic status on prevalence of IBS. There was a female preponderance, with a pooled odds ratio of 1.67 for IBS in women versus men.[2] Women with IBS were more likely to show IBS-C (odds ratio 2.38) and less likely to meet criteria for IBS-D (0.45) than men with IBS. Longitudinal follow-up studies suggest that IBS does not adversely affect survival in the community.[w4 w5]

What is the underlying pathophysiology of IBS?

There is no single unifying cause to explain the symptoms that sufferers report. However, numerous mechanisms have been proposed (fig). Presence of IBS is associated with increased levels of psychiatric distress, and maladaptive coping strategies.[w6] The condition aggregates in families,[w7] probably due to a combination of genetics and shared upbringing. Patients with IBS show abnormal small bowel and colonic transit compared with healthy controls, suggesting that changes in stool form or frequency could relate to disturbed gastrointestinal motility.[w8] The abdominal pain or discomfort could be due to a combination of an abnormal stimulus (for example, excessive gas production), visceral hypersensitivity, and abnormal central pain processing. Balloon distension of the gastrointestinal tract in patients leads to pain at lower thresholds than in those who do not have the disorder,[w9] as well as stimulating higher levels of brain activity in the regions associated with pain modulation and emotional arousal.[w10] Some investigators have reported perturbations of the gastrointestinal flora in patients.[w11] Chronic, low grade inflammation of the gastrointestinal mucosa, perhaps driven by inappropriate mast cell activation, has also been implicated as a potential aetiological factor.[w12] Biomarkers have been identified in the serum of some patients,[w13 w14] but are of uncertain significance.

How is IBS diagnosed?

In a patient without lower gastrointestinal alarm symptoms (box) who has longstanding typical symptoms of IBS (intermittent abdominal pain or discomfort associated with an erratic bowel habit, and often bloating), the diagnosis

---

SOURCES AND SELECTION CRITERIA

We searched Medline, Embase, the Cochrane Database of Systematic Reviews, and Clinical Evidence online using the search term "irritable bowel syndrome," as well as recent conference proceedings. We limited studies to those conducted in adults, and focused on systematic reviews, meta-analyses, and high quality randomised controlled trials published within the past five years, wherever possible.

SUMMARY POINTS

- Irritable bowel syndrome (IBS) affects up to one in five people at some point in their lives
- The condition is commoner in younger people and women, and is not associated with increased mortality
- A positive diagnosis of IBS should be reached using symptom based clinical criteria, not after excluding organic disease by exhaustive investigation
- Exclusion diets (for example, low levels of fermentable oligosaccharides, disaccharides, monosaccharides, and polyols) and exercise may be of benefit
- Soluble fibre, antispasmodics (including peppermint oil), antidepressants, agents acting on the 5-HT receptor, rifaximin, and probiotics are all more effective than placebo for treating IBS
- Psychological therapies should be reserved for patients failing these treatments

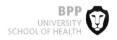

BMX BPP UNIVERSITY SCHOOL OF HEALTH

BOX: LOWER GASTROINTESTINAL ALARM SYMPTOMS

- ≥50 years with no previous colon cancer screening
- Family history of colon cancer
- Weight loss
- Rectal bleeding
- Recent change in bowel habit
- Abdominal mass
- Iron deficiency anaemia
- Haem positive stool

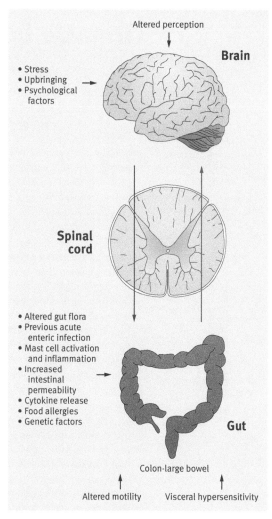

Proposed aetiological mechanisms in IBS

should be made on clinical grounds, without the need for recourse to invasive investigations. Symptom based diagnostic criteria facilitate this approach, which include the Manning criteria and the Rome criteria (table).[w2 w15] There have been three iterations of the Rome criteria to date, and the Rome III criteria are the current accepted diagnostic standard used among gastroenterologists for diagnosing IBS in clinical practice, as well as for recruiting patients into treatment trials for the disorder.

However, a recent systematic review and meta-analysis of observational studies, all of which were conducted in secondary care, showed that these criteria have not been validated extensively, and do not predict IBS with any great accuracy.[3] The Manning criteria, which had been validated in four studies, yielded pooled positive and negative likelihood ratios of 2.9 and 0.29, respectively. The first iteration of the Rome criteria had been validated in only one study (positive likelihood ratio 4.8, negative 0.34), and the Rome III criteria had not been validated at all. These differences may be of little relevance in primary care, where few physicians are familiar with these criteria or use them to make a diagnosis of IBS, yet can still diagnose the condition accurately using a symptom based approach.[w16] Longitudinal follow-up in patients with a positive diagnosis of IBS suggests that the development of subsequent organic disease is rare.[w17] Therefore, diagnostic testing is generally reserved for those with alarm features. No evidence supports undertaking a routine panel of blood tests,[w18] although clinicians often order tests such as a full blood count and C reactive protein. However, serological testing to exclude coeliac disease is probably worthwhile,[4] and is cost effective if the prevalence of coeliac disease among patients with suspected IBS is around 5%.[w19] An effective and empathetic doctor-patient relationship is essential once the diagnosis is reached, and is associated with increased patient satisfaction and reduced consultations.[w17]

What are the treatment options?

Diet and lifestyle

Theoretically, fibre should increase transit time in patients with IBS, but its role as a therapy remains controversial. A Cochrane review, updated recently, identified 12 randomised controlled trials of fibre, all conducted in secondary or tertiary care.[5] This review suggested no benefit for either soluble or insoluble fibre. However, another meta-analysis of the same trials showed that soluble fibre, used in six trials in the form of ispaghula, significantly improved symptoms compared with placebo, with a number needed to treat to prevent one patient with IBS remaining symptomatic of six.[6] This disparity in findings between meta-analyses probably results from the use of different endpoints to pool data when judging treatment success.[w20] The Cochrane review pooled data from eligible trials according to the effect of fibre on abdominal pain or global IBS symptoms separately,

whereas the second meta-analysis pooled data for both endpoints together. Adverse events were rare. A recent high quality trial conducted entirely in primary care also showed a significant benefit of ispaghula over placebo.[7]

Patients with IBS may report certain foodstuffs that trigger symptoms. In a randomised controlled trial conducted in tertiary care that performed IgG testing for foods, and which allocated patients to an elimination diet based on the results or a sham diet, symptom scores were significantly lower among patients receiving the elimination diet.[8] More recently, interest in the potential role of fermentable oligosaccharides, disaccharides, monosaccharides, and polyols (FODMAPs) in generating symptoms in IBS, via their fermentation and osmotic effects, has led to proposals of low FODMAP diets as a treatment. Foods with high levels of FODMAPs include some fruits (apples, cherries, peaches, and nectarines) artificial sweeteners, most lactose-containing foods, legumes, and many green vegetables (broccoli, Brussels sprouts, cabbage, and peas). In a crossover trial that switched 15 patients with IBS recruited in secondary care from diets that were either low or high in FODMAPs, symptoms such as abdominal pain or discomfort, bloating, and flatus were all significantly worse during the high FODMAP diet.[9] Evidence from a double blind, placebo controlled trial also suggests that a gluten free diet may benefit people with IBS who test negative for coeliac disease, with poorer control of symptoms among those randomised to gluten.[10]

84

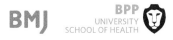

Exercise has been shown to improve symptoms in fibromyalgia and chronic fatigue syndrome, both of which may coexist with IBS. In a recent randomised controlled trial, 102 patients with IBS in secondary or tertiary care were instructed to increase their physical activity for 12 weeks, or to maintain current activity.[11] Patients allocated to increased physical exercise showed significant improvements in scores of IBS symptom severity compared with scores at baseline, while those who maintained current levels of activity were more likely to have worsening of their symptoms compared with the physical activity group.

Patient education also seems to provide some benefit. In one tertiary care study that administered a group education programme to a series of patients with IBS, resolution of symptoms was significantly commoner among attendees of the class, compared with non-attendees.[12] Advocating sleep hygiene helps patients with fibromyalgia, but whether this approach is also useful in IBS is unclear. However, evidence from a small randomised controlled trial conducted in tertiary care suggests that melatonin leads to significantly higher symptom response rates in women with IBS than placebo.[13]

Placebo
The placebo response rate in IBS is high. A meta-analysis of 73 randomised placebo controlled trials in IBS showed a pooled placebo response rate of almost 40%.[14] A recent trial conducted in tertiary care recruited and randomised 80 patients to either open label placebo, which they were told had "beneficial effects through mind-body self-healing processes," or no treatment.[15] Almost 50% of patients assigned to placebo reported adequate relief of symptoms, which was significantly higher than with no treatment. The authors suggested that this novel strategy allows the ethical use of placebo as a treatment, without the need for deception of the patient, which would otherwise undermine the patient-doctor relationship.

Antispasmodic drugs
Most antispasmodic drugs compete with acetylcholine at postganglionic parasympathetic nerve endings, inhibiting smooth muscle contraction. Peppermint oil also has antispasmodic properties, bringing about smooth muscle relaxation via calcium channel blockade. These drugs could therefore have beneficial effects on abdominal pain or discomfort. The efficacy of antispasmodics has been confirmed in two recent meta-analyses,[5][6] but both had substantial heterogeneity between randomised controlled trials, and none of the trials identified was conducted entirely in primary care. In one meta-analysis of 22 randomised

controlled trials,[6] the number needed to treat was five, and when the efficacy of individual antispasmodics was studied, otilonium, cimetropium, hyoscine, pinaverium, and dicycloverine were all more effective than placebo. Adverse events were summarised in one meta-analysis,[6] and were significantly commoner with active therapy, with a number needed to harm of 17.5. Data from four placebo controlled trials of peppermint oil, all conducted in secondary care, were pooled in one of these meta-analyses.[6] The number needed to treat to prevent one patient with IBS remaining symptomatic was 2.5. Adverse events were rare.

Antidepressants
Patients with IBS show higher levels of anxiety and depression than controls without IBS. Antidepressants are an effective therapy in chronic pain conditions, and alter gastrointestinal transit time. Evidence from two meta-analyses suggests that antidepressants are of benefit in IBS.[5][16] Both tricyclic antidepressants and selective serotonin reuptake inhibitors were more effective than placebo for the treatment of IBS. Again, none of the trials identified was conducted in primary care. When data from nine randomised controlled trials of tricyclic antidepressants were pooled, the number needed to treat was four, with no heterogeneity detected between studies. Selective serotonin reuptake inhibitors also showed a benefit, in five randomised controlled trials, with a number needed to treat of 3.5, but with significant heterogeneity between studies. Adverse events were not significantly commoner with antidepressants in the pooled trials,[16] but there remains a risk of harm with this class of agents.

Agents acting on the 5-hydroxytryptamine (5-HT) receptor
This class of drugs has the potential to ameliorate the smooth muscle spasm, abdominal pain, and change in bowel habit of patients with IBS. Alosetron, a 5-HT3 receptor antagonist, is licensed in the United States only for female patients with severe IBS-D. A meta-analysis of eight placebo controlled trials conducted in secondary or tertiary care showed a number needed to treat of eight, albeit with significant heterogeneity between studies.[17] However, the drug was associated with several cases of ischaemic colitis and severe constipation, and its use is now restricted by a prescribing programme from the US Food and Drug Administration. Prucalopride is a highly selective 5-HT4 agonist, and is effective for the treatment of chronic idiopathic constipation, with a number needed to treat of six.[18] It has yet to be tested in IBS, but theoretically should be of benefit in IBS-C.

Antibiotics and probiotics
In view of the proposed abnormalities of gastrointestinal flora in patients with IBS, antibiotics have the potential to modulate the bacterial composition of the gastrointestinal tract and alter the natural history of IBS in the short term. The non-absorbable antibiotic rifaximin has recently been tested in two large placebo controlled trials conducted in secondary and tertiary care in North America.[19] More than 1200 patients with IBS were randomised to two weeks of therapy, with follow-up at 12 weeks. Overall, adequate relief of global IBS symptoms and bloating were significantly more likely with rifaximin at four week follow-up; this effect seemed durable, being maintained at 12 weeks. Adverse events were no commoner with rifaximin and, importantly, there were no cases of *Clostridium difficile*.

Diagnostic criteria for IBS		
Criteria (year described)	Symptom items included	Minimum symptom duration required
Manning (1978)[w15]	Any of*: abdominal pain relieved by defecation, more frequent stools with onset of pain, looser stools with onset of pain, passage of mucus per rectum, feeling of incomplete emptying, visible abdominal distension reported by patients	None
Rome III (2006)[w2]	Recurrent abdominal pain or discomfort .3 days per month in the past 3 months associated with two or more of: improvement with defecation, onset associated with a change in frequency of stool, onset associated with a change in form of stool	Symptom onset .6 months before diagnosis

*No minimum number of symptom items is needed to meet criteria for IBS but, conventionally, the reporting of at least three items by the patient is used to increase specificity.

Probiotics are live or attenuated bacteria, or bacterial products, which, when ingested, have beneficial effects. There is evidence to suggest that some probiotics have anti-inflammatory properties or ameliorate visceral hypersensitivity. These effects could theoretically lead to an improvement in symptoms of IBS. A recent meta-analysis identified 18 randomised controlled trials that compared various probiotics with placebo.[20] Five of these trials were conducted in primary care. When data were pooled from the 10 trials that reported dichotomous data, probiotics were superior to placebo, with a number needed to treat of four. However, there was considerable heterogeneity between studies, and different strains and species were used, making it difficult to ascertain which, if any, were of particular benefit; however, a trend was seen towards bifidobacteria improving symptoms. Fifteen trials provided

continuous data, with analyses showing that probiotics had a beneficial effect on abdominal pain, and a trend towards a benefit for bloating. Adverse events were rare with active therapy in these trials.

Psychological and behavioural therapies

The rates of psychological disorders, such as anxiety, depression, and bipolar affective disorder are twofold to threefold higher in patients with IBS than in controls without IBS.[w21] There have been numerous randomised controlled trials of psychological and behavioural therapies such as cognitive behavioural therapy, hypnotherapy, and dynamic psychotherapy. Two separate meta-analyses have summarised these therapies.[16 21] A Cochrane review, which pooled continuous data from 25 eligible studies, suggested that these therapies are only marginally superior to no treatment,[21] and the authors questioned the clinical significance of any benefit.

In the second meta-analysis,[16] in which the original trial authors were asked to provide dichotomous data, the number needed to treat when all 20 eligible studies using psychological and behavioural therapies were pooled was four, although there was significant heterogeneity between studies and evidence of publication bias. Only one trial was conducted in primary care. There were benefits for cognitive behavioural therapy, hypnotherapy, multicomponent psychological therapy, and dynamic psychotherapy, but no benefit from relaxation therapy or self administered cognitive behavioural therapy. However, most of the trials assigned patients in the control arm to no treatment, other than joining a waiting list for the active intervention to be administered at study completion. Therefore, there is the possibility of a placebo effect in the active intervention arms, and the efficacy of these therapies may have been overestimated.

Further trials have been published since these two meta-analyses. A recent trial of hypnotherapy conducted in both secondary and tertiary care also showed a significant benefit over supportive treatment (in the form of dietary advice, relaxation training, and information about the pathophysiology of the disorder). This trial included the largest number of patients with IBS to date, but also noted that the efficacy of hypnotherapy was lower in secondary care, suggesting that it may be less reproducible outside of specialist centres.[22] Mindfulness training, which involves focusing on present-moment experience and non-judgmental awareness of body sensations, has also been studied in female patients with IBS.[23] In this tertiary care trial, patients were allocated to mindfulness training or a support group, and followed up for three months. Patients assigned to the active intervention had a significant reduction in severity of IBS symptoms and abdominal pain. Overall, psychological and behavioural therapies are probably of benefit in IBS, but they are time consuming to administer, and are probably best reserved for patients who fail more conventional treatments.

Alternative therapies

In a meta-analysis of 17 secondary and tertiary care based studies, acupuncture seemed to be superior to pharmacological therapy in several randomised controlled trials conducted in China.[24] However, it was no more effective, in terms of symptom improvement, than a sham acupuncture control, suggesting that the improvements observed may be based on Chinese patients' preconceived

---

TIPS FOR NON-SPECIALISTS

- Encourage patients to take regular exercise, and consider exclusion diets, although these diets need good patient compliance and dietitian support
- Try to tailor treatment according to either predominant stool form or the most troublesome symptom reported
- Consider antispasmodics or peppermint oil in patients for pain and diarrhoea, with tricyclic antidepressants as second line therapy
- Consider a soluble fibre supplement (ispaghula) as first line therapy in patients with IBS-C, possibly adding an osmotic laxative, with a trial of selective serotonin reuptake inhibitors as second line therapy
- In patients with bloating or diarrhoea as the predominant symptom consider the use of a probiotic (such as bifidobacteria or rifaximin)
- Consider referral to a specialist if first line or second line therapies are ineffective, or if there is doubt about the diagnosis on the part of either the patient or the physician

---

ADDITIONAL EDUCATIONAL RESOURCES

Resources for healthcare professionals

- Ruepert L, Quartero AO, de Wit NJ, van der Heijden GJ, Rubin G, Muris JW. Bulking agents, antispasmodics and antidepressants for the treatment of irritable bowel syndrome. *Cochrane Database Syst Rev* 2011;10:CD003460
- Ford AC, Vandvik PO. Irritable bowel syndrome. *Clin Evid* 2012;01:410
- Clinical practice guideline. Irritable bowel syndrome in adults: diagnosis and management of irritable bowel syndrome in primary care. February 2008. http://guidance.nice.org.uk/CG61/Guidance/pdf/English

Resources for patients

- Irritable bowel syndrome: NHS choices (www.nhs.uk/Conditions/Irritable-bowel-syndrome/Pages/Introduction.aspx)—a website providing advice on what IBS is, how it is diagnosed, and the treatments commonly used for the disorder
- IBS Network (www.theibsnetwork.org)—a website providing support and advice for people who think they may have IBS, as well as those with an established diagnosis

---

QUESTIONS FOR FUTURE RESEARCH

- Do antispasmodics or antidepressants have a benefit in patients with IBS in primary care?
- Do patients with IBS derive lasting reassurance following investigation to exclude organic illness?
- How does placebo exert a beneficial effect on IBS symptoms?
- What is the optimal dietary therapy for IBS?

HOW TO DISCUSS IBS AND ITS TREATMENT WITH PATIENTS

- Explain that IBS is likely to be a lifelong disorder, but that the symptoms come and go
- Explain that the cause of IBS is not known
- Explain that increasing soluble fibre, or excluding foods containing high levels of FODMAPs, may improve symptoms without the need for medical treatment
- Mention that increasing exercise levels may also help symptoms
- Where these measures fail and medical treatment is needed, make sure that the patient is aware that most drugs used to treat IBS are safe and well tolerated

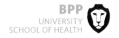

expectations of the relative efficacy of acupuncture compared to drugs. Herbal therapies such as iberogast (also known as STW 5), which is a combination of various plant extracts, and St John's wort, have also been the subject of placebo controlled trials in IBS,[25] [26] with STW 5 showing superiority over placebo, but St John's wort having no beneficial effect. Another trial of Chinese herbal therapy (a combination of 20 different herbs) suggested a benefit in IBS,[w22] but the formula's efficacy remains to be confirmed. In summary, any benefit of herbal therapies remains unclear.

Emerging therapies

Novel therapies for the treatment of IBS are emerging. Lubiprostone and linaclotide are drugs that act locally on chloride channels and guanylate cyclase receptors in the gastrointestinal tract, respectively. Both agents stimulate intestinal fluid secretion and accelerate transit, by increasing chloride concentration within the gastrointestinal lumen. These drugs are effective in the treatment of chronic idiopathic constipation,[18] and have also been tested in IBS-C. Results of two randomised trials conducted in secondary and tertiary care in the US showed significantly higher response rates with lubiprostone than placebo, although the overall effect was modest, with an absolute difference in treatment effect of only 8%.[27] The drug is now approved in the US for the treatment of IBS-C. More recently, the efficacy of linaclotide was studied in over 800 patients, again with response rates significantly greater than placebo.[28] Other emerging therapies include bile acid sequestrants (such as colesevelam), bile acid transporter inhibitors, and pancreatic enzyme supplements, all of which are under investigation,[29] [30] although convincing data from randomised controlled trials are currently lacking. These emerging therapies, which may act more selectively on the gastrointestinal tract, have the potential to improve symptoms, perhaps without causing the systemic side effects associated with more traditional pharmacological treatments.

Contributors: ACF and NJT conceived and designed the article, drafted the manuscript, approved the final version of the manuscript to be published. ACF is guarantor of the article.

Competing interests: All authors have completed the Unified Competing Interest form at www.icmje.org/coi_disclosure.pdf (available on request from the corresponding author) and declare: no support from any organisation for the submitted work; ACF has received speakers fees from Shire pharmaceuticals; NJT has consulted for ARYx, Astellenas Pharma, Boehringer Ingelheim, ConCERT Pharma, Forest, Ironwood Pharma, Janssen, Johnson & Johnson, Pfizer, Proctor and Gamble, Prometheus, Salix Pharma, Sanofi-Adventis, Theravance, Doyen, Care Capital, Edusa Pharma, Falk, Meritage Pharma, NicOx, Novaritis, Shire, Tranzyme, UptoDate, XenoPort, and Zeria; NJT has received speakers fees from Abbott, Focus Medical, Accreddit Ed, Astra Zeneca, Salix, and Ironwood; NJT has patents with Prometheus and separately for biomarkers, and has received research support from Falk, Forest, Janssen, and Takeda.

Provenance and peer review: Commissioned; peer reviewed.

1   Lovell RM, Ford AC. Global prevalence of, and risk factors for, irritable bowel syndrome: a meta-analysis. *Clin Gastroenterol Hepatol* 2012;10:712-21.

2   Lovell RM, Ford AC. Effect of gender on prevalence of irritable bowel syndrome in the community: systematic review and meta-analysis. *Am J Gastroenterol* 2012;107:991-1000.

3   Ford AC, Talley NJ, Veldhuyzen Van Zanten SJ, Vakil NB, Simel DL, Moayyedi P. Will the history and physical examination help establish that irritable bowel syndrome is causing this patient's lower gastrointestinal tract symptoms? *JAMA* 2008;300:1793-1805.

4   Ford AC, Chey WD, Talley NJ, Malhotra A, Spiegel BMR, Moayyedi P. Yield of diagnostic tests for celiac disease in subjects with symptoms suggestive of irritable bowel syndrome: systematic review and meta-analysis. *Arch Intern Med* 2009;169:651-8.

5   Ruepert L, Quartero AO, de Wit NJ, van der Heijden GJ, Rubin G, Muris JW. Bulking agents, antispasmodics and antidepressants for the treatment of irritable bowel syndrome. *Cochrane Database Syst Rev* 2011;10:CD003460.

6   Ford AC, Talley NJ, Spiegel BMR, Foxx-Orenstein AE, Schiller L, Quigley EMM, et al. Effect of fibre, antispasmodics, and peppermint oil in irritable bowel syndrome: systematic review and meta-analysis. *BMJ* 2008;337:1388-92.

7   Bijkerk CJ, de Wit NJ, Muris JW, Whorwell PJ, Knottnerus JA, Hoes AW. Soluble or insoluble fibre in irritable bowel syndrome in primary care? Randomised placebo controlled trial. *BMJ* 2009;339:b3154.

8   Atkinson W, Sheldon TA, Shaath N, Whorwell PJ. Food elimination based on IgG antibodies in irritable bowel syndrome: a randomised controlled trial. *Gut* 2004;53:1459-64.

9   Ong DK, Mitchell SB, Barrett JS, Shepherd SJ, Irving PM, Biesiekierski JR, et al. Manipulation of dietary short chain carbohydrates alters the pattern of gas production and genesis of symptoms in irritable bowel syndrome. *J Gastroenterol Hepatol* 2010;25:1366-73.

10 Biesiekierski JR, Newnham ED, Irving PM, Barrett JS, Haines M, Doecke JD, et al. Gluten causes gastrointestinal symptoms in subjects without celiac disease: a double-blind randomized placebo-controlled trial. *Am J Gastroenterol* 2011;106:508-14.

11 Johannesson E, Simren M, Strid H, Bajor A, Sadik R. Physical activity improves symptoms in irritable bowel syndrome: a randomized controlled trial. *Am J Gastroenterol* 2011;106:915-22.

12 Saito YA, Prather CM, Van Dyke CT, Fett S, Zinsmeister AR, Locke III GR. Effects of multidisciplinary education on outcomes in patients with irritable bowel syndrome. *Clin Gastroenterol Hepatol* 2004;2:576-84.

13 Lu WZ, Gwee KA, Moochhalla S, Ho KY. Melatonin improves bowel symptoms in female patients with irritable bowel syndrome: a double-blind placebo-controlled study. *Aliment Pharmacol Ther* 2005;15:927-34.

14 Ford AC, Moayyedi P. Meta-analysis: factors affecting placebo response rate in irritable bowel syndrome. *Aliment Pharmacol Ther* 2010;32:144-58.

15 Kaptchuk TJ, Friedlander E, Kelley JM, Sanchez MN, Kokkotou E, Singer JP, et al. Placebos without deception: a randomized controlled trial in irritable bowel syndrome. *PLoS One* 2010;5:e15591.

16 Ford AC, Talley NJ, Schoenfeld PS, Quigley EMM, Moayyedi P. Efficacy of antidepressants and psychological therapies in irritable bowel syndrome: systematic review and meta-analysis. *Gut* 2009;58:367-78.

17 Ford AC, Brandt LJ, Young C, Chey WD, Foxx-Orenstein AE, Moayyedi P. Efficacy of 5-HT3 antagonists and 5-HT4 agonists in irritable bowel syndrome: systematic review and meta-analysis. *Am J Gastroenterol* 2009;104:1831-43.

18 Ford AC, Suares NC. Effect of laxatives and pharmacological therapies in chronic idipathic constipation: systematic review and meta-analysis. *Gut* 2011;60:209-18.

19 Pimentel M, Lembo A, Chey WD, Zakko S, Ringel Y, Yu J, et al. Rifaximin therapy for patients with irritable bowel syndrome without constipation. *N Engl J Med* 2011;364:22-32.

20 Moayyedi P, Ford AC, Brandt LJ, Foxx-Orenstein AE, Cremonini F, Talley NJ, et al. The efficacy of probiotics in the treatment of irritable bowel syndrome: a systematic review. *Gut* 2010;59:325-32.

21 Zijdenbos IL, de Wit NJ, van der Heijden GJ, Rubin G, Quartero AO. Psychological treatments for the management of irritable bowel syndrome. *Cochrane Database Syst Rev* 2009;21:CD006442.

22 Lindfors P, Unge P, Arvidsson P, Nyhlin H, Bjornsson E, Abrahamsson H, et al. Effects of gut-directed hypnotherapy on IBS in different clinical settings—results from two randomized, controlled trials. *Am J Gastroenterol* 2012;107:276-85.

23 Gaylord SA, Palsson OS, Garland EL, Faurot KR, Coble RS, Mann JD, et al. Mindfulness training reduces the severity of irritable bowel syndrome in women: results of a randomized controlled trial. *Am J Gastroenterol* 2011;106:1678-88.

24 Manheimer E, Wieland LS, Cheng K, Li SM, Shen X, Berman BM, et al. Acupuncture for irritable bowel syndrome: systematic review and meta-analysis. *Am J Gastroenterol* 2012;107:835-47.

25 Saito YA, Rey E, Almazar-Elder AE, Harmsen WS, Zinsmeister AR, Locke GR, et al. A randomized, double-blind, placebo-controlled trial of St John's wort for treating irritable bowel syndrome. *Am J Gastroenterol* 2010;105:170-7.

26 Madisch A, Holtmann G, Plein K, Hotz J. Treatment of irritable bowel syndrome with herbal preparations: results of a double-blind, randomized, placebo-controlled, multi-centre trial. *Aliment Pharmacol Ther* 2004;19:271-9.

27 Drossman DA, Chey WD, Johanson JF, Fass R, Scott C, Panas R, et al. Clinical trial: lubiprostone in patients with constipation-associated irritable bowel syndrome—results of two randomized, placebo-controlled studies. *Aliment Pharmacol Ther* 2009;29:329-41.

28 Chey WD, Lembo AJ, MacDougall JE, Lavins BJ, Schneier H, Johnston JM. Efficacy and safety of linaclotide administered orally for 26 weeks in patients with IBS-C: results from a randomized, double-blind, placebo-controlled phase 3 trial. *Gastroenterology* 2011;5(suppl 1):S135.

29 Money ME, Walkowiak J, Virgilio C, Talley NJ. Pilot study: a randomised, double blind, placebo controlled trial of pancrealipase for the treatment of postprandial irritable bowel syndrome-diarrhoea. *Frontline Gastroenterol* 2011;2:48-56.

30 Odunsi-Shiyanbade ST, Camilleri M, McKinzie S, Burton D, Carlson P, Busciglio IA, et al. Effects of chenodeoxycholate and a bile acid sequestrant, colesevelam, on intestinal transit and bowel function. *Clin Gastroenterol Hepatol* 2010;8:159-65.

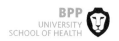

Related links

bmj.com/archive

Previous articles in this series

- Management of renal colic (2012;345:e5499)
- Diagnosis and management of peripheral arterial disease (2012;345:e5208)
- Diagnosis and management of cellulitis (2012;345:e4955)
- Management of osteoarthritis of the knee (2012;345:e4934)
- Management of difficult and severe eczema in childhood (2012;345:e4770)

bmj.com

- For all the latest BMJ Group articles on gastroenterology visit the gastroenterology portal

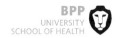

Chronic constipation in adults

Iain J D McCallum, specialty registrar, Sarah Ong, speciality registrar,
Mark Mercer-Jones, consultant colorectal surgeon

¹Colorectal Unit, Queen Elizabeth
Hospital, Gateshead Health NHS
Foundation Trust, Gateshead
NE9 6SX

Correspondence to: M Mercer-Jones
mark.mercer-jones@ghnt.nhs.uk

Cite this as: *BMJ* 2009;338:b831

DOI: 10.1136/bmj.b831

http://www.bmj.com/content/338/
bmj.b831

Chronic constipation in adults is a common and often debilitating problem that may present to almost any medical practitioner as it can have many causes. The most recent Rome criteria provide a useful research and clinical tool for defining chronic, functional constipation (box 1).[1] For the problem to be described as chronic, the Rome criteria need to have been met for the previous three months, with the onset of symptoms six months prior to diagnosis. We prefer a more inclusive definition of chronic constipation: any patient experiencing consistent difficulty with defecation. This review examines the evidence for the modern approach to treating chronic constipation and is based largely on systematic reviews and randomised controlled trials where these are available.

Who gets chronic constipation?

Since the most recent Rome criteria were published, a well conducted Spanish epidemiological study found that the prevalence of self reported constipation was 29.5% yet only half of those met the Rome criteria.[2] This study found that females had a higher incidence of constipation than males and that physical exercise and a high fibre diet were protective. The disparity between self reported incidence and failure to meet the Rome criteria highlights the difficulties in defining the condition. A systematic review of constipation in North America similarly found an average prevalence of 12-19%; increasing prevalence with increasing age; and female to male preponderance of 2.2:1.[3]

What causes constipation?

Box 2 summaries the simple causes of chronic constipation. Constipation resistant to simple measures may have both functional and organic causes. Careful investigation allows targeted treatment that will often be conservative. Causes include painful anorectal conditions unresponsive to simple measures; irritable bowel syndrome; obstructive defecation syndrome; and slow transit constipation.

What are the principles of managing constipation in primary care?

Many cases of constipation can be effectively managed in primary care. After exclusion of red flag symptoms, history and examination may guide initial management, which should be directed at the suspected cause.

Basic advice

Small series of comparative positions for defecation suggest that patients should be encouraged to adopt a "semi-squatting" position to defecate (figure).[7]

SOURCES AND SELECTION CRITERIA

We searched the Cochrane database for systematic reviews using the term constipation. We also searched Medline 1950 to April 2008, Embase, and PubMed, using the terms "chronic constipation", "slow-transit constipation", "irritable bowel syndrome", "levator ani syndrome", and "obstructive defecation" for titles and MESH headings. Two authors screened all abstracts and retrieved suitable articles for full critical appraisal.

Simple measures

Many patients may require only simple interventions to relieve constipation. Dietary modifications such as increasing fibre intake and ensuring good hydration are logical but do not have a formal evidence base.

Where dietary methods are unsuccessful simple treatments can be started. A recent systematic review of randomised controlled trials assessed the efficacy of simple interventions. It found good evidence for the use of polyethylene glycol and moderate evidence for lactulose and psyllium (isphagua) husk but few data on the use of other common agents such as senna, bisacodyl, and stool softeners.[8] Laxatives should be directed at the specific problem: bulking agents for those with poor dietary fibre intake; softeners for those with hard stools; and stimulant laxatives for poor colonic motility (such as with opiate use).

Investigations

A recent systematic review found no evidence to support the use of blood tests or abdominal radiography.[9] The British Society of Gastroenterology's guidelines advise that investigations in primary care should be limited to full blood count to exclude anaemia[5] and thyroid function assessment to exclude hypothyroidism. Other investigations may be relevant if other more unusual causes are suspected, but more complex investigations are undertaken in secondary care.

Local analgesia

Anal fissures may initially be treated with local application of 0.2-0.4% glyceryl trinitrate ointment, local application of calcium channel blocker ointment, or injection with botulinum toxin type A. A systematic review found that all of these agents were equally efficacious, but glyceryl trinitrate ointment has a higher side effect profile.[10] Stool softeners and local anaesthetic gels will also relieve pain and constipation.

Monitoring response to treatment

Scoring systems can be useful to monitor progress. The Bristol stool chart (developed by K W Heaton and S J Lewis, Bristol University) is widely available and can be used to monitor dietary manipulations or response to laxatives.

SUMMARY POINTS

- Chronic constipation is a common and debilitating condition
- Many cases can be managed in primary care with simple measures
- Investigations can often identify a cause for resistant constipation and thus guide treatment
- Targeted surgery can be of great benefit to carefully selected patients

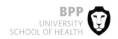

Irritable bowel syndrome in which constipation is predominant feature

Most investigations are likely to be normal in patients with irritable bowel syndrome. The British Society of Gastroenterology's guidelines include a full blood count as the only mandatory investigation in suspected cases of irritable bowel syndrome in which constipation is the predominant feature. Education and reassurance form the basis of management for this patient group. To encourage self management discuss possible symptom triggers, which may be physical, dietary, or psychological. A *BMJ* review[11] and recent NICE guidance[12] give detailed information about management of irritable bowel syndrome.

When to refer for specialist care

If dietary intervention, laxatives, and other approaches fail, referral to a specialist is indicated.

Psychological treatment for irritable bowel syndrome

Psychological referral is indicated for patients with irritable bowel syndrome who fail to respond to simple and pharmacological interventions after 12 months.[12]

Painful anorectal conditions

Conditions such as anal fissure, haemorrhoids, abscess, or fistula usually require specialised management when conservative measures fail. The management of haemorrhoids has recently been described in a *BMJ* clinical review.[13]

Levator ani syndrome is a condition characterised by recurrent chronic rectal pain without detectable organic cause. This pain is typically worse on walking and may be brought on by defecation. It is often reproducible with coccygeal traction with a specific trigger point on the levator muscle at digital rectal examination. Several theories of pathophysiology exist, but precise aetiology is yet to be defined.

Reports of treatment strategies vary and include digital massage, local anaesthetic injection, electrogalvanic stimulation, muscle relaxants, and biofeedback (an operant feedback technique where defecation retraining is achieved through simulated defecation). Small case series have recommended local anaesthetic injection,[14] although high quality evidence is not available.

Levator ani syndrome must be differentiated from proctalgia fugax, with the pain usually being more shortlived, lasting typically less than 30 minutes, often occurring at night. Treatment is with amitryptiline and gabapentin. When the condition is suspected, referral is usually indicated for both conditions to rule out organic causes such as fistula, abscess, proctitis, and rare presacral tumours.

Obstructed defecation

Obstructed defecation is a broad term for a pathophysiological condition describing the inability to evacuate contents from the rectum.[15] The causes may be anatomical or functional. Anatomical causes include ultrashort segment Hirschsprung's disease, rectocoele, intussusception, enterocoele, sigmoidocoele, and perhaps genital prolapse. Functional causes have confusing and varied nomenclature. The basic pathology behind these conditions is rectoanal neuromuscular malcoordination, hence proposal of the term dyssynergic defecation as a blanket term. Several terms have been used in the literature to specify individual types of malcoordination (anismus, paradoxical puborectalis contraction, pelvic floor dyssynergia).[16]

Symptoms include a feeling of incomplete evacuation, passage of hard stools, the need to self digitate rectally or vaginally, a need for laxative or enema for defecation, rectal discomfort, excessive straining and repeat visits to defecate. In some patients, symptoms of faecal or urinary incontinence may coexist.

Vaginal and rectal examination is necessary to assess for presence of a rectocoele, perineal descent, apical vaginal prolapse, cystocoele, full thickness rectal prolapse, and rectal mucosal ulceration. Common investigations are anorectal manometry (including a balloon expulsion test) to assess neuromuscular coordination and power, and defecating proctography. Dynamic magnetic resonance imaging of the pelvic floor and colonic transit time studies may be required.[15]

BOX 1 ROME CRITERIA*

- Presence of two or more of the following symptoms:
- -Straining during at least 25% of defecations
- -Lumpy or hard stools in at least 25% of defecations
- -Sensation of incomplete evacuations for at least 25% of defecations
- -Sensation of anorectal obstruction/blockage for at least 25% of defecations
- -Manual manoeuvres to facilitate at least 25% of defecations (such as digital evacuation, support of the pelvic floor)
- -Fewer than three bowel movements a week
- Loose stools are rarely present without the use of laxatives

*Criteria have to have been met for the previous three months, with the onset of symptoms six months prior to diagnosis

---

BOX 2 SIMPLE CAUSES OF CONSTIPATION

Dietary
- Low fibre, dieting, dementia, depression, anorexia, fluid depletion

Metabolic
- Diabetes mellitus, hypercalcaemia, hypokalaemia, hypothyroidism, porphyria

Neurological
- Parkinson's disease, spinal cord pathology, multiple sclerosis

Iatrogenic
- Antacids that contain aluminium, iron, anticholinergics, antidepressants, opiates for analgesia

Painful anorectal conditions
- Anal fissure, haemorrhoids, abscess, fistula, levator ani syndrome, proctalgia fugax

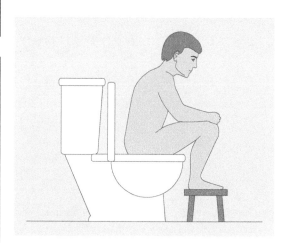

Fig 1 The correct position for defecation

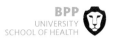

Treating obstructive defecation

Conservative treatment includes a high fibre diet, adequate hydration, regular physical activity, enemas, laxatives, and rectal irrigation.[15] Behavioural therapy with biofeedback training to teach patients to relax their pelvic floor can be useful.[17] The effectiveness and duration of the effects are variable, but the therapy has low morbidity. A *BMJ* clinical review discussed biofeedback for constipation.[18]

Paradoxical puborectalis contraction

Failure to relax the puborectalis muscle on attempted defecation causes this condition. If conservative treatment (usually biofeedback) has failed, it may be treated with an injection of type A botulinum toxin into puborectalis muscle and external anal sphincter. A case series found that this treatment was successful in 50-75% of cases but the effect was short lived, and therefore reinjection may be needed, as well as inducing temporary incontinence.[19]

Solitary rectal ulcer syndrome

This presents with tenesmus, straining, and passage of obvious blood or mucus. A biopsy of the ulcer is needed to exclude malignancy. Conservative treatments should be tried, but if they fail, surgery is recommended when there is full thickness rectal prolapse or intractable haemorrhage.[14]

Rectocoele

This is defined as herniation of the anterior rectal and posterior vaginal wall into the vaginal lumen. This is an important cause of anorectal symptoms, but most cases are asymptomatic. As before, conservative treatments should be tried before surgery.

Only the minority of rectocoeles need to be repaired, and indications for this are incomplete emptying of the rectocoele or the rectocoele causing obstruction to complete rectal emptying, assessed both clinically and on defecating proctography. Surgical repairs include traditional transvaginal posterior colporrhaphy, and transrectal or transperineal repair with prosthetic material. Newer techniques include the double stapled trans-anal rectal resection (commonly known as STARR) and single stapled trans-anal prolapsectomy with perineal levatorplasty (STAPL). A randomised controlled trial showed significant symptomatic improvement after each of these procedures in 88% and 76% of cases respectively two years after follow-up; however, concerns over continence of patients have been raised, and up to a third of patients develop urgency of defecation.[20]

Rectal intussusception and rectal prolapse

Dietary management and biofeedback are key to managing these patients. Surgery may be needed if there is additional faecal incontinence or associated full thickness rectal prolapse.[15] Surgery would be an abdominal procedure (open or laparoscopic) or a perineal procedure (especially in elderly patients). Traditional procedures involve full posterior rectal mobilisation and fixation to surrounding structures, often with concomitant segmental colonic resection. Major complications, worsening constipation, and recurrence are not uncommon. Laparoscopic ventral rectopexy for full thickness rectal prolapse or intussusception is a new procedure available at a few pelvic floor units in the United Kingdom. Initial results are encouraging with low recurrence rates and reduction in constipation symptoms.[21]

Sigmoidocoele and enterocoele

Sigmoidocoele and enterocoele involve the prolapse of a portion of terminal bowel into the rectovaginal pouch. They are confirmed on defecating proctography and classified according to the degree of descent into the pelvis.[22] Surgery is required for severe sigmoidocoeles and enterocoeles.

Slow transit constipation

Slow transit constipation is a delayed colorectal transit time and is usually measured with a radio-opaque marker study in which different shaped markers are ingested and their progress followed on serial abdominal radiography. Slow transit constipation may occur after pelvic trauma, usually either surgery or complicated childbirth, or may be idiopathic. The exact pathophysiology behind idiopathic cases is not known, although neuropathy, colonic myopathy, or mesenchymopathy have been proposed.[23]

Stimulant laxatives are a logical initial treatment, but we were unable to find evidence for the success or otherwise of this intervention. Reports of small numbers of cases with isolated slow transit constipation and successful biofeedback therapy do exist.[18]

Self administered antegrade colonic enemas may be possible if access to the proximal colon is fashioned usually by exteriorising the appendix as a stoma providing access for the patient to self administer antegrade enemas.[24]

Subtotal colectomy with ileorectal anastomosis has remained the intervention of choice for slow transit constipation that is unresponsive to other approaches. Patients' satisfaction rates have been reported as between 77%[25] and 90%,[26] confirming that this can be an appropriate management strategy for well informed patients having surgery in a unit with appropriate expertise. Patient selection is important. Segmental resection has been advocated by some authors for patients with isolated slow transit segments.

TIPS FOR NON-SPECIALISTS

- Most cases of constipation can be managed in primary care with attention to likely causative factors and simple targeted interventions
- Red flag symptoms mandate early specialist referral
- If simple interventions fail, consider specialist referral to evaluate possible unusual causes
- New non-surgical and surgical treatments are being developed constantly
- Many patients with debilitating symptoms can be helped greatly with specialist interventions

---

UNANSWERED QUESTIONS

- The efficacy of many commonly prescribed drugs, such as stool softeners, senna, and bisacodyl, remains to be defined
- The role and long term outcomes of new surgical procedures for obstructed defecation need further evaluation
- More work is required determining the efficacy of simple treatments such as botulinum toxin type A for obstructed defecation to define when and if these can be recommended to patients.
- The cause of slow transit constipation (and whether this is the same in all patients with slow transit) remains to found; an answer might guide therapeutic options, although all options in slow transit constipation are supported only by low level evidence
- Sacral nerve stimulation may present a therapeutic breakthrough, although evidence on this is extremely limited

---

ADDITIONAL EDUCATIONAL RESOURCES

- Rome Foundation (www.romecriteria.org)—Publishes guidelines on the diagnosis and management of a range of functional gastrointestinal disorders
- British Society of Gastroenterology (www.bsg.org.uk)—Publishes guidelines for the management of irritable bowel syndrome and other causes of chronic constipation
- Core (www.corecharity.org.uk)—This charity for research and information on gut and liver disease provides a useful information leaflet for patients on constipation

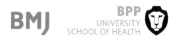

We thank Claire Egglestone (colorectal specialist nurse) for her help in preparation of the review.

Contributors: IJDMcC and SO performed the literature search and wrote the initial draft. MM-J supervised the project and revised the initial draft. All authors have seen and approved the manuscript. MM-J is the guarantor.

Funding: No special funding.

Competing interests: None declared.

Provenance and peer review: Not commissioned; externally peer reviewed.

1   Longstreth GF, Thompson WG, Chey WD, Houghton LA, Mearin F, Spiller RC. Functional bowel disorders. *Gastroenterology* 2006;130:480-91.
2   Garrigues V, Gálvez C, Ortiz V, Ponce M, Nos P, Ponce J. Prevalence of constipation: agreement among several criteria and evaluation of the diagnostic accuracy of qualifying symptoms and self-reported definition in a population-based survey in Spain. *Am J Epidemiol* 2004;159:520-6.
3   Higgins PD, Johanson JF. Epidemiology of constipation in North America: a systematic review. *Am J Gastroenterol* 2004;99:750-9.
4   Thompson WG, Heaton KW, Smyth GT, Smyth C. Irritable bowel syndrome in general practice: prevalence, characteristics, and referral. *Gut* 2000;46:78-82.
5   Spiller R, Aziz Q, Creed F, Emmanuel A, Houghton F, Hungin P, et al. Guidelines on irritable bowel syndrome. *Gut* 2007;56:1770-98.
6   National Institute for Health and Clinical Excellence (NICE). Irritable bowel syndrome in adults: diagnosis and management of irritable bowel syndrome in primary care. (Clinical guideline 27.) 2008. www.nice.org.uk/CG27.
7   Sikirov D. Comparison of straining during defecation in three positions: results and implications for human health. *Dig Dis Sci* 2003 Jul;48:1201-5.
8   Ramkumar D, Rao SS. Efficacy and safety of traditional medical therapies in chronic constipation: a systematic review. *Am J Gastroenterol* 2005;100:936-71.
9   Rao SS, Ozturk R, Laine L. Clinical utility of diagnostic tests for constipation in adults: a systematic review. *Am J Gastroenterol* 2005;100:1605-15.
10 Nelson RL. Non-surgical therapy for anal fissure. *Cochrane Database Syst Rev* 2006;(4):CD003431.
11 Agarwal A, Whorwell PJ. Irritable bowel syndrome: diagnosis and management. *BMJ* 2006;332:280-3.
12 National Institute for Health and Clinical Excellence (NICE). *Irritable bowel syndrome in adults: diagnosis and management of irritable bowel syndrome in primary care* . (Clinical guideline 61.) 2008. www.nice.org.uk/CG61
13 Acheson AG, Scholefield JH. Management of haemorrhoids. *BMJ* 2008;336:380-3.
14 Park DH, Yoon SG, Kim KU, Hwang DY, Kim HS, Lee JK, et al. Comparison study between electrogalvanic stimulation and local injection therapy in levator ani syndrome. *Int J Colorectal Dis* 2005;20:272-6.
15 Khaikin M, Wexner SD. Treatment strategies in obstructed defecation and faecal incontinence. *World J Gastroenterol* 2006;12:3168-73.
16 Rao SS. Dyssynergic defecation. *Gastroenterol Clin North Am* 2001;30:97-112.
17 Koh CE, Young CJ, Young JM, Solomon MJ. Systematic review of randomized controlled trials of the effectiveness of biofeedback for pelvic floor dysfunction. *Br J Surg* 2008;95:1079-87.
18 Bassotti G, Chistolini F, Sietchiping-Nzepa F, de Roberto G, Morelli A, Chiarioni G. Biofeedback for pelvic floor dysfunction in constipation. *BMJ* 2004;328:393-6.
19 Ron Y, Avni Y, Lukovetski A, Wardi J, Geva D, Birkenfeld S, et al. Botulinum toxin type-A in therapy of patients with anismus. *Dis Colon rectum* 2001;44:1821-6.
20 Boccasanta P, Venturi M, Salamina G, Cesana BM, Bernasconi F, Roviaro G. New trends in the surgical treatment of outlet obstruction: clinical and functional results of two novel transanal stapled techniques from a randomised controlled trial. *Int J Colorectal Dis* 2004;19:359-69.
21 D'Hoore A, Penninck F. Laparoscopic ventral recto(colpo)pexy for rectal prolapse: surgical technique and outcome for 109 patients. *Surg Endosc* 2006;20:1919-23.
22 Jorge JM, Yang YK, Wexner SD. Incidence and clinical significance of sigmidocoeles as determined by new classification system. *Dis Colon Rectum* 1994;37:1112-7.
23 Knowles CH, Martin JE. Slow transit constipation: a model of human gut dysmotility. Review of possible aetiologies. *Neurogastroenterol Motil* 2000;12:181-96.
24 Rongen MJ, van der Hoop AG, Baeten CG. Cecal access for antegrade colon enemas in medically refractory slow-transit constipation: a prospective study. *Dis Colon Rectum* 2001;44:1644-9.
25 Zutshi M, Hu, T, Trzcinski R, Arvelakis A, Xu M. Surgery for slow transit constipation: are we helping patients? *Int J Colorectal Dis* 2007;22:265-9.
26 Lubowski DZ, Chen FC, Kennedy ML, King DW. Results of colectomy for severe slow transit constipation. *Dis Colon Rectum* 1996;39:23-9.

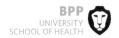

Outpatient parenteral antimicrobial therapy

Ann L N Chapman, consultant in infectious diseases

¹Department of Infection and Tropical Medicine, Royal Hallamshire Hospital, Sheffield Teaching Hospitals NHS Foundations Trust, Sheffield S10 2JF, UK

ann.chapman@sth.nhs.uk

Cite this as: *BMJ* 2013;346:f1585

DOI: 10.1136/bmj.f1585

http://www.bmj.com/content/346/bmj.f1585

Outpatient parenteral antimicrobial therapy (OPAT) allows patients to be given intravenous antibiotics in the community rather than as an inpatient. First developed in the 1970s in the US for the treatment of children with cystic fibrosis,[1] OPAT has expanded substantially and is now standard practice in many countries.[2][3] In the UK, uptake has been much slower, although OPAT is now being increasingly used in both primary and secondary care, driven by a national focus on efficiency savings in healthcare, improving patient experience, and provision of care closer to home. It is important that medical practitioners are aware both of the opportunities that OPAT presents and of the potential risks of treatment outside hospital for patients with serious and often complex infections. This article aims to describe the clinical practice of OPAT, highlight potential risks, and explore how these may be reduced.

What is OPAT?

OPAT is the administration of intravenous antimicrobial therapy to patients in an outpatient setting or in their own home. It can be used for patients with severe or deep seated infections who require parenteral treatment but are otherwise stable and well enough not to be in hospital; these patients may be discharged early to an OPAT service or may avoid hospital admission altogether.

What type of infections can be treated?

Cellulitis

OPAT is most widely used for patients with soft tissue sepsis, mainly cellulitis.[4][5] Cellulitis accounts for 1-2% of emergency hospital admissions in England and Wales, or about 80 000 admissions annually.[6] Around 30% of patients presenting to hospital with cellulitis have moderately severe infection that requires intravenous antibiotics but do not have severe systemic sepsis necessitating inpatient care.[7][8] One randomised controlled trial of twice daily intravenous cefazolin administered by a nurse at home compared with standard inpatient care showed no significant difference in duration of intravenous or subsequent oral antibiotic therapy, patient functional outcomes, or complications but reported improved patient satisfaction with home treatment.[9]

Data from several large retrospective case series show that outpatient treatment with once daily ceftriaxone is also safe and effective, with good short and long term clinical outcomes, and this is now the predominant antibiotic used for outpatient intravenous treatment of cellulitis in the UK.[4][5][10] If there is concern about possible meticillin resistant *Staphylococcus aureus* (MRSA) infection, teicoplanin or daptomycin are alternatives.[5] Increasingly a nurse led model of care is being used for management of cellulitis outside hospital, with treatment set out in a protocol and limited input from doctors.[11]

Bone and joint infections

Patients with bone and joint infections invariably require prolonged parenteral antibiotic courses, and several large retrospective case series have shown that outpatient treatment can be used successfully in this group.[12][13][14] Patients may receive outpatient antibiotics within a two stage revision of an infected joint or as sole therapy for septic arthritis or osteomyelitis. One UK study reported outcomes for 198 patients with a range of bone and joint infections treated by OPAT. Seventy three per cent of patients were disease free at median follow-up of 60 weeks; patients with advanced age, MRSA infection, and diabetic foot infections were more likely to have a relapse or recurrence.[12]

Infective endocarditis

US, European, and UK guidelines now recommend OPAT as part of routine clinical care for patients with infective endocarditis.[15][16][17] Although initially recommended only for uncomplicated native valve infections with low risk organisms, there is increasing evidence that OPAT is safe in more complex patients after an initial period of inpatient care, as long as the potential risks are assessed on a case by case basis and treatment is administered through a formal OPAT service with the appropriate safeguards to minimise risk.[18][19] Such safeguards include daily nurse review, once or twice weekly physician review, and the establishment of an escalation pathway for medical staff familiar with the case to be informed of potential problems.[15][16]

Other uses

Use of OPAT has been described for numerous other infections, including resistant urinary tract infections, central nervous system infections, and low risk neutropenic sepsis.[20][21][22] The availability of long acting antibiotics such as ceftriaxone, teicoplanin, and daptomycin and the diversity of models for delivering OPAT allows most stable patients requiring intravenous antimicrobials to be considered for outpatient treatment. However, there are some situations where it is less useful—for example, patients with pneumonia are best managed either with outpatient oral therapy for mild infection or intravenous antibiotics in hospital for more severe cases.[23]

SOURCES AND SELECTION CRITERIA

References were sourced through a systematic review of the literature undertaken for the UK OPAT Good Practice Recommendations in 2012. The search included all English language articles between 1998 and 2010, and was further updated with a search of PubMed, Medline, and Cochrane databases. Published OPAT guidelines from other countries and key reviews were also used, as well as the author's knowledge of the literature.

SUMMARY POINTS

- Outpatient parenteral antimicrobial therapy (OPAT) allows patients requiring intravenous antibiotics to be treated outside hospital
- OPAT is suitable for many infections, especially cellulitis, bone and joint infections, and infective endocarditis
- Antibiotics can be administered in an outpatient unit, at home by a nurse, or at home by the patient or a carer
- Patients should be assessed by a doctor and specialist nurse to determine medical and social suitability
- Evidence suggests that OPAT is safe as long as it is administered through a formal service structure to minimise risk

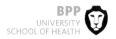

Which patients are suitable?

Patients referred for outpatient treatment need to be clinically stable, both in terms of their general condition and their infection. Thus they should have stable vital signs and be at low risk of their infection progressing or developing serious complications.[2] [3] [24] Patients with a diagnosis of cellulitis, for example, need to be assessed by a healthcare practitioner competent to exclude other more serious conditions that could potentially be confused with cellulitis, such as septic arthritis or necrotising fasciitis. Patients with endocarditis are more likely to develop potentially life threatening complications in the first two weeks of therapy, and outpatient administration is therefore not recommended until after this period.[16] Determination of suitability will generally require a medical review, unless a protocol is in place for assessment by another trained healthcare practitioner.[11]

Other health and social issues also need to be explored. OPAT requires the patient to engage actively and reliably with therapy, and thus patients with substance misuse or serious mental health problems may not be suitable. In addition, there must be no other barrier to discharge from hospital. For example, although diabetic foot infections may be suitable for OPAT, many patients will require other care that has to be provided in hospital, including adjustment of diabetic control, vascular assessment, and surgical intervention.[25] Finally, home based care must be suitable from a social perspective—for example, an acceptable home environment, access to a telephone, adequate transport, and support from family or carers. In general the OPAT nurse, in collaboration with other professional teams, is best placed to assess these additional factors, and current OPAT guidelines recommend that patients should be assessed by both a doctor and nurse before being accepted for outpatient administration.[2] [3] [24]

How is OPAT delivered?

Three service models can be used to deliver OPAT, all of which have been shown to be effective: an ambulatory care centre, a nurse attending the patient's home, or self administration. The approach used varies among countries—for example, infusion centres have been the dominant model in the US whereas services in Australia tend to follow the "hospital in the home" visiting nurse model. However, it is becoming increasingly common for individual OPAT services to offer all three models, allowing treatment to be tailored to each patient's circumstances.[2] Most OPAT services described in the literature are based in acute hospitals, predominantly in specialist infectious diseases units.[4] [5] [13] [18] Services may also be established by other inpatient specialist teams or in frontline emergency or acute medicine units[9]: in the UK, the Society of Acute Medicine has recently established a working group to promote the development of OPAT in this setting.

In the ambulatory care centre model, the patient attends a healthcare facility daily, or as required, with antibiotics administered by a healthcare practitioner. Treatment in the patient's home may be administered by community nurses, outreach nurses from the acute hospital, or nurses provided through a private healthcare company. In the third model patients (or carers) are taught to administer therapy; this has the advantages of engaging patients in their care, allowing more flexibility of dose frequency and timing, and reducing staffing costs. Despite theoretical concerns about line infections, two large retrospective studies have shown

that self administration is as safe as administration by a healthcare worker in the community.[14] [26]

The model of OPAT used largely determines the type of intravenous access. Options include temporary "butterfly" needles that are inserted and removed for each dose, short term peripheral cannulas, or, for longer antibiotic courses, peripherally inserted central cannulas or tunnelled central lines. Bolus injections or infusions may be used, depending on the choice of antimicrobial agent(s). Infusions allow higher doses to be administered but require additional administration time and training.[27] Novel delivery devices allow patients greater freedom to continue normal daily activities. For example, portable elastomeric infusion devices can be carried in the patient's pocket or a carrying pouch and deliver continuous infusions over 24 hours.[3]

What are the benefits?

The clinical effectiveness of OPAT has been established for a wide range of infections through numerous retrospective case series, as outlined above. However, there have been few randomised controlled trials comparing OPAT with inpatient care. Furthermore, there are no published data on clinical efficacy of OPAT services based entirely in a community setting, although there are descriptions of collaborative services across primary and secondary care sectors.[9]

OPAT has been shown to be cost effective in many healthcare contexts. One retrospective study from a UK service compared the actual costs of OPAT over two years with the theoretical costs of inpatient care for the same patient cohort and found that OPAT cost 47% of equivalent inpatient national average costs.[4] However, in reality there is a wide range of funding arrangements for OPAT in operation across the UK, and in some instances OPAT may offer little cost advantage to commissioners over inpatient care. A national tariff for OPAT would allow consistency and equity and support wider use.

In addition to reducing direct costs, OPAT frees inpatient capacity, which can then be used either to admit further patients or as part of a planned reduction in bed capacity. More detailed modelling of these downstream benefits has not been undertaken but might provide added evidence of OPAT's cost effectiveness.

Finally, there is increasing evidence that OPAT is associated with a very low rate of healthcare associated infection. Despite theoretical concerns about the use of broad spectrum agents such as ceftriaxone, the risk of *Clostridium difficile* infection seems to be low: a meta-analysis of three large UK OPAT cohorts found the rate of *C difficile* infection to be 0.1%,[10] although there are no published prospective data.

What are the risks?

Despite these benefits, OPAT is associated with increased clinical risk compared with inpatient care because of the reduced level of supervision. At least 25% of patients having OPAT experience an adverse reaction of some type, ranging from mild antibiotic associated diarrhoea to severe line infections.[24] The treatment pathway—from patient selection, determination of the therapeutic regimen and intravenous access device to communication with other teams and ongoing monitoring during therapy—provides numerous opportunities for error.[28] In addition, as OPAT is used increasingly for more complex infections in patients with serious comorbidities, the likelihood of adverse events unrelated to the infection increases. A retrospective survey of US physi-

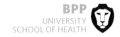

cians involved in OPAT found that 68% had seen at least one major adverse event in their patients in the preceding year,[29] highlighting the importance of a formal governance structure. The adverse events included unexpected death, line related bacteraemia, air embolism, drug hypersensitivity, and drug induced blood dyscrasia.

About 10% of patients will require readmission, with higher rates for patients with more complex infections.[4] [5] [14] [18] [19] In addition, many patients require further unplanned input during therapy: one study found that 12% of OPAT patients needed urgent advice or an unscheduled home visit.[30] Thus it is essential that the service has an established system for 24 hour access to clinical support and a formal (re)admission pathway to secondary care.

One further potential risk is overuse of intravenous antimicrobial therapy as an alternative to oral agents purely because an OPAT service exists. Similarly, there is also a risk that a broad spectrum once daily parenteral antimicrobial agent could be chosen in preference to a potentially more efficacious agent requiring multiple daily doses for reasons of convenience alone. OPAT should therefore operate within the context of an antibiotic stewardship programme, and it is essential that a microbiologist or infectious diseases physician is involved in both the initial design of antibiotic protocols and ongoing patient care. Several studies have found that assessment of referred patients by an infection specialist results in reduced use of intravenous therapy, improved clinical care, and substantial cost savings.[31] [32] [33]

How can the risks be reduced?

It is clear that OPAT delivered through a formal service structure is safer than when delivered through ad hoc arrangements. Several bodies have published recommendations on delivery of OPAT[2] [3] [34] and the aim of these is to ensure that the risks associated with OPAT are minimised. In the UK a consensus statement on the use of OPAT was recently published as a joint initiative between the British Society for Antimicrobial Chemotherapy and the British Infection Association.[24] It covers service structure, patient selection criteria, antimicrobial selection and delivery, frequency and type of clinical and blood test monitoring, monitoring of outcomes, and clinical governance. It recommends the core OPAT team should comprise, as a minimum, an OPAT specialist nurse, doctor, infection specialist (either an infectious diseases physician or a microbiologist), and a pharmacist. A doctor with suitable training and experience (who may also be the infection specialist, when he or she delivers hands-on clinical care) should take responsibility for management decisions for each patient, in collaboration with the team. Although patients on prolonged courses of antimicrobials can be reviewed weekly, or less frequently if stable, those receiving treatment for cellulitis should be reviewed daily to allow switching from intravenous to oral therapy as soon as clinically appropriate.

What is the future of OPAT in the UK?

OPAT offers a rare opportunity not only to improve patient choice while maintaining service quality but also to reduce healthcare costs and improve service efficiency. Use of OPAT is likely to continue to expand in the UK, as in many other countries, driven by enthusiasm for increasing care delivery in the community as well as by cost pressures and patient choice. OPAT was recently cited as one of five antimicrobial prescribing decision options in Department of Health guidance on antibiotic stewardship.[35] Services will continue

---

ADDITIONAL EDUCATION RESOURCES

E-OPAT (http://e-opat.com)—an online resource for setting up OPAT services from the British Society for Antimicrobial Chemotherapy

---

to be developed both in primary and secondary care, and it is likely that integrated services across sectors will be established in order to combine primary care's capacity and expertise in home treatment with the specialist knowledge and back-up of secondary care.

Competing interests: The author has completed the ICMJE uniform disclosure form at www.icmje.org/coi_disclosure.pdf (available on request from her) and declares: no support from any organisation for the submitted work; no financial relationships with any organisations that might have an interest in the submitted work in the previous 3 years. The author co-chaired the development of the 2012 UK OPAT good practice recommendations.

Provenance and peer review: Not commissioned; externally peer reviewed.

1   Rucker RW, Harrison GM. Outpatient intravenous medications in the management of cystic fibrosis. *Pediatrics* 1974;54:358-60.
2   Tice AD, Rehm SJ, Dalovisio JR, Bradley JS, Martinelli LP, Graham DR, et al. Practice guidelines for outpatient parenteral antibiotic therapy. IDSA guidelines. *Clin Infect Dis* 2004;38:1651-72.
3   Howden BP, Grayson ML. Hospital-in-the-home treatment of infectious diseases. *Med J Aust* 2002;176:440-5.
4   Chapman ALN, Dixon S, Andrews D, Lillie PJ, Bazaz R, Patchett JD. Clinical efficacy and cost effectiveness of outpatient parenteral antibiotic therapy (OPAT): a UK perspective. *J Antimicrob Chemother* 2009;64:1316-24.
5   Barr DA, Semple L, Seaton RA. Outpatient parenteral antimicrobial therapy (OPAT) in a teaching hospital-based practice: a retrospective cohort study describing experience and evolution over 10 years. *Int J Antimicrob Agents* 2012;39:407-13.
6   Phoenix G, Das S, Joshi M. Diagnosis and management of cellulitis. *BMJ* 2012;345:e4955.
7   CREST (Clinical Resource Efficiency Support Team). Guidelines on the management of cellulitis in adults. 2005. www.acutemed.co.uk/docs/Cellulitis%20guidelines,%20CREST,%2005.pdf.
8   Marwick C, Broomhall J, McCowan C, Phillips G, Gonzalez-McQuire S, Akhras K, et al. Severity assessment of skin and soft tissue infections: cohort study of management and outcomes for hospitalised patients. *J Antimicrob Chemother* 2011;66:387-97.
9   Corwin P, Toop L, McGeoch G, Than M, Wynn-Thomas S, Wells JE, et al. Randomised controlled trial of intravenous antibiotic treatment for cellulitis at home compared to hospital. *BMJ* 2005;330:129-32.
10   Duncan CJA, Barr DA, Seaton RA. Outpatient parenteral antimicrobial therapy with ceftriaxone, a review. *Int J Clin Pharm* 2012;34:410-7.
11   Seaton RA, Bell E, Gourlay Y, Semple L. Nurse-led management of uncomplicated cellulitis in the community: evaluation of a protocol incorporating intravenous ceftriaxone. *J Antimicrob Chemother* 2005;55:764-7.
12   Mackintosh CL, White HA, Seaton RA. Outpatient parenteral antibiotic therapy (OPAT) for bone and joint infections: experience from a UK teaching hospital-based service. *J Antimicrob Chemother* 2011;66:408-15.
13   Esposito S, Leone S, Noviello S, Ianniello F, Fiore M, Russo M, et al. Outpatient parenteral antibiotic therapy for bone and joint infections: an Italian multicenter study, *J Chemother* 2007;19:417-22.
14   Matthews PC, Conlon CP, Berendt AR, Kayley J, Jefferies L, Atkins B, et al. Outpatient parenteral antimicrobial therapy (OPAT): is it safe for selected patients to self-administer at home? A retrospective analysis of a large cohort over 13 years. *J Antimicrob Chemother* 2008;61:226-7.
15   Gould FK, Denning DW, Elliott TSJ, Foweraker J, Perry JD, Prendergast BD, et al. Guidelines for the diagnosis and antibiotic treatment of endocarditis in adults: a report of the working party of the British Society for Antimicrobial Chemotherapy. *J Antimicrob Chemother* 2012;67:269-89.
16   Habib G, Hoen B, Tornos P, Thuny F, Prendergast B, Vilacosta I, et al. Guidelines on the prevention, diagnosis, and treatment of infective endocarditis. *Eur Heart J* 2009;30:2369-413.
17   Baddour LM, Wilson WR, Bayer AS, Fowler Jr VG, Bolger AF, Levison ME, et al. Infective endocarditis: diagnosis, antimicrobial therapy, and management of complications: a statement for healthcare professionals from the Committee on Rheumatic Fever, Endocarditis, and Kawasaki Disease, Council on Cardiovascular Disease in the Young, and the Councils on Clinical Cardiology, Stroke, and Cardiovascular Surgery and Anesthesia, American Heart Association: endorsed by the Infectious Diseases Society of America. *Circulation* 2005;111:e394-434.
18   Amodeo MR, Clulow T, Lainchbury J, Murdoch DR, Gallagher K, Dyer A, et al. Outpatient intravenous treatment for infective endocarditis: safety, effectiveness and one-year outcomes. *J Infect* 2009;59:387-93.

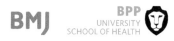

19 Partridge DG, O'Brien E, Chapman ALN. Outpatient parenteral antibiotic therapy for infective endocarditis: a review of 4 years' experience at a UK centre. *Postgrad Med J* 2012;88:377-81.

20 Bazaz R, Chapman ALN, Winstanley TG. Ertapenem administered as outpatient parenteral antibiotic therapy for urinary tract infections caused by extended-spectrum-β-lactamase-producing Gram-negative organisms. *J Antimicrob Chemother* 2010;65:1510-3.

21 Tice AD, Strait K, Ramey R, Hoaglund PA. Outpatient parenteral antimicrobial therapy for central nervous system infections. *Clin Infect Dis* 1999;29:1394-9.

22 Teuffel O, Ethier MC, Alibhai SM, Beyene J, Sung L. Outpatient management of cancer patients with febrile neutropenia: a systematic review and meta-analysis. *Ann Oncol* 2011;22:2358-65.

23 Ingram PR, Cerbe L, Hassell M, Wilson M, Dyer JR. Limited role for outpatient parenteral antibiotic therapy for community-acquired pneumonia. *Respirology* 2008;13:893-6.

24 Chapman ALN, Seaton RA, Cooper MA, Hedderwick S, Goodall V, Reed C, et al. Good practice recommendations for outpatient parenteral antimicrobial therapy (OPAT) in adults in the UK: a consensus statement. *J Antimicrobial Chemother* 2012;67:1053-62.

25 Lipsky BA, Berendt AR, Cornia PB, Pile JC, Peters EJG, Armstrong DG, et al. Infectious Diseases Society of America clinical practice guideline for the diagnosis and treatment of diabetic foot infections. *Clin Infect Dis* 2012;54:132-73.

26 Barr DA, Semple L, Seaton RA. Self-administration of outpatient parenteral antibiotic therapy and risk of catheter-related adverse events: a retrospective cohort study. *Eur J Clin Microbiol Infect Dis* 2012;31:2611-9.

27 Royal College of Nursing. Standards for infusion therapy. 3rd ed. 2010. www.rcn.org.uk/__data/assets/pdf_file/0005/78593/002179.pdf.

28 Gilchrist M, Franklin BD, Patel JP. An outpatient parenteral antibiotic therapy (OPAT) map to identify risks associated with an OPAT service. *J Antimicrob Chemother* 2009;64:177-83.

29 Chary A, Tice AD, Martinelli LP, Liedtke LA, Plantenga MS, Strausbaugh LJ. Experience of infectious diseases consultants with outpatient parenteral antimicrobial therapy: results of an emerging infections network survey. *Clin Infect Dis* 2006;43:1290-5.

30 Montalto M. How safe is hospital-in-the-home care? *Med J Aust* 1998;168:277-80.

31 Sharma R, Loomis W, Brown RB. Impact of mandatory inpatient infectious disease consultation on outpatient parenteral antibiotic therapy. *Am J Med Sci* 2005;330:60-4.

32 Heintz BH, Halilovic J, Christensen CL. Impact of a multidisciplinary team review of potential outpatient parenteral antimicrobial therapy prior to discharge from an academic medical centre. *Ann Pharmacother* 2011;45:1329-37.

33 Shrestha NK, Bhaskaran A, Scalera NM, Schmitt SK, Rehm SJ, Gordon SM. Contribution of infectious disease consultation toward the care of inpatients being considered for community-based parenteral anti-infective therapy. *J Hosp Med* 2012;7:365-9.

34 Nathwani D, Zambrowski JJ. Advisory group on home-based and outpatient care (AdHOC): an international consensus statement on non-inpatient parenteral therapy. *Clin Microbiol Infect* 2000;6:464-76.

35 Department of Health. Antimicrobial stewardship: start smart—then focus. DH, 2011. http://e-opat.com/wp-content/uploads/2012/07/DH-guidance-on-Antimicrobial-Stewardship-Start-Smart-then-Focus-Nov11.pdf.

Related links

bmj.com

- Diagnosis and management of carotid atherosclerosis (2013;346:f1485)
- Achilles tendon disorders (2013;346:f1262)
- Malignant and premalignant lesions of the penis (2013;346:f1149)
- Postpartum management of hypertension (2013;346:f894)
- Diagnosis and management of pulmonary embolism (2013;346:f757)
- Anaphylaxis: the acute episode and beyond (2013;346:f602)

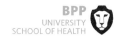

BMJ   BPP UNIVERSITY SCHOOL OF HEALTH

Management of people with diabetes wanting to fast during Ramadan

E Hui, specialist registrar[1], V Bravis, academic research fellow[1],
M Hassanein, consultant physician[2], W Hanif, consultant physician[3],
R Malik, professor of medicine[4], T A Chowdhury, consultant physician[5],
M Suliman, consultant physician[6], D Devendra, consultant community diabetologist[1][7]

[1]Department of Investigative Science, Imperial College London, London

[2]Department of Diabetes, Glan Clwyd Hospital, Rhyl

[3]Department of Diabetes and Endocrinology, University Hospital Birmingham, Birmingham

[4]Cardiovascular Research Group, University of Manchester, Manchester

[5]Department of Diabetes, Barts and the London NHS Trust, London

[6]Department of Medicine, Royal Preston Hospital, Preston

[7]Northwest London NHS Trust and Brent Community Services, London

Correspondence to: D Devendra, Jeffrey Kelson Diabetes Centre, Central Middlesex Hospital, London NW10 7NS d.devendra@imperial.ac.uk

Cite this as: *BMJ* 2010;340:c3053

DOI: 10.1136/bmj.c3053

http://www.bmj.com/content/340/bmj.c3053

The holy month of Ramadan is one of five main pillars of being a Muslim. Most Muslims are passionate about fasting during this month. Although the Koran exempts sick people from the duty of fasting,[1][2] many Muslims with diabetes may not perceive themselves as sick and are keen to fast. A large epidemiological study of Muslims with diabetes in 13 Muslim countries (n=12914)—the EPIDIAR study—showed that 43% of patients with type 1 and 79% of those with type 2 diabetes fasted during Ramadan.[3]

As the month of Ramadan follows the lunar calendar, the fasting month is brought forward by about 10 days each year, which means that over time the season in which Ramadan falls changes. For the next decade Ramadan will fall in the summer in the northern hemisphere. As daylight hours vary considerably between summer and winter months in non-equatorial countries, the length of the fast (which lasts from dawn to sunset) increases in the summer (to about 16-20 hours). People with diabetes who fast are at risk of adverse events, and the risks may increase with longer fasting periods. We review the evidence for optimum management of diabetic patients who wish to fast during Ramadan, drawing on a small evidence base comprising randomised trials, non-randomised comparison studies, and observational studies. We combine this with recommendations based on expert consensus. To reduce complications experienced by diabetic patients who fast during Ramadan, health professionals should aim to educate Muslim patients about safe fasting, not only before Ramadan but also at their annual diabetic review and at diagnosis.

> **SOURCES AND SELECTION CRITERIA**
>
> We searched Embase, Medline, and the Cochrane Library from January 1970 to May 2010 for systematic reviews, randomised trials, large population based studies, case-control studies, observational studies, and published consensus statements. We used the search terms "Ramadan", "fasting", and "diabetes mellitus".

> **SUMMARY POINTS**
>
> - Ramadan is one of the five main pillars of Islam
> - Muslims are obliged to abstain from food and drink from dawn to sunset during the month of Ramadan
> - Muslims with diabetes may be exempted from fasting during Ramadan, although a high proportion fast
> - Patients with diabetes who fast risk hypoglycaemia, hyperglycaemia, and dehydration
> - Guidelines from the National Institute for Health and Clinical Excellence emphasise the importance of individualising care on the basis of patients' social, cultural, and religious needs
> - Diabetic patients who want to fast need an assessment before Ramadan and education to increase their awareness of the risks of fasting

What does fasting during Ramadan involve?

Fasting during Ramadan involves abstaining from food and drink from dawn to sunset for about 30 days. Most people take two meals a day during Ramadan—suhur (the meal before dawn) and iftar (the meal after sunset).

What are the risks of fasting for people with diabetes?

Most Muslim religious authorities accept that if a person is advised by a trusted health professional (such as a doctor or nurse) that fasting is harmful to his or her health, then that person is exempted from fasting.[4] The risks of fasting include hypoglycaemia, hyperglycaemia, and dehydration. The EPIDIAR study found that the change in eating patterns during Ramadan increased the risk of severe hypoglycaemia 4.7-fold (from 3 to 14 events per 100 people per month) in type 1 diabetes and 7.5-fold (from 0.4 to 3 events per 100 people per month) in type 2 diabetes. It also found a fivefold increase in the incidence of severe hyperglycaemia in patients with type 2 diabetes during Ramadan. A small observational study (n=41) conducted in 1998 found an increase in symptomatic hypoglycaemia,[5] but other studies have not found a significant increase in the risk of hypoglycaemia during Ramadan in patients treated with oral hypoglycaemic medications or insulin.[6][7] One explanation for different findings among studies is that because Ramadan occurs in a different season every nine years, and the duration and temperature of fasting days change, rates of hypoglycaemia may vary according to the year in which the study was performed. The differences in methods and the small number of patients included in these studies would also explain the disparity of the results.

Over the coming decade, the number of fasting hours will progressively increase in the northern hemisphere as Ramadan falls in the summer months. This will have important implications for Muslims with diabetes who wish to fast.

How should patients with diabetes who fast for Ramadan be managed?

Assessment before Ramadan

Expert opinion recommends that if a patient has made it clear that they wish to fast during Ramadan their primary physicians and/or diabetes care specialists should assess whether they increase their health risk by doing so.[8] Box 1 outlines how patients planning to fast during Ramadan may be categorised as either high, moderate, or low risk of adverse events. Patients classed as high risk are advised not to fast as it can lead to worsening diabetes control, resulting in, for example, severe hypoglycaemia and diabetes ketoacidosis. Patients at moderate risk can reduce their level of risk if they see a healthcare professional several months before Ramadan and make necessary changes to their diabetes treatment. Those at low risk can fast without healthcare advice. Patients who choose to fast despite advice not to do so need support to help them fast as safely as possible.

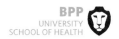

In case patients miss the opportunity for assessment before Ramadan, discussion with patients and provision of information packs (see the "Additional educational resources" box) that include advice on Ramadan fasting can be made available at diagnosis and also at annual diabetic review.

Ramadan focused education

Structured education interventions have been endorsed by the National Institute for Health and Clinical Excellence as important in empowering patients to improve their journey with diabetes. In a large observational study, patients who fasted during Ramadan without attending a structured education session had a fourfold increase in hypoglycaemic events, whereas those who attended an education programme focusing on Ramadan had a significant decrease in hypoglycaemic events.[9] We therefore recommend that Muslim patients with diabetes attend some form of structured education intervention to increase their chance of being well when fasting during Ramadan. Patients at high risk who plan to fast despite medical advice not to are also invited to attend structured education to support their self management and decision to fast. Box 2 outlines suggested content of Ramadan focused education.

How should fasting patients with type 2 diabetes be managed?

Patients taking oral hypoglycaemic agents

Metformin

Hypoglycaemia occurs in patients with type 2 diabetes taking metformin who are not fasting.[14] A systematic review reported that levels of risk for hypoglycaemia among people taking metformin who are not fasting range from 0% to 21%.[15] No data exist for the incidence of hypoglycaemia in people who fast for prolonged periods and take only metformin.

As iftar is usually the largest meal during Ramadan, expert consensus suggests that the metformin dose should be split such that two thirds of the dose is taken at iftar and one third at suhur (as the lunchtime dose during the daytime fast is not allowed). So for a regimen of, for example, metformin 500 mg three times a day, we recommend 500 mg at suhur and 1000 mg at iftar.

Acarbose

Acarbose inhibits the action of intestinal brush border alpha-glucosidases, which retards glucose absorption and modifies the secretion of insulin.[16] A randomised double blind study showed that the risk of hypoglycaemia is low with this class of drugs,[17] although we could not find any evidence that this is so during Ramadan. We suggest that it is acceptable to continue with the prescribed dose(s) of acarbose taken only with meals during fasting.

Rapid acting insulin secretogogues

An open label, multicentre, randomised study showed that repaglinide, a rapid acting insulin secretogogue, contributed to improved glycaemic control, with a lower number of hypoglycaemic events among fasting patients during Ramadan when compared with glibenclamide. Patients taking repaglinide lowered their fructosamine levels from baseline, and there were 0.03 hypoglycaemic events per patient per month in this group versus 0.05 events per patient per month in the glibenclamide group.[18]

A small study compared repaglinide (n=27) with a group of patients taking a sulphonylurea (glimepiride (n=23) or gliclazide (n=17)). Fructosamine, HbA1c, and body weight did not change significantly in either group from before to after Ramadan. Hypoglycaemia was documented in only one patient who took glimepiride during Ramadan.[19] The evidence cited suggests that rapid acting insulin secretogogues taken at suhur and iftar are a safer alternative than glibenclamide for patients who fast.

Sulphonylureas

Early studies examined the use of glibenclamide or glimepiride during Ramadan.[20] A more recent, large prospective observational study (n=332) showed that changing once daily glimepiride from a morning dose taken with breakfast before Ramadan to an evening dose taken at iftar during Ramadan did not alter rates of hypoglycaemia or glycaemic control.[21] However, the rate of hypoglycaemia in patients taking glimepiride in the mornings during Ramadan was not studied, so whether that rate is higher than the rate in those taking glimepiride in the evenings is unknown. The incidence of hypoglycaemic events did not differ between a group of patients taking once daily glimepiride (n=21) and a group taking twice daily repaglinide (n=20) (taken at suhur and iftar).[22] More recently, gliclazide has been compared with newer agents, such as dipeptidyl peptidase-4 inhibitors.[23]

On the basis of the prospective study by the GLIRA study group[21] we recommend that during Ramadan clinicians change the timing of the once daily dose of sulphonylurea (such as glimepiride) from the usual morning dose to the evening (at iftar). With regard to gliclazide, we recommend that patients take a larger dose at iftar than at suhur and that clinicians consider reducing the prescribed dose for suhur if the patient's glycaemic control before Ramadan is stable (for example, change gliclazide 160 mg twice daily to 80 mg in the morning and 160 mg in the evening).

Thiazolidenediones

A randomised controlled trial that compared pioglitazone 30 mg once daily with placebo in patients already taking other oral hypoglycaemic agents or alone, found no increase in hypoglycaemia during Ramadan fasting.[24] No studies have been reported on the use of rosiglitazone use during Ramadan. Continuing with thiazolidenediones during fasting is considered safe.

BOX 1 EXPERT RECOMMENDATIONS FOR RISK STRATIFICATION IN PATIENTS WITH TYPE 1 OR TYPE 2 DIABETES WHO FAST DURING RAMADAN[8]

Patients at high risk
- Those with severe and recurrent episodes of hypoglycaemia and unawareness
- Those with poor glycaemic control
- Those with ketoacidosis in the three months before Ramadan
- Those who experience hyperosmolar hyperglycaemic coma within the three months before Ramadan
- Those with acute illness
- Those who perform intense physical labour
- Pregnant women
- Those with comorbidities such as advanced macrovascular complications, renal disease on dialysis, cognitive dysfunction, uncontrolled epilepsy (particularly precipitated by hypoglycaemia)

Moderate risk
- Well controlled patients treated with short acting insulin secretogogue, sulphonylurea, insulin, or taking combination oral or oral plus insulin treatment

Low risk
- Well controlled patients treated with diet alone, monotherapy with metformin, dipeptidyl peptidase-4 inhibitors, or thiazolidinediones who are otherwise healthy

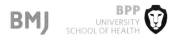

Dipeptidyl peptidase-4 inhibitors

A retrospective audit of Muslim patients with type 2 diabetes showed that adding vildagliptin to metformin treatment was associated with a reduced incidence of hypoglycaemic events and improved glucose control compared with patients treated with gliclazide and metformin during Ramadan.[23] This low grade evidence suggests that it may be safer to combine dipeptidyl peptidase-4 inhibitors, rather than sulphonylureas, with metformin in patients who are not well controlled when taking metformin alone and are planning to fast during Ramadan.

Glucagon-like peptide-1 mimetics

Glucagon-like peptide-1 mimetics are currently used in combination with other oral hypoglycaemic agents. In non-Ramadan studies, hypoglycaemic events associated with glucagon-like peptide-1 mimetics occurred primarily in patients taking a sulphonylurea.[25] The findings of an audit suggested that its dosage does not need to be adjusted during Ramadan but that other agents, such as sulphonylureas, may need dose reductions when used as a combination treatment.[26]

Patients taking insulin

Single basal insulin and oral combined treatment

A multicentre, prospective, observational study compared fasting patients taking metformin combined with glimepiride (n=21), repaglinide (n=18), or glargine (n=10).[7] Although the rate of hypoglycaemia was higher in the glimepiride group (14.3%) than in the repaglinide (11%) and glar-

gine (10%) groups, the increased rate was not significant. Glimepiride was given before iftar; repaglinide was given with both meals; and glargine at 10.00 pm. No studies have compared the incidence of hypoglycaemic events in patients taking insulin detemir or isophane insulin (NPH) (such as Insulatard, Novo Nordisk; or Humulin I, Lilly).

In a small prospective non-randomised study of 19 patients who had type 2 diabetes, were at low risk of diabetic complications, and had a pre-Ramadan HbA1c concentration of <8%, neither fasting (n=11) nor non-fasting (n=8) patients who were taking repaglinide three times a day and glargine experienced hypoglycaemic events, and both groups maintained stable glycaemic control.[6] Those who fasted took repaglinide at iftar, at midnight, and at suhur, and the doses of repaglinide and glargine remained unchanged throughout Ramadan. We advise patients who take long acting basal insulin, such as glargine, to reduce the dose by 20% to avoid hypoglycaemia. Patients taking repaglinide and single dose glargine may continue taking the same doses of repaglinide but to be safer should consider reducing glargine by 20%. The timing of repaglinide can be rearranged to coincide with suhur and iftar.

Premixed insulins

A randomised, open labelled, crossover study comparing Humalog Mix25 (Lilly) (25% short acting insulin lispro and 75% intermediate acting neutral lispro protamine) and Humulin M3 (Lilly) (human insulin 30% soluble, 70% isophane) given in identical doses showed that the former offered better control of postprandial blood glucose after iftar and a lower occurrence of hypoglycaemic events.[27] However, the findings of an observational study suggested that using Humalog Mix50 (Lilly) at ifta instead of Mix30 reduced postprandial glucose excursions and reduced hypoglycaemia.[28] We suggest that patients taking twice daily insulin should reduce the suhur dose by 30% if they are well controlled, and consider switching to a Mix 50 preparation if their postprandial glucose remains raised.

Is fasting safe for pregnant women with diabetes?

Pregnant women with diabetes, including gestational diabetes, are exempted from fasting and are strongly cautioned against fasting because clear maternal and fetal risks are associated with poor glycaemic control in pregnancy.[29] However, no outcome study of women with diabetes specifically related to Ramadan fasting has been conducted. Preconception counselling for diabetic Muslim women must include education about the substantial risks associated with poor glycaemic control to help to dissuade them from trying to fast.

How should fasting patients with type 1 diabetes be managed?

A small study examined the use of glargine and insulin lispro or aspart, divided in a 6:4 ratio of the total 24 hour insulin dose in nine patients with type 1 diabetes.[30] Of seven patients who started to fast, five continued for the whole month, and two broke the fast owing to hypoglycaemia. None of the patients had any episodes of severe hypoglycaemia or diabetic ketoacidosis requiring admission to hospital, and the patients' HbA1c concentrations remained stable at the end of Ramadan. As the insulin requirement in this study group decreased by 28% from baseline (P=0.002), the authors suggested a reduced dose (70% of a patient's usual dose) during the fast.

BOX 2 FOUR KEY AREAS IN RAMADAN FOCUSED EDUCATION[9]

Meal planning and dietary advice

- The diet during Ramadan should be a healthy balanced diet
- Slow energy release foods (such as wheat, semolina, beans, rice) should be taken before and after fasting, whereas foods high in saturated fat (such as ghee, samosas, and pakoras) should be minimised[10]
- Advise patients to use only a small amount of monounsaturated oils (such as rapeseed or olive oil) in cooking
- Before and after fasting include high fibre foods such as wholegrain cereals, granary bread, brown rice; beans and pulses; fruit, vegetables, and salads

Exercise

- Regular light and moderate exercise is safe in type 2 diabetes patients[11]
- Rigorous exercise is not recommended as the risk of hypoglycaemia may be increased, particularly in patients taking sulphonylureas or insulin
- Encourage patients to continue their usual physical activity, especially during non-fasting periods
- Tarawaih prayers (a series of prayers after the sunset meal) should be considered as part of the daily exercise regimen as they involve standing, bowing, prostrating, and sitting

Blood glucose monitoring

- Blood glucose monitoring does not constitute the break of fast[12]
- All patients who fast should be provided with the means to monitor their blood glucose[13]
- Capillary blood glucose testing should be done when:
- -The patient suspects they have symptoms of hypoglycaemia (subjective to the individual). Patients should be advised to break their fast if hypoglycaemia is confirmed on blood glucose testing
- -The patient is unwell (eg has a fever)
- Testing at other times may be useful only if patients are able and willing to adjust their diabetes treatment regimens, such as insulin dosage titration

Recognising and managing complications

- Patients should be aware of the warning symptoms of dehydration, hypoglycaemia, and hyperglycaemia and should stop the fast as soon as any complications or acute illness occur

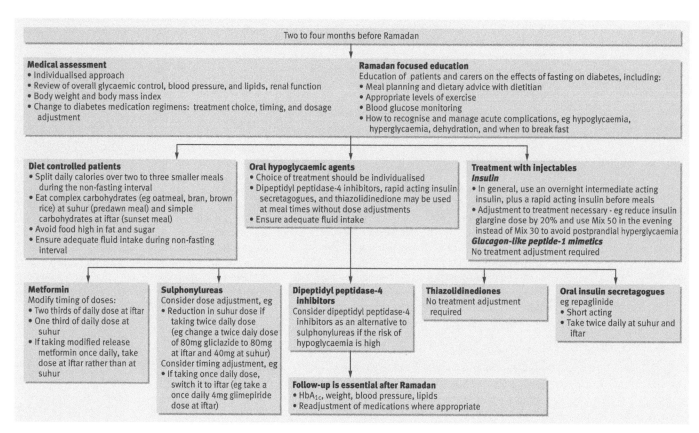

An approach to oral treatment of type 2 diabetes during Ramadan for patients planning to fast

An open label, comparative, crossover study of 64 patients with type 1 diabetes found significantly lower (P=0.026) two hour, postprandial glucose concentrations after iftar and fewer hypoglycaemic events with insulin lispro than with regular human insulin.[31] In both arms isophane insulin (Humulin I) was given as the basal insulin.

Most studies of patients with type 1 diabetes have comprised small numbers of patients and some have excluded adolescents, elderly patients, or patients with comorbidities such as renal impairment. Suggested treatments, therefore, may not be generalised to all fasting patients with type 1 diabetes, and no good evidence exists to allow us to give clear guidance for those who are not on a basal bolus regimen (basal insulins are intermediate or long acting insulins; bolus is rapid acting insulin taken with meals).

We suggest that patients with type 1 diabetes who are on a basal bolus regimen four times daily should be discouraged from fasting owing to the risks of poor glycaemic control. If patients choose to fast despite medical advice, it will help if they are familiar with carbohydrate counting. We suggest they reduce their background insulin by 20% and omit the midday rapid acting insulin if their capillary blood glucose concentration is ≤7 mmol/l. If their blood glucose concentration is >7 mmol/l, patients will need to calculate their insulin correction dose as determined by their specialists.

Conclusion

The figure summarises the recommendations given in this article, based on the best available and most current evidence and on our collective experience in managing patients who fast during Ramadan. Overall, the evidence available for guiding management of patients with diabetes who wish to fast during Ramadan is poor, and well designed studies

are lacking. An assessment of a patient's individual risk and a tailored approach to treatment seems to be the best management strategy. Offering structured education to enable patients to manage their condition better themselves during Ramadan is essential.

ADDITIONAL EDUCATIONAL RESOURCES

For healthcare professionals

- Al-Arouj M, Bouguerra R, Buse J, Hafez S, Hassanein M, Ibrahim MA, et al. American Diabetes Association recommendations for management of diabetes during Ramadan. *Diabetes Care* 2005;28:2305-11

- Karamat MA, Syed A, Hanif W. Review of diabetes management and guidelines during Ramadan. *J R Soc Med* 2010;103:139-47.

- Benaji B, Mounib N, Roky R, Aadil N, Houti IE, Moussamih S, et al. Diabetes and Ramadan: review of the literature. *Diabetes Res Clin Pract* 2006;73:117-25.

- Ramadan health factsheet 2009 (from Muslim Spiritual Care Provision in the NHS, PO box 57330, London E1 2WJ; nhsspiritualcare@mcb.org.uk)—Provides a brief summary of issues for doctors, healthcare staff, and patients

For patients

- LeicestershireDiabetes (www.leicestershirediabetes.org.uk)—Website with information on fasting and insulin treatment during Ramadan

- United Kingdom Ramadan Diabetes Network (www.ukRamadandiabetes.net)—Has a useful publication on diabetes and fasting

- Ramadan health guide: a guide to healthy fasting. 2007. www.ramadan.co.uk/RamadhanHealth_Guide.pdf (Useful Department of Health document on healthy fasting, but not specifically about diabetes)

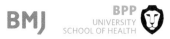

Contributors: DD had the idea for the article. EH and VB did the literature search and wrote the first draft. MH, WH, RM, TAC, MS, and DD redrafted the article and produced the final draft. DD and MH are the guarantors.

Funding: No special funding.

Competing interests: All authors have completed the Unified Competing Interest form at www.icmje.org/coi_disclosure.pdf (available on request from the corresponding author) and declare that (1) No authors have support from any company for the submitted work; (2) MS had speaker honorariums with Novo Nordisk and MSD; DD had speaker honorariums and research grants with Lilly, Novartis, and Daichii Sankyo that might have an interest in the submitted work in the previous 3 years; (3) their spouses, partners, or children have no financial relationships that may be relevant to the submitted work; and (4) All authors have no non-financial interests that may be relevant to the submitted work.

Provenance and peer review: Not commissioned; externally peer reviewed.

1   Rashed AH. The fast of Ramadan. *BMJ* 1992;304:521-2.
2   Koran 2:183-5.
3   Salti I, Be'nard E, Detournay B, Bianchi-Biscay M, Le Brigand C, Voinet C, et al. Results of the Epidemiology of Diabetes and Ramadan 1422/2001 (EPIDIAR) study. *Diabetes Care* 2004;27:2306-11.
4   Beshyah SA. Fasting during the month of Ramadan for people with diabetes: medicine and Fiqh united at last. *Ibnosina Journal of Medicine and Biomedical Sciences* 2009;1:58-60.
5   Uysal A, Erdogan MF, Sahin G, Kamel N, Erdogan G. Clinical and metabolic effects of fasting in 41 type 2 patients during Ramadan. *Diabetes Care* 1998;21:2033-34.
6   Bakiner O, Ertorer ME, Bozkirli E, Tutuncu NB, Demirag NG. Repaglinide plus single-dose insulin glargine: a safe regimen for low-risk type 2 diabetic patients who insist on fasting in Ramadan. *Acta Diabetologia* 2009;46:63-5.
7   Cesur M, Corapcioglu D, Gursoy A, Gonen S, Ozduman M, Emral R, et al. A comparison of glycemic effects of glimepiride, repaglinide, and insulin glargine in type 2 diabetes mellitus during Ramadan fasting. *Diabetes Research and Clinical Practice* 2007;75:141-7.
8   Al-Arouj M, Bouguerra R, Buse J, Hafez S, Hassanein M, Ibrahim MA, et al. American Diabetes Association recommendations for management of diabetes during Ramadan. *Diabetes Care* 2005;28:2305-11.
9   Bravis V, Hui E, Salih S, Mehar S, Hassanein M, Devendra D. Ramadan education and awareness in diabetes programme for Muslims with type 2 diabetes who fast during Ramadan. *Diabetes Medicine* 2010;27:327-31.
10   Mojaddidi M, Hassanein M, Malik R. Ramadan and diabetes: evidence-based guidelines. *Prescriber* 2006;Sep:38-41.
11   Benaji B, Mounib N, Roky R, Aadil N, Houti IE, Moussamih S, et al. Diabetes and Ramadan: review of the literature. *Diabetes Res Clin Pract* 2006;73:117-25.
12   Muslim Spiritual Care Division in the NHS. Ramadan Health Factsheet 2009. A project of the Muslim Council in Partnership with the department of Health. Available from Muslim Spiritual Care Provision in the NHS, PO box 57330, London E1 2WJ; nhsspiritualcare@mcb.org.uk
13   National Institute for Health and Clinical Excellence. Type 2 diabetes—newer agents (partial update of CG66). (Clincal guideline 87.) 2009. http://guidance.nice.org.uk/CG87.
14   UK Prospective Diabetes Study (UKPDS) Group. Effect of intensive blood-glucose control with metformin on complications in overweight patients with type 2 diabetes (UKPDS 34). *Lancet* 1998;352:854-65.
15   Bolen S, Feldman L, Vassy J, Wilson L, Yeh HC, Marinopoulos S, et al. Systematic review: comparative effectiveness and safety of oral medications for type 2 diabetes mellitus. *Ann Intern Med* 2007;147:386-99.
16   Rosak C, Mertes G. Effects of acarbose on proinsulin and insulin secretion and their potential significance for the intermediary metabolism and cardiovascular system. *Current Diabetes Review* 2009;5:157-64.
17   Pan C, Yang W, Barona JP, Wang Y, Niggli M, Mohideen P, et al. Comparison of vildagliptin and acarbose monotherapy in patients with type 2 diabetes: a 24-week, double-blind, randomized trial. *Diabetes Medicine* 2008;25:435-41.
18   Mafauzy M. Repaglinide versus glibenclamide treatment of type 2 diabetes during Ramadan fasting. *Diabetes Res Clin Pract* 2002;58(1):45-53.
19   Sari R, Balci MK, Akbas SH, Avci B. The effects of diet, sulfonylurea and repaglinide therapy on clinical and metabolic parameters in type 2 diabetic patients during Ramadan. *Endocrine Research* 2004;30:169-77.
20   Belkhadir J, El-Ghomari H, Klocker N, Mikou A, Nasciri M, Sabri M. Muslims with noninsulin-dependent diabetes fasting during Ramadan: treatment with glibenclamide. *BMJ* 1993;307:292-5.
21   Glimeperide in Ramadan (GLIRA) Study Group. The efficacy and safety of glimepiride in the management of type 2 diabetes in Muslim patients during Ramadan. *Diabetes Care* 2005;28:421-422.
22   Anwar A, Azmi KN, Hamidon BB, Khalid BA. An open label comparative study of glimepiride versus repaglinide in type 2 diabetes mellitus Muslim subjects during the month of Ramadan. *Medical Journal of Malaysia* 2006;61:28-35.
23   Devendra D, Gohel B, Bravis V, Hui E, Salih S, Mehar S, et al. Vildagliptin therapy and hypoglycaemia in Muslim type 2 diabetes patients during Ramadan. *Int J Clin Pract* 2009;63:1446-50.
24   Vasan S, Thomas N, Bharani, Ameen M, Abraham S, Job V, et al. A double-blind, randomized, multicenter study evaluating the effects of pioglitazone in fasting Muslim subjects during Ramadan. *Int J Diabetes Dev Ctries* 2006;26:70-6.
25   Norris SL, Lee N, Thakurta S, Chan BKS. Exenatide efficacy and safety: a systematic review. *Diabetes Medicine* 2009;26:837-46.
26   Bravis V, Hui E, Salih S, Hassanein M, Devendra D. A comparative analysis of exenatide and gliclazide during the month of Ramadan. *Diabetic Medicine* 2010;27(suppl 1):130.
27   Mattoo V, Milicevic Z, Malone JK, Schwarzenhofer M, Ekangaki A, Levitt LK, et al. A comparison of insulin lispro Mix25 and human insulin 30/70 in the treatment of type 2 diabetes during Ramadan. Ramadan Study Group. *Diabetes Res Clin Pract* 2003;59:137-43.
28   Hui E, Bravis V, Salih S, Hassanein M, Devendra D. Comparison of Humalog Mix 50 with human insulin Mix 30 in type 2 diabetes patients during Ramadan. *Int J Clin Pract* 2010;March 10 (epub ahead of print; www3.interscience.wiley.com/journal/123318627/abstract).
29   Metzger BE, Lowe LP, Dyer AR, Trimble ER, Charovarindr U, Coustan DR, et al. Hyperglycemia and adverse pregnancy outcomes. *New Engl J Med* 2008;358:1991-2002.
30   Azar ST, Khairallah WG, Merheb MT, Zantout MS, Fliti F. Insulin therapy during Ramadan fast for patients with type 1 diabetes mellitus. *Journal Medical Libanais* 2008;56(1):46.
31   Kadiri A, Al-Nakhi A, El-Ghazali S, Jabbar A, Al Arouj M, Akram J, et al. Treatment of type 1 diabetes with insulin lispro during Ramadan. *Diabetes Metabolism* 2001;27:482-6.

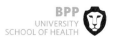

Assessment and management of non-visible haematuria in primary care

John D Kelly, senior lecturer[1], Derek P Fawcett, consultant urologist[2],
Lawrence C Goldberg, consultant nephrologist[3]

[1]Department of Oncology, Cambridge University, Addenbrooke's Hospital, Cambridge CB2 0QQ

[2]Harold Hopkins Department of Urology, Royal Berkshire Hospital, Reading RG1 5AN

[3]Sussex Kidney Unit, Brighton and Sussex University Hospitals NHS Trust, Royal Sussex County Hospital, Brighton BN2 5BE

Correspondence to: J D Kelly jk334@cam.ac.uk

Cite this as: BMJ 2008;337:a3021

DOI: 10.1136/bmj.a3021

http://www.bmj.com/content/338/bmj.a3021

Many clinicians are not sure what constitutes clinically relevant haematuria; they are also unsure about when patients with haematuria should be referred for specialist assessment and whether they should be referred to a urologist, nephrologist, or both.

In 2006 the National Institute for Health Research, Health Technology Assessment (NIHR HTA) commissioned a systematic review of the evidence for the investigation of microscopic haematuria, with a view to developing an algorithm for assessing patients in primary care.[1] They concluded that, "Given the paucity of evidence . . . it is not possible to derive an algorithm of the diagnostic pathway for haematuria that would be solely supported by existing evidence." None the less, the investigation of microscopic haematuria is important because serious underlying conditions are present in a proportion of patients.

In the absence of definitive evidence, guidelines based on consensus agreement and expert opinion would be useful and have been proposed.[3][4] However, the terminology and definitions used have not been standardised, so the appropriate baseline assessment of patients is still unclear. In this review, we discuss the rationale for introducing the terms "visible haematuria" and "non-visible haematuria" (symptomatic and asymptomatic) (box 1). The figure shows an algorithm for the assessment of patients with non-visible haematuria.

What causes non-visible haematuria?
The presence of non-visible blood in the urine can have a transient or spurious cause; if it persists it may indicate underlying pathology.

Causes of transient non-visible haematuria
The causes of transient non-visible haematuria should be considered and excluded before further assessment (box 2). Transient non-visible haematuria is commonly associated with urinary tract infection, and a repeat dipstick test after treatment for infection will determine whether haematuria is persistent. Urinary tract infection can be the first presentation of important urinary pathology, so recurrent infections are an indication for further investigation, regardless of haematuria.[5][6] Observational studies in

SOURCES AND SELECTION CRITERIA
We drew on evidence published in the systematic reviews of the National Institute for Health and Clinical Excellence, Health Technology Assessment (microscopic haematuria),[1] and guidelines for the early diagnosis and management of chronic kidney disease.[1][2] We searched electronic databases, including Medline and the Cochrane database, to identify recent publications and studies that were deemed relevant but outside the inclusion criteria of the systematic review. We included the evidence presented in published guidelines for the investigation of haematuria published by the American Urological Association and the Scottish Intercollegiate Guidelines Network.

athletes confirm that repeated foot striking, such as in long distance running, can cause haematuria,[7] and urine testing should be repeated at least three days after such activity.

Spurious causes
Menstruation can lead to urinary contamination with erythrocytes, so testing when menstruation has ended is recommended. Discoloration of urine (by drugs or foods) and myoglobin released from necrotic muscle cells (rhabdomyolysis) are other considerations when haematuria is detected on dipstick testing.[8]

Causes of persistent non-visible haematuria
Persistent non-visible haematuria can have urological or nephrological causes (box 3). The most important urological causes include cancer and calculus disease, which are seen in about 5% and 8% of patients, respectively.[9][10] Urothelial cell carcinoma is the most common cancer detected. It is present in about 4% of cases overall but is more prevalent in males and increases with age to 10% in men over 60 with risk factors for disease.[9][10] In young people (<40 years), especially young females, cancer is an uncommon cause of asymptomatic non-visible haematuria, and a glomerular cause is more likely. It is unclear what proportion of patients with haematuria have nephrological as opposed to urological haematuria, because many patients with negative urological investigations do not have a renal biopsy. However, the most common causes are IgA nephropathy and thin membrane nephropathy.[11]

How common is non-visible haematuria and should testing for haematuria be performed routinely?
Non-visible haematuria is present in about 2.5% of the general population, although it can be as high as 20%, depending on features of the study population, such as age, sex, the presence of risk factors for disease, and the definition used.[12][13][14] Within cohorts of patients with asymptomatic non-visible haematuria detected by screening, the overall incidence of serious conditions such as urological malignancy is <1.5%,[12] so the consensus is that population screening is not warranted. In contrast, a cause for non-visible haematuria is found in about 15% of cases selected for referral from primary care to haematuria

SUMMARY POINTS
- The terms visible haematuria should replace macroscopic or gross haematuria, and non-visible haematuria (both symptomatic and asymptomatic) should replace microscopic haematuria or dipstick positive haematuria
- Urine testing for haematuria should be performed for clinical reasons only—current evidence does not support opportunistic testing
- The test of choice for diagnosing haematuria is urine dipstick analysis—scores of ≥1+ are positive
- Transient or spurious causes of haematuria need to be excluded
- All patients aged ≥40 with haematuria should be investigated for urological disease
- All patients with no identified urological cause should be monitored long term

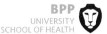

clinics.[9] [10] These cases will usually have had an indication for urine testing, such as urinary tract symptoms.[15] There is currently no evidence to support opportunistic testing for haematuria without a clinical reason.

How should we test for non-visible haematuria in primary care?

Urine dipstick

Chemical dipsticks detect haem (intact red cells, free haemoglobin, or free myoglobin); they provide an instant result and are used to detect non-visible haematuria in primary care.[10] Chemical dipsticks are available from several manufacturers and are read visually or using automated systems on a semi-quantitative scale. Although it is difficult to interpret studies on the efficiency of this test because of inherent design and reporting bias, analysis of pooled data sets indicates that it is a reasonable way to detect non-visible haematuria in primary care (positive likelihood ratio 5.99 (95% confidence interval 4.04 to 8.89), negative likelihood ratio 0.21 (0.17 to 0.26)).[1] The detection of trace haematuria can be considered negative because the threshold for significance is probably less than three to five red blood cells per high power field.[16] A positive result in a haemolysed sample should be treated the same as in a non-haemolysed sample because we have no evidence that the clinical relevance differs.

Urine microscopy

Red blood cell counts have been used to define microscopic haematuria, and cut-off points have varied (including ≥2 cells per high power field and ≥5 cells per high power field).[17] [18] Microscopy provides an accurate measure of red blood cells when assessed by trained technicians or nephrologists in fresh voided early morning midstream specimens of urine.[19] [20] However, time to analysis affects the integrity of red blood cells.[21] In a prospective multicentre study, red blood cell counts dropped by 5-9% at five hours, 11-28% at 24 hours, and 29-35% at 72 hours.[22] Because immediate microscopy is not feasible in primary care, the accuracy of quantitative red blood cell microscopy is questionable. In general practice, it is therefore not logical, and rarely necessary, to validate dipstick haematuria by urine microscopy.

BOX 1 NEW TERMINOLOGY FOR HAEMATURIA AND ITS DIAGNOSIS

Terminology
- Visible haematuria—replaces macroscopic and gross haematuria
- Non-visible haematuria—replaces microscopic and dipstick positive haematuria
- Symptomatic non-visible haematuria—non-visible haematuria plus lower urinary tract symptoms (hesitancy, frequency, urgency, dysuria) or upper urinary tract symptoms
- Asymptomatic non-visible haematuria—incidental detection of non-visible haematuria in the absence of upper or lower urinary tract symptoms

Diagnosis of haematuria
- Exclude transient causes, such as urinary tract infection, before further assessment
- A urine dipstick test for blood is generally sufficient. It is sensitive when performed on fresh voided urine with no preservatives. A score of ≥1+ is positive; a trace amount is considered negative
- A positive result for haemolysed red blood cells should be treated the same as for non-haemolysed red cells
- Further assessment is warranted in patients with urinary tract symptoms and non-visible haematuria and a score of ≥1+ on a single blood dipstick test
- In patients with asymptomatic non-visible haematuria confirm persistence of blood in at least two out of three dipstick tests
- It is not necessary to confirm the dipstick result by microscopy

---

BOX 2 TRANSIENT OR SPURIOUS NON-VISIBLE HAEMATURIA

Transient
- Urinary tract infection
- Exercise related

Spurious
- Menstrual contamination
- Sexual intercourse
- Foods such as beetroot, blackberries, and rhubarb
- Rhabdomyolysis
- Drugs such as doxorubicin, chloroquine, and rifampicin
- Chronic lead or mercury poisoning

BOX 3 CAUSES OF PERSISTENT NON-VISIBLE HAEMATURIA

Urological causes

Common
- Benign prostatic hyperplasia
- Cancer (bladder, kidney, prostate, ureter)
- Calculus disease or nephrolithiasis
- Cystitis or pyelonephritis
- Prostatitis or urethritis
- *Schistosoma haematobium* infection

Less common
- Radiation cystitis
- Urethral strictures
- Tuberculosis
- Medullary sponge kidney
- Cyclophosphamide induced cystitis

Rare
- Arteriovenous malformation
- Renal artery thrombosis
- Polycystic kidney disease
- Papillary necrosis of any cause
- Loin pain haematuria syndrome

Nephrological causes

Common
- IgA nephropathy (Berger's disease)
- Thin basement membrane disease

Less common
- Acute glomerular disease:
- Postinfectious glomerulonephritis
- Rapidly progressive glomerulonephritis
- Systemic lupus nephritis
- Vasculitis
- Goodpasture's disease
- Henoch-Schönlein purpura syndrome
- Haemolytic-uraemic syndrome
- Chronic primary glomerulonephritis:
- Focal segmental glomerulonephritis
- Mesangio-capillary glomerulonephritis
- Membranous nephropathy
- Mesangial proliferative glomerulonephritis
- Familial causes:
- Polycystic kidney disease (autosomal dominant or recessive)
- Hereditary nephritis (Alport's syndrome)
- Fabry's disease
- Nail-patella syndrome

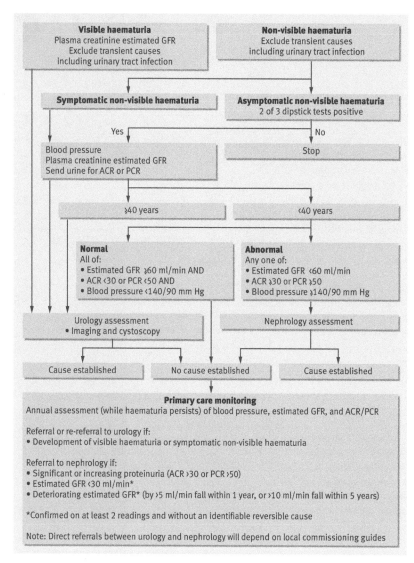

Decision algorithm for the investigation of non-visible haematuria and the referral criteria adopted by the British Association of Urological Surgeons and the Renal Association. GFR, glomerular filtration rate; PCR, protein:creatinine ratio; ACR, albumin:creatinine ratio

How can glomerular haematuria be distinguished from urinary tract haematuria?

Urine microscopy for red cell morphology and casts

The detection of red cell casts is virtually pathognomonic for a glomerular pathology. Casts are fragile, however, and can be very rare or absent even when glomerular disease is present. The test therefore has low sensitivity, particularly for routine samples sent from primary or secondary care clinics to the laboratory.

The relevance of dysmorphic red cells as indicators of glomerular disease is unclear. Samples often contain a mixture of isomorphic (normal shaped) and dysmorphic cells, and the term dysmorphic includes cells with a variety of different shapes. In an observational study to evaluate urinary particles, the presence of acanthocytes (erythrocytes with ring form blebs) was significantly associated with glomerular disease, but other shapes did not distinguish renal disease from urological disease.[23] Urine microscopy relies on the examination of fresh urine by a skilled person and is most useful in specialist clinics rather than as a screening test in primary care.

Proteinuria

Proteinuria is a marker of glomerular damage, particularly as the amount of protein increases (low amounts can result from tubular disease or dysfunction). The presence of proteinuria and haematuria increases the likelihood that the underlying disease is glomerular and is an indication for a referral to the nephrology department.[24] The threshold for significant proteinuria in the presence of non-visible haematuria is 0.5 g/d and equivalent to a protein:creatinine ratio ≥50 mg/mmol or albumin:creatinine ratio ≥30 mg/mmol (NICE guidelines).

Hypertension

Renal disease is strongly associated with hypertension,[25] and it must be considered in patients with hypertension and non-visible haematuria. However, the prevalence of essential hypertension increases with age and hypertension is often an unrelated comorbidity.[26] It is of most discriminatory use in people under 40, where the prevalence of hypertension is low, as is the risk of urological malignancy.[9] [10]

Do anticoagulants and antiplatelet agents cause haematuria?

Visible haematuria in patients taking warfarin or aspirin is caused by underlying pathology in up to 25% of cases.[27] Few detailed studies have assessed non-visible haematuria in patients taking these drugs. In a subgroup analysis of a prospective randomised trial to determine the effects of warfarin and aspirin on the heart, non-visible haematuria was detected in about 10% of patients taking the drugs, and an underlying cause including bladder cancer was detected in 10% of cases.[28] Although not adjusted for age and other risk factors, the incidence of non-visible haematuria in anticoagulated patients is similar to non-anticoagulated patients, and bleeding cannot be attributed solely to these agents.

What level of non-visible haematuria warrants further investigation?

The term non-visible haematuria best describes a clinical entity and avoids the uncertainties of either microscopic or dipstick test definitions. We define symptomatic non-visible haematuria as haematuria in patients with voiding lower urinary tract symptoms—hesitancy, frequency, urgency, dysuria, and loin or suprapubic pain in the absence of a transient cause such as urinary tract infection. A single symptomatic episode should prompt further assessment—in these patients serious pathology is more likely to be present and may cause intermittent bleeding. Asymptomatic non-visible haematuria is haematuria in the absence of these symptoms. When incidental haematuria is detected in asymptomatic patients it must be confirmed as persistent in two of three isolated dipstick tests assessed at an interval of two to three weeks. Patients with asymptomatic disease are least likely to have an underlying urological condition, especially if they are under 40 years.

Who should patients be referred to?

Primary referral

A urological cause is more likely in patients with either visible haematuria or symptomatic non-visible haematuria, whatever their age, and all those with symptomatic non-visible haematuria aged 40 or more.[9] [10] In all these cases,

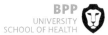

initial referral to urology is important to exclude malignancy. An exception is young adults who present with cola coloured (rather than red or pink) urine, particularly after a respiratory tract infection, who are more likely to have acute glomerulonephritis than urological disease.

Patients under 40 with asymptomatic non-visible haematuria are more likely to have renal rather than urological disease, particularly IgA nephropathy or thin membrane disease.[11] A urology referral is unnecessary in such patients, and a specialist nephrology opinion is often not required either. A definitive diagnosis requires renal biopsy, and unless the management of the patient would be altered by such a diagnosis, it is hard to justify the

associated risks. In patients under 40, only the presence of other risk factors for severe glomerulonephritis should trigger a specialist nephrology assessment, namely:

- Proteinuria ≥0.5 g/d (albumin:creatinine ratio ≥30 mg/mmol or protein:creatinine ratio ≥50 mg/mmol)
- Estimated glomerular filtration rate <60 ml/min
- Hypertension.

Management after negative urological investigations and long term follow-up

If no abnormalities are found on initial assessment, routine urological follow-up is not needed.[29] Patients with haematuria need a nephrological assessment if they have or develop manifestations of kidney disease, namely[24]:

- Evidence of deteriorating renal function (fall in estimated glomerular filtration rate of >5 ml/min within previous year or >10 ml/min any time within past five years)
- Chronic kidney disease stage 4 or 5 (estimated glomerular filtration rate <30 ml/min)
- Proteinuria (≥0.5 g/d).

The development or presence of hypertension in people over 40 is not a good discriminator because of the increasing prevalence of essential hypertension with age, although it should be checked routinely.

Persistent non-visible haematuria needs to be followed up, usually in primary care. Important but undiagnosed urological disease may become more apparent through the development of urinary tract symptoms in previously asymptomatic patients or the development of visible haematuria.[29] If haematuria is caused by low grade chronic glomerulonephritis (such as IgA nephropathy), this may progress over time and result in new or increasing proteinuria or worsening renal function (or both).[30][31] Patients should therefore have at least an annual review to check for new symptoms and measure the estimated glomerular filtration rate, urinary protein, and blood pressure. The algorithm (figure) lists criteria for referral or re-referral.

The joint working party of the British Association of Urological Surgeons and the Renal Association that developed the haematuria guidelines on which this article is based consisted of the authors and John Anderson, consultant urologist, Royal Hallamshire Hospital, Sheffield; John Feehally, professor of nephrology, Leicester General Hospital; and Robert MacTier, consultant nephrologist, Glasgow Royal Infirmary.

Contributors: DF had the idea for the article and helped write the review. JK and LG searched the literature and wrote the review. JK is guarantor.

Funding: No special funding.

Competing interests: None declared.

Provenance and peer review: Offered and encouraged but not commissioned; externally peer reviewed.

INITIAL INVESTIGATIONS FOR PATIENTS WITH SYMPTOMATIC NON-VISIBLE HAEMATURIA AND PERSISTENT ASYMPTOMATIC NON-VISIBLE HAEMATURIA

- Measure plasma creatinine and estimated glomerular filtration rate
- Measure proteinuria—send a random sample of urine for protein:creatinine ratio or albumin:creatinine ratio (according to local practice). Twenty four hour urine collections for protein are rarely needed—24 hour urine protein or albumin excretion (in mg) can be approximated by multiplying the ratio (in mg/mmol) by 10
- Measure blood pressure

TIPS FOR NON-SPECIALISTS

- Non-visible haematuria can be an indication of an underlying nephrological or urological condition, but exclude transient causes (such as urinary tract infection) or spurious causes (such as menstruation) before investigating
- Baseline assessment of renal function (estimated glomerular filtration rate), proteinuria, and blood pressure are recommended before referring from primary to secondary care
- All patients with visible or non-visible haematuria who have urinary tract symptoms should be referred for urological assessment
- Patients aged ≥40 with asymptomatic non-visible haematuria should be referred for urological assessment
- Patients under 40 with asymptomatic non-visible haematuria need urological assessment only if the estimated glomerular filtration rate is reduced (<60 ml/min) or proteinuria is >0.5 g/d
- Patients with no abnormal findings on urological assessment need long term observation, usually in primary care. Patients should be reassessed if they develop visible haematuria or urinary tract symptoms. Nephrology assessment is recommended for falling renal function or new or increasing proteinuria

---

ADDITIONAL EDUCATIONAL RESOURCES

- Rodgers M, Nixon J, Hempel S, Aho T, Kelly J, Neal D, et al. *Diagnostic tests and algorithms used in the investigation of haematuria: systematic reviews and economic evaluation.* 2006. www.hta.ac.uk/execsumm/summ1018.shtml
- National Institute for Health and Clinical Excellence. *Referral for suspected cancer.* 2005. www.nice.org.uk/guidance/index.jsp?action=byID&o=10968
- Joint Specialty Committee on Renal Medicine of the Royal College of Physicians of London and the Renal Association. *Chronic kidney disease in adults: UK guidelines for identification, management and referral.* 2006. www.rcplondon.ac.uk/pubs/contents/54942fe5-ef23-4dc7-aeb8-ed60354ffb23.pdf
- NHS. *Urology: 18 week commissioning pathway.* 2008. www.18weeks.nhs.uk/Content.aspx?path=/achieve-and-sustain/Specialty-focussed-areas/Urology
- National Institute for Health and Clinical Excellence. Chronic kidney disease guidelines. 2008. www.nice.org.uk/Guidance/CG73

FUTURE RESEARCH

- Is targeted screening for haematuria effective in at risk populations, such as smokers and those with a history of occupational exposure to chemicals, urological disease, urinary tract infection, analgesic abuse, and pelvic irradiation?
- Future studies that define whether patients have symptomatic or asymptomatic non-visible haematuria may help redefine the indications for referral and appropriate assessment of patients with asymptomatic non-visible haematuria
- Is there an appropriate threshold for semi-quantitative dipstick analysis of non-visible haematuria in symptomatic and asymptomatic cases?
- How do new preservation fluids affect the results of quantitative and qualitative microscopy?

1 Rodgers MA, Hempel S, Aho T, Kelly JD, Kleijnen J, Westwood M. Diagnostic tests used in the investigation of adult haematuria: A systematic review and economic evaluation. *Health Technol Assess* 2006;10:1-276.
2 National Institute for Health and Clinical Excellence. *Chronic kidney disease guidelines.* 2008. www.nice.org.uk/Guidance/CG73.
3 Grossfeld GD, Litwin MS, Wolf JS Jr, Hricak H, Shuler CL, Agerter DC, et al. Evaluation of asymptomatic microscopic hematuria in adults: the American Urological Association best practice policy—part I: definition, detection, prevalence, and etiology. *Urology* 2001;57:599-603.
4 Scottish Intercollegiate Guidelines Network. *Investigation of asymptomatic microscopic haematuria in adults .* 1997. http://intranet.alemana.cl/lac_intraclinica/Mbe/GPC/Guidelines/Urologia/Hematuria.pdf.
5 González CA, Errezola M, Izarzugaza I, López-Abente G, Escolar A, Nebot M, et al. Urinary infection, renal lithiasis and bladder cancer in Spain. *Eur J Cancer* 1991;27:498-500.
6 Kantor AF, Hartge P, Hoover RN, Narayana AS, Sullivan JW, Fraumeni JF Jr. Urinary tract infection and risk of bladder cancer. *Am J Epidemiol* 1984;119:510-5.
7 Bellinghieri G, Savica V, Santoro D. Renal alterations during exercise. *J Ren Nutr* 2008;18:158-64.

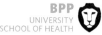

8   Sinert R, Kohl L, Rainone T, Scalea T. Exercise-induced rhabdomyolysis.
     Ann Emerg Med 1994;23:1301-6.
9   Khadra MH, Pickard RS, Charlton M, Powell PH, Neal DE. A prospective
     analysis of 1,930 patients with hematuria to evaluate current
     diagnostic practice. *J Urol* 2000;163:524-7.
10   Edwards TJ, Dickinson AJ, Natale S, Gosling J, McGrath JS. A
     prospective analysis of the diagnostic yield resulting from the
     attendance of 4020 patients at a protocol-driven haematuria clinic.
     BJU Int 2006;97:301-5.
11   Tiebosch AT, Wolters J, Frederik PF, van der Wiel TW, Zeppenfeldt
     E, van Breda Vriesman PJ. Epidemiology of idiopathic glomerular
     disease: a prospective study. *Kidney Int* 1987;32:112-6.
12   Hiatt RA, Ordoñez JD. Dipstick urinalysis screening, asymptomatic
     microhematuria, and subsequent urological cancers in a population-
     based sample. *Cancer Epidemiol Biomarkers Prev* 1994;3:439-43.
13   Woolhandler S, Pels RJ, Bor DH, Himmelstein DU, Lawrence RS.
     Dipstick urinalysis screening of asymptomatic adults for urinary tract
     disorders. I. Hematuria and proteinuria. *JAMA* 1989;262:1215-9.
14   Mohr DN, Offord KP, Owen RA, Melton LJ 3rd. Asymptomatic
     microhematuria and urologic disease. A population-based study. *JAMA*
     1986;256:224-9.
15   Friedman GD, Hiatt RA, Quesenberry CP Jr, Selby JV, Weiss NS.
     Problems in assessing screening experience in observational studies
     of screening efficacy: example of urinalysis screening for bladder
     cancer. *J Med Screen* 1995;2:219-23.
16   Freni SC, Heederik GJ, Hol C. Centrifugation techniques and
     reagent strips in the assessment of microhaematuria. *J Clin Pathol*
     1977;30;336-40.
17   Cohen RA, Brown RS. Clinical practice. Microscopic hematuria. *N Engl J
     Med* 2003;348:2330-8.
18   Sutton JM. Evaluation of hematuria in adults. *JAMA* 1990;263:2475-80.
19   Venkat Raman G, Pead L, Lee HA, Maskell R. A blind controlled trial of
     phase-contrast microscopy by two observers for evaluating the source
     of haematuria. *Nephron* 1986;44:304-8.
20   Tsai JJ, Yeun JY, Kumar VA, Don BR. Comparison and interpretation
     of urinalysis performed by a nephrologist versus a hospital-based
     clinical laboratory. *Am J Kid Dis* 2005;46:820-9.
21   Dowell AC, Britton JP. Microhaematuria in general practice: is urine
     microscopy misleading? *Br J Gen Pract* 1990;40:67-8.
22   Kouri T, Malminiemi O, Penders J, Pelkonen V, Vuotari L, Delanghe J.
     Limits of preservation of samples for urine strip tests and particle
     counting. *Clin Chem Lab Med* 2008;46:703-13
23   Köhler H, Wandel E, Brunck B. Acanthocyturia—a characteristic marker
     for glomerular bleeding. *Kidney Int* 1991;40:115-20.
24   Joint Specialty Committee on Renal Medicine of the Royal College
     of Physicians and the Renal Association, and the Royal College of
     General Practitioners. *Chronic kidney disease in adults: UK guidelines
     for identification, management and referral* . London: Royal College of
     Physicians, 2006.
25   Buckalew VM Jr, Berg RL, Wang SR, Porush JG, Rauch S, Schulman
     G. Prevalence of hypertension in 1,795 subjects with chronic renal
     disease: the modification of diet in renal disease study baseline
     cohort. Modification of Diet in Renal Disease Study Group. *Am J Kidney
     Dis* 1996;28:811-21.
26   Wolf-Maier K, Cooper RS, Banegas JR, Giampaoli S, Hense HW,
     Joffres M, et al. Hypertension prevalence and blood pressure levels
     in 6 European countries, Canada, and the United States. *JAMA*
     2003;289:2363-9.
27   Van Savage JG, Fried FA. Anticoagulant associated hematuria: a
     prospective study. *J Urol* 1995;153:1594-6.
28   Hurlen M, Eikvar L, Seljeflot I, Arnesen H. Occult bleeding in three
     different antithrombotic regimes after myocardial infarction. A
     WARIS-II subgroup analysis. *Thromb Res* 2006;118:433-8.
29   Mishriki SF, Nabi G, Cohen NP. Diagnosis of urologic malignancies in
     patients with asymptomatic dipstick hematuria: prospective study
     with 13 years' follow-up. *Urology* 2008;71:13-6.
30   Geddes CC, Rauta V, Gronhagen-Riska C, Bartosik LP, Jardine AG,
     Ibels LS, et al. A tricontinental view of IgA nephropathy. *Nephrol Dial
     Transplant* 2003;18:1541-8.
31   D'Amico G. Natural history of idiopathic IgA nephropathy: role
     of clinical and histological prognostic factors. *Am J Kidney Dis*
     2000;36:227-37.

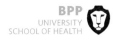

Gout

Edward Roddy, senior lecturer in rheumatology[1],
Christian D Mallen, professor of general practice research[1],
Michael Doherty, professor of rheumatology[2]

[1]Arthritis Research UK Primary Care Centre, Primary Care Sciences, Keele University, Keele ST5 5BG, UK

[2]Academic Rheumatology, University of Nottingham, Clinical Sciences Building, City Hospital, Nottingham, UK

Correspondence to: E Roddy
e.roddy@keele.ac.uk

Cite this as: BMJ 2013;347:f5648

DOI: 10.1136/bmj.f5648

http://www.bmj.com/content/347/bmj.f5648

Gout is the most common inflammatory arthritis, affecting 1-2% of the population. Acute gout is one of the most painful forms of arthritis and is characterised by the abrupt onset of severe joint pain (classically the first metatarsophalangeal joint), swelling, and erythema. The major risk factor is a raised serum urate concentration (hyperuricaemia), which results in the deposition of monosodium urate crystals in and around joints. Untreated, continuing crystal deposition can result in irreversible joint damage. Although effective treatments are available for acute and chronic gout, uptake is poor, and many patients experience repeated acute attacks and reduced quality of life. This clinical review summarises current evidence for the diagnosis and management of acute and chronic gout.

What is gout?

The pathogenesis of gout is well understood. If serum urate concentrations persistently exceed the physiological saturation threshold of urate (around 380 µmol/L; 1 µmol/L=0.02 mg/dL), monosodium urate crystals form and deposit, particularly in cartilage, bone, and periarticular tissues of peripheral joints. Continuing crystal deposition is clinically silent, with about 10% of people with hyperuricaemia developing clinical gout.[1]

The first acute attack of gout occurs when crystals are shed from the articular cartilage into the joint space. It is usually monoarticular and typically affects the lower limb. Involvement of the first metatarsophalangeal joint ("podagra") is common and occurs in 56-78% of first attacks.[2] The mid-foot, ankle, knee, finger joints, wrist, and elbow are also commonly affected.[2] The shoulder, hips, and spine are rarely affected. Acute attacks are characterised by sudden onset, severe joint pain—which reaches peak intensity within 12-24 hours and is associated with swelling and erythema—and then complete resolution within one to two weeks.[3]

SOURCES AND SELECTION CRITERIA

We searched Medline, Embase, PubMed, Cochrane Controlled Trials Register, ISI Web of Science, and AMED (Allied and Complementary Medicine Database) using the search terms "gouty arthritis", "podagra", "tophus", "monosodium urate crystals" and "hyperuricaemia". We also used personal archived references. Priority was given to systematic reviews, meta-analyses, randomised controlled trials, and prospective epidemiological studies where possible.

SUMMARY POINTS

- Gout is associated with serious comorbidity and increased risk of cardiovascular disease

- The definitive diagnosis of gout requires microscopic identification of monosodium urate crystals

- A clinical diagnosis can be made when typical features of inflammation affect the first metatarsophalangeal joint; serum urate values have limited diagnostic value

- First line medical treatment options for acute gout are a non-steroidal anti-inflammatory drug or low dose colchicine

- Long term management requires full patient education, dealing with any modifiable risk factors (such as overweight or obesity, chronic diuretic intake), and urate lowering drugs

- Start allopurinol at a low dose (such as 100 mg daily) and increase gradually with the aim of lowering then maintaining serum urate below 360 µmol/L

The time between acute attacks is termed the intercritical period. If untreated, a second acute attack often occurs within two years. Recurrent attacks may become more frequent and affect different joints or more than one joint. Chronic tophaceous gout can be a consequence of untreated gout and is associated with progressive joint damage, chronic pain and disability, and clinically evident subcutaneous tophi (hard, impacted monosodium urate crystals (fig 1). Tophi mainly occur on the fingers, olecranon processes, toes, Achilles' tendons, knees, and occasionally the helix of the ears.

Who gets gout?

Gout usually affects men aged 40 years and over and women over 65 years.[4] It increases with age, affecting 7% of men aged over 75 in the United Kingdom.[4] The incidence and prevalence of gout are rising because of an ageing population, increasing prevalence of the metabolic syndrome, and possibly dietary changes.

Uric acid is the relatively insoluble endproduct of purine metabolism. Around 70% of uric acid derives from the breakdown of endogenous purines, with the remaining 30% from dietary purines. Most uric acid (around 70%) is excreted through the kidney, the remainder through the gut.[5] Hyperuricaemia is caused by reduced renal elimination (most commonly) or increased production (or both). Epidemiological studies show that the metabolic syndrome and its components (insulin resistance, obesity, hyperlipidaemia, and hypertension) are strongly associated with gout (box 1).[4 6 7] A large cross-sectional study found a 62.8% prevalence of the metabolic syndrome in people with gout compared with 25.4% in those without gout (adjusted odds ratio 3.05, 95% confidence interval 2.0 to 4.6).[8]

Although associations between gout and dietary factors—including alcoholic drinks and purine-rich foods—have been recognised for centuries, these have only recently been examined in high quality prospective studies (box 1).[9 10] The risk of developing gout is directly related to alcohol consumption (multivariate relative risk 1.17 per 10 g alcohol intake/day, 95% confidence interval 1.11 to 1.22).[9] The risk is high for beer (2.51, 1.77 to 3.55) and spirit consumption (1.60, 1.19 to 2.16), but not for wine (1.05). Compared with the lowest fifth of consumption, the relative risk of developing gout in the highest fifth was 1.41 (1.07 to 1.86) for red meat and 1.51 (1.17 to 1.95) for seafood.[10] Dairy products are protective (0.54, 0.42 to 0.74). Sugar sweetened soft drinks, especially those with fructose (1.85, 1.08 to 3.16) increase the risk of gout, whereas consumption of caffeinated and decaffeinated coffee (0.41, 0.19 to 0.88) is thought to be protective.[11 12]

Gout often runs in families, and this is possibly related to lifestyle and genetic factors. Patients may inherit a genetic predisposition to gout, with several rare enzymatic defects known to be a cause. A twin study estimated the hereditability of renal clearance and fractional excretion of urate to be 60% and 87%, respectively.[13] Putative mutations

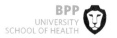

affecting several genes involved in renal urate transport have been proposed to influence developing hyperuricaemia and gout including *SLC22A12*, *SLC2A9* (*GLUT9*), *ABCG2*, and *SLC17A3*, although work is ongoing.[14]

Drugs are often implicated in the pathogenesis of gout (box 1). A recent systematic review including 13 original studies found a trend towards a higher risk for acute gout in patients taking loop and thiazide diuretics, although the magnitude of risk and independence were not consistent.[15] Although no randomised controlled trials (RCTs) have tested cessation of chronic diuretic use in people with gout, consider cessation or reduction when the indication is hypertension rather than cardiac or renal failure.[16 17] Low dose aspirin (75-150 mg/day) has well recognised urate retaining properties, but this is thought to be clinically insignificant, and low dose aspirin should continue if needed for cardiovascular prophylaxis.

Is gout associated with any other diseases?

Gout is increasingly being viewed as more than just a joint disease. Comorbidity including hypertension (74%), hyperlipidaemia, chronic kidney disease (20%), osteoarthritis, obesity (53%), diabetes (26%), congestive heart failure (11%), and ischaemic heart disease (14%) is common and often unrecognised and undertreated.[6 7 8 18] Comorbidity may adversely affect diagnosis, limit management options, and contribute to long term adverse clinical outcomes.

How is gout diagnosed and assessed?

For patients presenting with classic symptoms (rapid onset, podagra, swelling, erythema) a clinical diagnosis is usually accurate.[3] Figure 2 shows likelihood ratios for different clinical features. Podagra has high sensitivity (0.96, 0.91 to 1.01) and specificity (0.97, 0.96 to 0.98), performing better than pain, swelling, and erythema. A definitive diagnosis requires confirmation of the presence of monosodium urate

crystals in synovial fluid or tophi. Although joint aspiration is not needed when the presentation is classic, aspiration and examination of synovial fluid for crystals can be useful when presentation is atypical or involves other joints, during either the acute attack or the intercritical period. It also allows differentiation from the main differential diagnoses of acute calcium pyrophosphate crystal arthritis (pseudogout) and septic arthritis.[3] A systematic review highlights the high degree of interobserver reliability (κ 0.35-0.63) for identifying monosodium urate crystals in synovial fluid, emphasising the need for training and quality control.[19]

Serum uric acid concentrations, although important when "treating to target," are less useful in the diagnosis of gout. Two large population based cohorts found that, although the risk of clinical gout increases with increasing concentrations of serum urate, not all people with hyperuricaemia develop gout.[20 21] There is no evidence to support drug treatment of people with asymptomatic hyperuricaemia. Patients with confirmed gout may have normal serum urate concentrations, especially during an acute attack, when concentrations are often reduced because renal urate excretion increases during the acute phase.[22]

It is also useful to screen for comorbidity by requesting urea and electrolytes, estimated glomerular filtration rate, glucose, and lipids. Measuring and dealing with problems of blood pressure, body mass index, smoking, alcohol use, and cardiovascular risk should form part of a comprehensive gout assessment.

Imaging is not usually needed to diagnose gout. Plain radiographs are often normal, although radiographic evidence of asymmetrical swelling and subcortical cysts without erosion may be useful to diagnose chronic gout.[3] A systematic review concluded that ultrasound is a promising diagnostic tool, but further research is needed to assess the responsiveness, reliability, and feasibility of using this modality routinely.[23] The "double contour" sign—hyperechoic enhancement of the superficial margin of the articular cartilage—is an ultrasound finding thought to be specific to gout (sensitivity 44%, specificity 99%) that is also seen in 25% of patients with asymptomatic hyperuricaemia.[23 24 25]

How are acute attacks of gout treated?

Treatment of acute gout aims to provide rapid relief of joint pain and swelling. First line oral drugs are usually non-steroidal anti-inflammatory drugs (NSAIDs) or colchicine.[16] There is no evidence that any one NSAID is more effective than another. A systematic review commented on the poor quality of existing NSAID trials in acute gout, with the

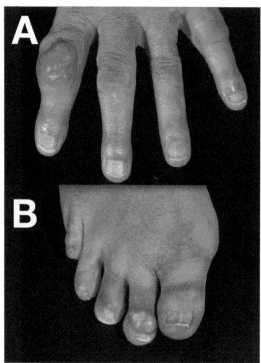

Fig 1 Tophi affecting the interphalangeal joints of the left hand (A) and right second toe (B). Note asymmetry of swelling and yellow-white discoloration

---

BOX 1 CLINICALLY IMPORTANT RISK FACTORS FOR GOUT

- Male sex
- Older age
- Genetic factors (mainly reduced excretion of urate)
- Metabolic syndrome
- Obesity (reduced excretion of urate)
- Hypertension (reduced excretion of urate)
- Hyperlipidaemia (reduced excretion of urate)
- Loop and thiazide diuretics (reduced excretion of urate)
- Chronic kidney disease (reduced excretion of urate)
- Osteoarthritis (enhanced crystal formation)
- Dietary factors (increased production of uric acid):
- Excess purine-rich foods, fructose, sugar sweetened soft drinks
- Excess alcohol consumption, particularly beer

exception of two moderately sized RCTs, which found an equivalent effect of indometacin 50 mg three times daily and etoricoxib 120 mg daily on pain.[26] [27] [28] More recently, two well conducted trials have found indometacin (50 mg three times daily for two days, then 25 mg three times daily for three days) and naproxen 500 mg twice daily to be as effective as oral prednisolone.[29] [30] Indometacin was associated with more gastrointestinal adverse events, however, and is best avoided.[29]

British Society for Rheumatology and American College of Rheumatology guidelines suggest using a fast acting NSAID, such as naproxen, at full dose. Caution is needed, however, in people with heart failure, ischaemic heart disease, renal insufficiency, or a history of gastrointestinal ulcers, bleeds, or perforations.[17] [31] Continue treatment until the attack has resolved (typically a few days to two weeks).

Colchicine is a naturally occurring alkaloid that inhibits leucocytic phagocytosis of monosodium urate crystals, the inflammasome, and cell mediated immune responses. It has traditionally been used in high doses (1 mg initially, followed by 500 µg every two to three hours until pain relief is obtained). Although a small trial showed the effectiveness of high dose regimens over placebo, all participants randomised to receive colchicine developed diarrhoea or vomiting (or both).[32] Lower doses of colchicine are as effective and better tolerated than high dose regimens.

A recent well conducted moderately sized RCT found at least a 50% reduction in pain within 24 hours in 33% of participants treated with high dose colchicine (1.2 mg initially and then 600 µg hourly for six hours). There was also a 38% reduction in those treated with low dose colchicine (1.2 mg initially, followed by 600 µg after one hour) and a 16% reduction in those receiving placebo.[33] Diarrhoea affected 77% of the high dose group, 23% of the low dose group, and 14% receiving placebo. The *British National Formulary* recommends 500 µg two to four times daily.[34] Although no head to head comparison between colchicine and a NSAID exists, oral NSAIDs are generally considered to be the first line treatment for acute gout, with colchicine reserved for those with contraindications to, or intolerance of, NSAIDs.[17] Several drugs can increase the risk of colchicine toxicity (box 2).

Corticosteroids provide a further treatment option. Although there are no RCTs,[35] expert consensus agrees that joint aspiration and intra-articular injection of corticosteroids is a rapid and highly effective treatment for acute gout.[16] [17] The diagnosis can be confirmed by microscopy of aspirated fluid, and such treatment is probably best practice in a hospital setting. However, the necessary skills to perform aspiration and injection might not be present in all settings, particularly primary care. Intramuscular or oral corticosteroids provide a useful option, particularly when there are contraindications to NSAIDs and colchicine and more than one joint is affected or joint injection is not possible.[16] [31] Two high quality RCTs found that oral prednisolone at doses of 30-35 mg daily for five days are as effective as NSAIDs.[29] [30]

Rest and cooling of the joint are also effective for acute gout. A small RCT found that the application of topical ice in combination with oral prednisolone and colchicine reduces pain more effectively than combined prednisolone and colchicine alone.[36]

How is gout managed in the long term?
Long term management of gout aims to prevent formation of new monosodium urate crystals and cause existing crystals to dissolve by lowering serum urate below the physiological saturation threshold. This will cause acute attacks to cease and tophi to resolve, as well as prevent long term joint damage. Urate lowering is best achieved by combining non-drug based and drug based interventions. Individualised patient education is a fundamental component of management and should focus on the causes and consequences of hyperuricaemia and gout,[37] the importance of urate lowering, and how this can be achieved.

What does non-drug based management of gout consist of?
Non-drug based management consists of risk factor modification, including lifestyle factors. Dietary modification comprises restriction of, but not total abstinence from, purine-rich foods (including red meat and seafood) and alcohol (particularly beer).[16] [17] Weight loss is recommended if appropriate. Uncontrolled intervention studies have confirmed modest effects of weight loss and low purine diet on urate lowering and frequency of attacks.[38] [39] Although there is currently insufficient evidence to support modification of other dietary factors—such as consumption of cherries, dairy products, vitamin C, and coffee, and restriction of fructose and sugar sweetened soft drinks— patients are often aware of the preliminary evidence for each of these. Patients should therefore be advised that although these factors may influence the risk of developing gout, the effectiveness of modifying these factors is unclear.

How and when should urate lowering drugs be used?
There is debate about the indications for urate lowering therapy. Expert consensus advocates offering such drugs to patients with recurrent acute gout, tophi, radiographic damage, renal insufficiency, or uric acid urolithiasis.[16] [17] The precise threshold at which recurrence of acute attacks warrants treatment is controversial. Opinions vary from starting these drugs after the first attack, when the

Likelihood ratio (95% CI)

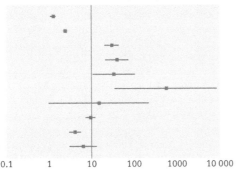

Pain and swelling
Erythema
Podagra
Definite tophus
Possible tophus
MSU crystals during acid attack
MSU crystals during intercritical period
Hyperuricaemia
Radiographic asymmetrical swelling
Radiographic subcortical cysts, no erosion

0.1   1   10   100   1000   10 000

Fig 2 Likelihood ratio and 95% confidence interval (CI) for various features in the diagnosis of gout. MSU=monosodium urate. Reproduced, with permission, from the *Annals of the Rheumatic Diseases*[3]

BOX 2 DRUGS THAT MIGHT INCREASE THE RISK OF COLCHICINE TOXICITY

- Amiodarone
- Ciclosporin
- Digoxin
- Diltiazem
- Fibrates
- Antifungals (itraconazole, ketoconazole)
- Macrolide antibiotics
- Protease inhibitors
- Statins
- Verapamil

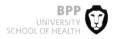

crystal load is small and substantial joint damage has not yet occurred, to waiting until two or more attacks have occurred over 12 months. Because most patients experience recurrent attacks, it is best to discuss treatment options early on. Urate lowering therapy is usually started two to four weeks after resolution of an acute attack to reduce the risk of the drug exacerbating the attack. However, one RCT of 51 patients found no difference in pain between those started on allopurinol during an attack and those given placebo.[40] Delaying initiation of allopurinol also allows a rational discussion about treatment when the patient is no longer in pain. When fully informed about urate lowering therapy, most people wish to receive it, and subsequent adherence can be excellent.[37]

The most commonly used drug is allopurinol—a purine, non-specific xanthine oxidase inhibitor. Allopurinol should be started at low dose (usually 100 mg daily) and increased in 100 mg increments monthly until serum uric acid is below 360 µmol/L. Two small observational studies reported that the effect on cessation of acute attacks, resolution of tophi, and reduction of crystal load is greatest if uric acid

is reduced below this value.[41] [42] Some expert consensus groups recommend reducing uric acid further, to below 300 µmol/L,[17] at least for the first one to two years of treatment, because this speeds up the rate of crystal elimination and tophus reduction.[43]

The maximum permitted dose of allopurinol in the UK is 900 mg per day. Although such doses are rarely needed, many patients need doses of 400-500 mg daily to reduce uric acid.[37] During the dose escalation phase, measure full blood count, renal function, liver function, and serum uric acid monthly. The active metabolite of allopurinol (oxypurinol) is excreted through the kidney, so lower doses and more cautious upward titration are recommended in people with renal failure because of the risk of the rare but potentially life threatening allopurinol hypersensitivity syndrome, which involves severe skin reactions and hepatic and renal dysfunction.[44] [45] Clinical risk factors for allopurinol hypersensitivity syndrome include renal failure, diuretic use, and higher allopurinol dose at initiation.[44] [45]

Ninety per cent of people tolerate allopurinol without problems. As with all urate lowering drugs, patients may experience an acute attack of gout when they start allopurinol because it encourages crystal shedding through partial crystal dissolution. Although the likelihood of this is reduced by gradual dose escalation, prophylactic low dose colchicine or an NSAID can be coprescribed for up to six months until a stable dose is reached. One small placebo controlled RCT showed fewer gout flares when allopurinol was coprescribed with colchicine 600 µg twice daily.[46] Allopurinol should not be discontinued if an acute attack occurs.

The main alternative to allopurinol is the specific non-purine xanthine oxidase inhibitor, febuxostat. A recent systematic review found that target serum urate values are more often achieved with febuxostat at either of its licensed doses (80 mg or 120 mg daily) than with allopurinol.[47] However, allopurinol was used at a fixed dose of 300 mg daily rather than best practice dose escalation. Only 70% of participants taking 120 mg febuxostat achieved the therapeutic target. Febuxostat is largely metabolised by the liver, does not require dose reduction in mild-moderate renal impairment, and does not interact with warfarin. In England and Wales, the National Institute for Health and Care Excellence (NICE) has approved febuxostat as an option for the management of chronic hyperuricaemia in gout for people who are intolerant of allopurinol or for whom allopurinol is contraindicated.[48] It is not recommended in people with ischaemic heart disease, congestive cardiac failure, organ transplant recipients, or, like allopurinol, those taking azathioprine.[49]

Urate lowering therapy in patients who cannot tolerate or have contraindications to allopurinol and febuxostat is challenging. Options include uricosuric drugs such as sulfinpyrazone, probenecid, and benzbromarone, but these have limited availability. Such patients are best referred to a rheumatologist for specialist care.

Treatment is life long. Once a stable target serum urate concentration has been achieved, measurements must be repeated about every six months to ensure the therapeutic target is being maintained. Once the patient is considered crystal free and "cured" (no attacks, resolution of tophi—usually achieved after two years of treatment), the dose may be adjusted to maintain uric acid concentrations of 300-360 µmol/L and monitored every one to two years. Treating to target is a new concept, but when combined with appropriate patient education it can result in "cure" and considerable[13] improvements in patient centred outcomes.

QUESTIONS FOR FUTURE RESEARCH

- Are cardiovascular and renal risk reduced by lowering serum urate in people with gout?
- Which is the most effective and safest treatment for acute gout—a non-steroidal anti-inflammatory drug or low dose colchicine?
- How effective are dietary modification and weight loss at lowering serum urate and treating gout?
- How effective is cessation of diuretics at lowering serum urate and treating gout?
- When starting a urate lowering drug such as allopurinol that can be slowly uptitrated from a low dose, is prophylaxis against acute attacks (with colchicine or a non-steroidal anti-inflammatory drug) needed?
- When starting urate lowering therapy, what is the optimum target to which serum urate levels should be lowered?

TIPS FOR NON-SPECIALISTS

- The diagnosis of typical gout can usually be made clinically
- When assessing patients with gout, screen for common comorbidities including hypertension, diabetes, renal disease, and hyperlipidaemia
- Urate lowering therapy is safe and effective yet underused in primary care. Treating to target can reduce and eventually eliminate acute attacks and prevent longer term joint damage
- Don't forget about non-drug based approaches when managing chronic gout, including dietary modification and weight loss if relevant

---

ADDITIONAL EDUCATIONAL RESOURCES

Resources for healthcare professionals

- Jordan KM, Cameron JS, Snaith M, Zhang W, Doherty M, Seckl J, et al. British Society for Rheumatology and British Health Professionals in Rheumatology guideline for the management of gout. *Rheumatol (Oxford)* 2007;46:1372-4.
- Zhang W, Doherty M, Pascual E, Bardin T, Barskova V, Conaghan P, et al. EULAR evidence based recommendations for gout. Part I: Diagnosis. Report of a task force of the Standing Committee for International Clinical Studies Including Therapeutics (ESCISIT). *Ann Rheum Dis* 2006;65:1301-11
- Zhang W, Doherty M, Bardin T, Pascual E, Barskova V, Conaghan P, et al. EULAR evidence based recommendations for gout. Part II: Management. Report of a task force of the EULAR Standing Committee for International Clinical Studies Including Therapeutics (ESCISIT). *Ann Rheum Dis* 2006;65:1312-24
- Khanna D, Fitzgerald JD, Khanna PP, Bae S, Singh MK, Neogi T, et al. 2012 American College of Rheumatology guidelines for management of gout. Part 1: systematic non-pharmacologic and pharmacologic therapeutic approaches to hyperuricemia. *Arthritis Care Res* 2012;64:1431-46
- Khanna D, Khanna PP, Fitzgerald JD, Singh MK, Bae S, Neogi T, et al. 2012 American College of Rheumatology guidelines for management of gout. Part 2: therapy and antiinflammatory prophylaxis of acute gouty arthritis. *Arthritis Care Res* 2012;64:1447-61

Resources for patients

- Arthritis Research UK (www.arthritisresearchuk.org/arthritis-information/conditions/gout. aspx)—Booklet with information on what gout is, what causes it, how it presents, and how it is diagnosed and treated

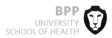

A PATIENT'S PERSPECTIVE

During my early 50s I suddenly woke up one night with severe pain in one of my big toes. My doctor sent me up to the hospital where they said I had gout, but I wasn't prescribed any treatment. I'd heard of gout, although I didn't know much about it or know that it was a form of arthritis. I thought that possibly it was seen in older men who liked drinking alcohol.

Because I hate taking tablets I wanted to avoid long term medication. I asked my GP if I could try to control my gout by watching what I ate. He allowed me to do what I was comfortable with. I was later prescribed naproxen to deal with the attacks as and when they occurred.

Watching my diet worked reasonably well for a while. It didn't stop me getting gout, but at least I felt I was a bit in control of it. That was basically the case for 10 years or so, but the flare-ups started to become more frequent.

Gout is extremely painful—I can't possibly describe what the pain is like. I can only say it is excruciating. When I get a flare-up, I often can't walk or drive the car, and I occasionally wasn't able to go to work. It is exhausting because you can't sleep and you can't move or have the bedclothes on the affected joint because of the pain. I enjoy competing in agility competitions with my dogs, but when I had a flare-up of gout I couldn't do this. As the years went by, I got better at recognising when I was going to have a flare-up and starting my anti-inflammatory drugs quickly, but I decided that I needed to do something more than just managing my diet and dealing with episodes when they occurred.

I went to see my doctor last year and agreed to start on a low dose of allopurinol. Because I was still getting attacks, my GP increased the dose from 200 mg to 300 mg. I had a blood test six weeks later and was told that my uric acid concentration (281 µmol/L) was now within the target range and lower than before I started taking the allopurinol (555 µmol/L). Touch wood, I haven't had an attack since.

I feel positive about the future. Gout doesn't cause me lots of worry any more. Maybe I should have bitten the bullet long ago and gone straight on to allopurinol. If I could turn the clocks back, yes, I probably would have taken allopurinol sooner.

Thanks to Michelle Hui for help with the literature search, and to Jenny Liddle and Carole Smailes for providing the patient story, which was recorded as part of the "Understanding and improving patient experience of gout in primary care" study funded by the National Institute for Health Research School for Primary Care Research, and reproduced with consent.

Contributors: ER and CDM drafted the manuscript. All authors planned the manuscript, commented on further drafts, and approved the final version. MD was commissioned to write the article and is guarantor.

Competing interests: We have read and understood the BMJ policy on declaration of interests and declare the following interests: MD has received honorariums for ad hoc advisory boards for Menarini, Novartis, and Ardea. ER and MD are expert clinical advisers on gout for the National Institute for Health and Care Excellence. All authors are members of the gout guideline development groups of the British Society for Rheumatology and European League Against Rheumatism. CDM is funded by an Arthritis Research UK clinician scientist award.

Provenance and peer review: Commissioned; externally peer reviewed.

Patient consent obtained.

1   Vitart V, Rudan I, Hayward C, Gray NK, Floyd J, Palmer CN, et al. SLC2A9 is a newly identified urate transporter influencing serum urate concentration, urate excretion and gout. Nat Genet 2008;40:437-42.
2   Roddy E. Revisiting the pathogenesis of podagra: why does gout target the foot? J Foot Ankle Res 2011;4:13.
3   Zhang W, Doherty M, Pascual E, Bardin T, Barskova V, Conaghan P, et al; EULAR Standing Committee for International Clinical Studies Including Therapeutics. EULAR evidence based recommendations for gout. Part I: diagnosis. Report of a task force of the Standing Committee for International Clinical Studies Including Therapeutics (ESCISIT). Ann Rheum Dis 2006;65:1301-11.
4   Roddy E, Doherty M. Epidemiology of gout. Arthritis Res Ther 2010;12:223.
5   Edwards NL. The role of hyperuricemia and gout in kidney and cardiovascular disease. Cleveland Clin J Med 2008;75:S13-16.
6   Mikuls TR, Farrar JT, Bilker WB, Fernandes S, Schumacher HR Jr, Saag KG. Gout epidemiology: results from the UK General Practice Research Database, 1990-1999. Ann Rheum Dis 2005;64:267-72.
7   Zhu Y, Pandya BJ, Choi HK. Comorbidities of gout and hyperuricemia in the US general population: NHANES 2007-2008. Am J Med 2012;125:679-687.e1.
8   Choi HK, Ford ES, Li C, Curhan G. Prevalence of the metabolic syndrome in patients with gout: the third national health and nutrition examination survey. Arthritis Rheum 2007;57:109-15.
9   Choi HK, Atkinson K, Karlson EW, Willett W, Curhan G. Alcohol intake and risk of incident gout in men: a prospective study. Lancet 2004;363:1277-81.
10 Choi HK, Atkinson K, Karlson EW, Willett W, Curhan G. Purine-rich foods, dairy and protein intake, and the risk of gout in men. N Engl J Med 2004;350:1093-103.
11 Choi HK, Curhan G. Soft drinks, fructose consumption, and the risk of gout in men: prospective cohort study. BMJ 2008;336:309-12.
12 Choi HK, Willett W, Curhan G. Coffee consumption and risk of incident gout in men: a prospective study. Arthritis Rheum 2007;56:2049-55.
13 Emmerson BT, Nagel SL, Duffy DL, Martin NG. Genetic control of the renal clearance of urate: a study of twins. Ann Rheum Dis 1992;51:375-7.
14 Merriman TR, Dalbeth N. The genetic basis of hyperuricaemia and gout. Joint Bone Spine 2011;78:35-40.
15 Hueskes BA, Roovers EA, Mantel-Teeuwisse AK, Janssens HJ, van de Lisdonk EH, Janssen M. Use of diuretics and the risk of gouty arthritis: a systematic review. Semin Arthritis Rheum 2012;41:879-89.
16 Zhang W, Doherty M, Pascual E, Bardin T, Barskova V, Conaghan P, et al; EULAR Standing Committee for International Clinical Studies Including Therapeutics. EULAR evidence based recommendations for gout. Part II: management. Report of a task force of the Standing Committee for International Clinical Studies Including Therapeutics (ESCISIT). Ann Rheum Dis 2006;65:1312-24.
17 Jordan KM, Cameron JS, Snaith M, Zhang W, Doherty M, Seckl J, et al. British Society for Rheumatology and British Health Professionals in Rheumatology Standards, Guidelines and Audit Working Group (SGAWG). British Society for Rheumatology and British Health Professionals in Rheumatology guideline for the management of gout. Rheumatol (Oxford) 2007;46:1372-4.
18 Roddy E, Mallen CD, Hider SL, Jordan KP. Prescription and comorbidity screening following consultation for acute gout in primary care. Rheumatol (Oxford) 2010;49:105-11.
19 Swan A, Amer H, Dieppe P. The value of synovial fluid assays in the diagnosis of joint disease: a literature survey. Ann Rheum Dis 2002;61:493-8.
20 Brauer GW, Prior IA. A prospective study of gout in New Zealand Maoris. Ann Rheum Dis 1978;37:466-72.
21 Goldthwait JC, Butler CF, Stillman JS. The diagnosis of gout; significance of an elevated serum uric acid value. N Engl J Med 1958;259:1095-9.
22 Urano W, Yamanaka H, Tsutani H, Nakajima H, Matsuda Y, Taniguchi A, et al. The inflammatory process in the mechanism of decreased serum uric acid concentrations during acute gouty arthritis. J Rheumatol 2002;29:1950-3.
23 Chowalloor PV, Keen HI. A systematic review of ultrasonography in gout and asymptomatic hyperuricaemia. Ann Rheum Dis 2013;72:638-45.
24 Pineda C, Amezcua-Guerra LM, Solano C, et al. Joint and tendon subclinical involvement suggestive of gouty arthritis in asymptomatic hyperuricemia: an ultrasound controlled study. Arthritis Res Ther 2011;13:R4.
25 De Miguel E, Puig JG, Castillo C, et al. Diagnosis of gout in patients with asymptomatic hyperuricaemia: a pilot ultrasound study. Ann Rheum Dis 2012;71:157-8.
26 Sutaria S, Katbamna R, Underwood M. Effectiveness of interventions for the treatment of acute and prevention of recurrent gout--a systematic review. Rheumatol (Oxford) 2006;45:1422-31.
27 Schumacher HR Jr, Boice JA, Daikh DI, Mukhopadhyay S, Malmstrom K, Ng J, et al. Randomised double blind trial of etoricoxib and indometacin in treatment of acute gouty arthritis. BMJ 2002;324:1488-92.
28 Rubin BR, Burton R, Navarra S, Antigua J, Londoño J, Pryhuber KG, et al. Efficacy and safety profile of treatment with etoricoxib 120 mg once daily compared with indomethacin 50 mg three times daily in acute gout: a randomized controlled trial. Arthritis Rheum 2004;50:598-606.
29 Man CY, Cheung IT, Cameron PA, Rainer TH. Comparison of oral prednisolone/paracetamol and oral indomethacin/paracetamol combination therapy in the treatment of acute goutlike arthritis: a double-blind, randomized, controlled trial. Ann Emerg Med 2007;49:670-7.
30 Janssens HJ, Janssen M, van de Lisdonk EH, van Riel PL, van Weel C. Use of oral prednisolone or naproxen for the treatment of gout arthritis: a double-blind, randomised equivalence trial. Lancet 2008;371:1854-60.
31 Khanna D, Khanna PP, Fitzgerald JD, Singh MK, Mae S, Neogi T et al. 2012 American College of Rheumatology guidelines for management of gout. Part 2: therapy and antiinflammatory prophylaxis of acute gouty arthritis. Arthritis Care Res 2012;64:1447-61.
32 Ahern MJ, Reid C, Gordon TP, McCredie M, Brooks PM, Jones M. Does colchicine work? The results of the first controlled study in acute gout. Aust N Z J Med 1987;17:301-4.
33 Terkeltaub RA, Furst DE, Bennett K, Kook KA, Crockett RS, Davis MW. High versus low dosing of oral colchicine for early acute gout flare: twenty-four-hour outcome of the first multicenter, randomized, double-blind, placebo-controlled, parallel-group, dose-comparison colchicine study. Arthritis Rheum 2010;62:1060-8.
34 British National Formulary. 10.1.4. Gout and cytotoxic-induced hyperuricaemia. Colchicine. June 2013.
35 Wechalekar MD, Vinik O, Schlesinger N, Buchbinder R. Intra-articular glucocorticoids for acute gout. Cochrane Database Syst Rev 2013;4:CD009920.
36 Schlesinger N, Detry MA, Holland BK, Baker DG, Beutler AM, Rull M, et al. Local ice therapy during bouts of acute gouty arthritis. J Rheumatol 2002;29:331-4.

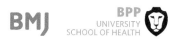

37 Rees F, Jenkins W, Doherty M. Patients with gout adhere to curative treatment if informed appropriately: proof-of-concept observational study. *Ann Rheum Dis* 2013;72:826-30.

38 Dessein PH, Shipton EA, Stanwix AE, Joffe BI, Ramokgadi J. Beneficial effects of weight loss associated with moderate calorie/carbohydrate restriction, and increased proportional intake of protein and unsaturated fat on serum urate and lipoprotein levels in gout: a pilot study. *Ann Rheum Dis* 2000;59:539-43.

39 Kullich W, Ulreich A, Klein G. [Changes in uric acid and blood lipids in patients with asymptomatic hyperuricemia treated with diet therapy in a rehabilitation procedure]. *Rehabilitation (Stuttg)* 1989;28:134-7.

40 Taylor TH, Mecchella JN, Larson RJ, Kerin K, MacKenzie TA. Initiation of allopurinol at first medical contact for acute attacks of gout: a randomized clinical trial. *Am J Med* 2012;125:1126-3e7.

41 Li-Yu J, Clayburne G, Sieck M, Beutler A, Rull M, Eisner E, et al. Treatment of chronic gout. Can we determine when urate stores are depleted enough to prevent attacks of gout? *J Rheumatol* 2001;28:577-80.

42 Shoji A, Yamanaka H, Kamatani N. A retrospective study of the relationship between serum urate level and recurrent attacks of gouty arthritis: evidence for reduction of recurrent gouty arthritis with antihyperuricemic therapy. *Arthritis Rheum* 2004;51:321-5.

43 Perez-Ruiz F, Calabozo M, Pijoan JI, Herrero-Beites AM, Ruibal A. Effect of urate-lowering therapy on the velocity of size reduction of tophi in chronic gout. *Arthritis Rheum* 2002;47:356-60.

44 Stamp LK, Taylor WJ, Jones PB, Dockerty JL, Drake J, Frampton C, et al. Starting dose is a risk factor for allopurinol hypersensitivity syndrome: a proposed safe starting dose of allopurinol. *Arthritis Rheum* 2012;64:2529-36.

45 Dalbeth N, Stamp L. Allopurinol dosing in renal impairment: walking the tight-rope between adequate urate-lowering and adverse events. *Semin Dial* 2007;20:391-5.

46 Borstad GC, Bryant LR, Abel MP, Scroggie DA, Harris MD, Alloway JA. Colchicine for prophylaxis of acute flares when initiating allopurinol for chronic gouty arthritis. *J Rheumatol* 2004;31:2429-32.

47 Tayar JH, Lopez-Olivo MA, Suarez-Almazor ME. Febuxostat for treating chronic gout. *Cochrane Database Syst Rev* 2012;11:CD008653.

48 National Institute for Health and Care Excellence. Febuxostat for the management of hyperuricaemia in people with gout. TA164. 2011. www.nice.org.uk/nicemedia/live/12101/42738/42738.pdf.

49 Electronic Medicines Compendium (eMC). Summary of product characteristics: adenuric film-coated tablets. 2013. www.medicines.org.uk/emc/medicine/22830/SPC.

Related links

bmj.com/archive
- Testicular germ cell tumours (BMJ 2013;347:f5526)
- Managing cows' milk allergy in children (BMJ 2013;347:f5424)
- Personality disorder (BMJ 2013;347:f5276)
- Dyspepsia (BMJ 2013;347:f5059)
- Tourette's syndrome (BMJ 2013;347:f4964)

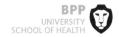
The management of ingrowing toenails

Derek H Park, specialist registrar in trauma and orthopaedics,
Dishan Singh, consultant orthopaedic surgeon, clinical lead

¹Foot and Ankle Unit, Royal
National Orthopaedic Hospital,
Stanmore HA7 4LP, UK

Correspondence to: D H Park
derekpark@doctors.net.uk

Cite this as: *BMJ* 2012;344:e2089

DOI: 10.1136/bmj.e2089

http://www.bmj.com/content/344/
bmj.e2089

Ingrowing toenails are a common condition that causes pain and disability in the foot. The condition occurs when the nail plate traumatises the nail fold, giving rise to pain, inflammation, or infection (or a combination thereof). It commonly occurs in the great toe but can also affect the lesser toes. Patients with ingrowing toenails are usually male, between the ages of 15 and 40 years; they are often encountered in general practice, with an estimated 10 000 new cases presenting in the United Kingdom each year.[1] The condition is managed by a wide variety of healthcare professionals including general practitioners, podiatrists, dermatologists, general surgeons, and orthopaedic surgeons. The surgical treatments for ingrowing toenails include procedures on the nail plate, the nail bed (germinal matrix), and the surrounding soft tissues. Historically, a recurrence rate of 13-50% has been reported after surgical treatment,[2] although more recent papers have reported recurrence rates of less than 5%, particularly with the use of wedge resection of the nail and phenol ablation of the nail matrix.[3] [4] A Cochrane review of nine randomised clinical trials of surgical treatments concluded that simple nail avulsion combined with phenol ablation was most effective in reducing symptomatic recurrence.[5] It is important to recognise, however, that the presentation and disease process of ingrowing toenails covers a wide spectrum, and that management options will depend on the stage at which a patient presents. We review the management of ingrowing toenails, focusing on the effectiveness of the procedures most commonly used.

Anatomy of the nail and surrounding area

Figure 1 depicts the anatomy of the nail and the surrounding area.

How does an ingrowing toenail occur?

The term ingrowing toenail is used to describe a sharp spike of nail growing into an overlapping nail fold. This condition is caused by a combination of extrinsic and intrinsic factors, such as poorly fitting shoes, improperly trimmed nails, tight socks, excessive sweating, soft tissue abnormalities of the toe, and inherent nail deformity.[9] Normal nails vary greatly in shape, and the nail walls are adaptable to marked curvature of the nails. Ingrowing toenails can occur in the context of normal nail shape or abnormal nail shape. In normal nails the nail plate is slightly convex from side to side; in people with normal nails, improper nail trimming can lead to a nail spike

SOURCES AND SELECTION CRITERIA

We searched Medline (PubMed), the *Cochrane Database of Systematic Reviews*, Cochrane central register of controlled trials, and CINAHL using the search terms "ingrowing toenails", "ingrown toenails", and "onychocryptosis". We identified additional literature from the references of identified papers. In addition, we consulted standard orthopaedic textbooks on the subject and reviewed the main references quoted.

that traumatises soft tissue. This provides a port of entry for bacterial and fungal skin flora, resulting in tenderness, inflammation, and infection. Poorly fitting shoes can exacerbate the situation. Ingrowing toenails can also occur in people with abnormal nail shapes, such as incurvated nails or a wide nail plate. In this situation, the condition can occur congenitally or in adults, where increased pressure on the nail leads to increased transverse curvature that causes the edge of the nail to dig into the toe.[6] [9] [10] [11]

What are the clinical features of an ingrowing toenail?

The clinical presentation of an ingrowing toenail has traditionally been divided into three stages (fig 2; box):

- Stage I: Pain, swelling, and erythema
- Stage II: Signs of inflammation together with active or acute infection
- Stage III: Chronic infection leading to formation of hypergranulation tissue at the nail folds.[7] [12] [13]

It can be difficult to determine the clinical stage, however, and it is simpler to consider the presentation as being on a spectrum of the disease process. The initial clinical presentation is of pain, swelling, erythema, and hyperhidrosis in the affected toe. After the initial inflammation and infection, a draining abscess causes further erythema, oedema, hyperhidrosis, and tenderness. Attempts at healing lead to the formation of hypertrophic granulation tissue, which is slowly covered by epithelium; this inhibits drainage and promotes oedema, leading to chronic infection and hypertrophy of the nail wall.

What are the treatment options for ingrowing toenails?

Traditionally, management has been dictated by the clinical stage of presentation.[7] [12] [13] [14] With the recent evaluation of treatment methods such as partial nail avulsion and segmental phenol ablation, however, the management of this condition has changed, and it is simpler to classify ingrowing toenails into those that occur in normal nails and those occurring in abnormally wide or incurvated edge toenails (fig 3).

Normal nails

Ingrowing toenails in normal nails tend to present in younger people and are usually a result of improper nail trimming of the lateral edge, which leaves a sharp nail spike that traumatises the nail fold. Evidence from observational studies indicates that the initial treatment should be conservative, with the patient given general instructions in

SUMMARY POINTS

- Ingrowing toenails are common, cause serious disability, and affect mainly young men
- There is a spectrum to the clinical presentation with pain progressing to infection, hypergranulation, and finally chronic infection
- Ingrowing toenails can occur in normal or abnormally shaped nails
- Cases in abnormally shaped nails are more difficult to manage conservatively and usually require surgery
- Symptoms are less likely to recur after partial nail avulsion and segmental phenol ablation than after simple nail avulsion or wedge excisions alone

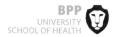

foot care and footwear.[9][12] The nail should be trimmed at right angles to the long axis of the toe and patients are able to carry this out at home. A chiropodist can gently retract the nail fold and trim the offending nail spike.

Abnormal nails

Ingrowing toenails most commonly develop in adults with abnormally wide toenails or those with an incurvated edge. Incurvated (or involuted) toenails can be caused by a bony malformation of the dorsum of the distal phalanx,[15] or by secondary changes in the toenail as a result of irritation and pressure.[16] There is no consensus on standard non-operative treatment of ingrowing toenails in abnormally shaped nails, but failure of conservative management should lead to consideration of surgical options. These patients are best offered partial nail avulsion with segmental phenol ablation. Phenol has potent antiseptic properties, so the procedure can be carried out even in the presence of infection without risk of wound infection. Patients with severe involuted nails on both the tibial and fibular sides (pincer nails) would be left with a too thin nail after wedge excision and may be better treated with a total nail avulsion.[14]

What are the different types of surgical treatments?

The surgical options consist of procedures that are temporary or permanent.

Temporary procedures

A Cochrane review has shown that recurrence of symptoms is high after temporary measures, such as simple (or partial) nail avulsion without chemical or surgical ablation, and this may lead to low patient satisfaction.[2] Therefore, we prefer to perform the procedure in selected patients only. However, removal of the nail spike is curative if followed by appropriate aftercare, as detailed above.

Permanent procedures

Historically, ablation of the germinal matrix centre (Zadik's procedure) or reductive procedures to the lateral nail fold (Winograd's procedure) were popular.[17][18] In Zadik's (sometimes mistakenly called Zadek's) procedure, the nail forming part of the nail bed is removed and adequate skin

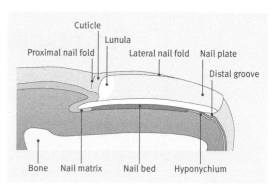

Fig 1 Anatomy of the nail and surrounding area. The nail plate inserts proximally into the proximal nail fold and consists of modified skin epithelium composed mainly of keratin. The cuticle is a thin membranous extension of the proximal nail fold. The nail bed matrix lies beneath the nail plate and is conventionally divided into the germinal matrix proximally and the sterile matrix distally; the germinal matrix is the regenerative part of the nail, whereas the sterile matrix adds thickness to the nail as the nail grows longitudinally along the nail bed. The hyponychium is the area under the free edge of the nail plate.[6][7][8] The lunula is a white crescent shaped area seen in the posterior fifth of the nail plate, distal to the cuticle: it marks the distal part of the less vascular germinal centre

cover is provided without shortening the distal phalanx.[17] Winograd's technique of wedge excision involves partial removal of the nail plate and matrix,[18] as well as removal of a wedge of the lateral nail fold. In essence, these procedures attempt to prevent nail recurrence by destroying the germinal matrix by surgical ablation, but are less commonly performed than procedures that combine partial nail avulsion with ablation of the nail matrix using electrocauterisation, laser surgery, or agents such as phenol or sodium hydroxide.

A Cochrane review of surgical treatments suggests that simple nail avulsion combined with phenol ablation should be the treatment of choice.[5] A recent randomised clinical trial also showed lower rates of recurrence with partial nail avulsion and phenol ablation compared with partial avulsion with nail matricectomy.[19] The success of phenol matricectomy depends on the use of good quality phenol and satisfactory haemostasis. Individually packed and sealed sterile containers of 90% liquid phenol with

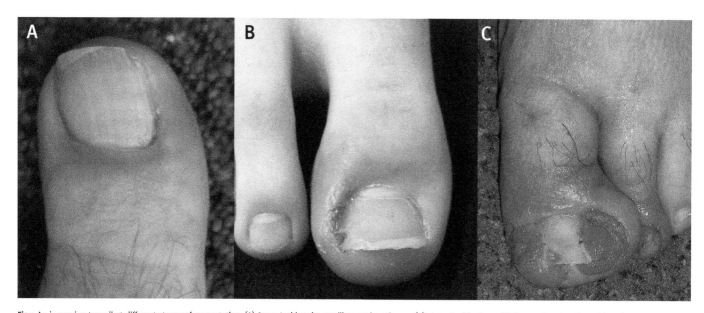

Fig 2 An ingrowing toenail at different stages of presentation. (A) Stage I with pain, swelling, and erythema; (B) stage II with signs of inflammation together with active or acute infection; (C) stage III with chronic infection leading to granulation tissue formation at the nail folds

appropriately sized cotton tips are now available, and these are safer to use than phenol in brown bottles, which usually come from pharmaceutical suppliers. These individually packed containers also reduce the risk of spillage.

Partial nail avulsion with segmental phenol ablation

We use the following technique when performing this procedure (fig 4). The toe is cleaned with an appropriate skin preparation, such as povidone-iodine or chlorhexidine. A ring block with 1% plain lidocaine is injected at the base of the toe and a coloured ring tourniquet with a tag is applied—flesh coloured glove tourniquets are no longer used because of the risk of failing to remove them at the end of the procedure. Blunt dissection is carried out to separate the edge of the appropriate nail plate from the soft tissues. A cut is made with a straight Beaver mini-blade to isolate an appropriate (usually 3-5 mm) section of the affected nail segment extending under the proximal nail fold, which is lifted off by grasping with an artery clip and using a central to lateral twisting motion to avulse the germinal centre. Good haemostasis should be achieved before application of phenol because the presence of blood prevents a proper matricectomy. Denatured matrix looks white as opposed to the black colour of denatured blood. The surrounding skin is protected by application of paraffin jelly. A one minute application of phenol is usually performed twice, followed by a washout with normal saline. A washout with alcohol is commonly performed but is unnecessary. The chemical action of phenol is self limiting as a result of the process of cellular destruction, not the change in solvents after the application of alcohol.[20] A postoperative dressing is applied (fig 4E) and the patient is asked to remove the dressing in 48 hours and soak the foot in tepid salt baths daily. This is done to prevent debris from accumulating in the nail folds because this can lead to infection. Patients usually experience very little postoperative pain and can return to work the next day. Warn the patient that a serous discharge often occurs but usually settles within two weeks, although it can sometimes persist for several weeks.

The rate of recurrence after phenol ablation is low and is usually treated by repeat application of phenol.[3 4 19 21 22 23 24] An added advantage of this procedure is that it can be carried out even in the presence of acute infection. We advise against making an incision in the skin to remove the nail segment in the presence of acute infection.

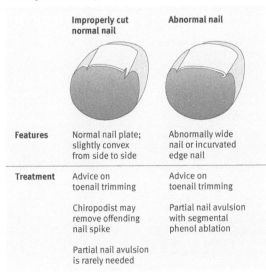

	Improperly cut normal nail	Abnormal nail
Features	Normal nail plate; slightly convex from side to side	Abnormally wide nail or incurvated edge nail
Treatment	Advice on toenail trimming	Advice on toenail trimming
	Chiropodist may remove offending nail spike	Partial nail avulsion with segmental phenol ablation
	Partial nail avulsion is rarely needed	

Fig 3 Management options for normal and abnormal toenails

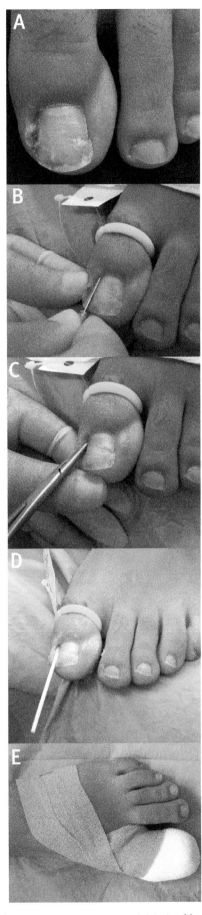

Fig 4 (A) An ingrowing toenail causing chronic infection; (B) a cut is made in the isolated nail segment to allow partial nail avulsion; (C) partial nail avulsion with removal of a nail segment that extends under the eponychium; (D) application of phenol; (E) postoperative dressing

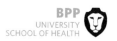

ADDITIONAL EDUCATIONAL RESOURCES FOR PATIENTS

- Patient.co.uk (www.patient.co.uk/health/Ingrowing-Toenails-(Ingrown-Toenails).htm)—Patient website that provides health information to patients
- British Orthopaedic Foot and Ankle Society (www.bofas.org.uk/PatientAdvice/Ingrowingtoenail.aspx)—Information for patients on how to detect, prevent, and care for ingrowing toenails, in addition to when to seek professional advice
- American Academy of Orthopaedic Surgeons (http://orthoinfo.aaos.org/topic.cfm?topic=a00154)—Information on surgical treatments for ingrowing toenails

CLINICAL FEATURES

- Pain, swelling, erythema, and hyperhidrosis of the affected toe
- ↓
- Inflammation and infection lead to a draining abscess with discharge
- ↓
- Development of hypertrophic granulation tissue, epithelial lining inhibits drainage, chronic infection results

Conclusion

The treatment of ingrowing toenails has traditionally been blighted by high recurrence rates and poor patient satisfaction,[2] but with the increasing use of chemical ablation of the nail matrix in combination with partial nail avulsion reported recurrence rates have decreased. On the basis of the Cochrane review and our review of the current literature, fig 3 sets out a simple approach to the management of this common but poorly treated condition.

Contributors: Both authors helped in the conception of the manuscript, the analysis of the relevant literature, the drafting and revision the manuscript, and the final approval of the version to be published. DS is guarantor.

Funding: None received.

Competing interests: Both authors have completed the ICMJE uniform disclosure form at www.icmje.org/coi_disclosure.pdf (available on request from the corresponding author) and declare: no support from any organisation for the submitted work; no financial relationships with any organisations that might have an interest in the submitted work in the previous three years; no other relationships or activities that could appear to have influenced the submitted work.

Provenance and peer review: Not commissioned; externally peer reviewed.

Patient consent not required (patient anonymised, dead, or hypothetical).

1 Sykes PA. Ingrowing toenails: time for critical appraisal? *J R Coll Surg Edinb* 1986;31:300-4.
2 Laxton C. Clinical audit of forefoot surgery performed by registered medical practitioners and podiatrists. *J Public Health Med* 1995;17:311-7.
3 Herold N, Houshian S, Riegels-Nielsen P. A prospective comparison of wedge matrix resection with nail matrix phenolization for the treatment of ingrown toenail. *J Foot Ankle Surg* 2001;40:390-5.
4 Shaikh FM, Jafri M, Giri SK, Keane R. Efficacy of wedge resection with phenolization in the treatment of ingrowing toenails. *J Am Podiatr Med Assoc* 2008;;98:118-22.
5 Rounding C, Bloomfield S. Surgical treatments for ingrowing toenails. *Cochrane Database Syst Rev* 2005;2:CD001541.
6 Pardo Castello V, Pardo Sanson OA. Diseases of the nails. 3rd ed. Thomas, 1960.
7 Zaias N. The nail in health and disease. MTP, 1980.
8 Zook EG, Van Beek AL, Russell RC, Beatty ME. Anatomy and physiology of the perionychium: A review of the literature and anatomic study. *J Hand Surg Am* 1980;5:528-36.
9 Lloyd-Davies RW, Brill GC. The aetiology and out-patient management of ingrowing toe-nails. *Br J Surg* 1963;50:592-7.
10 Fowler AW. Excision of the germinal matrix: a unified treatment for embedded toe-nail and onychogryphosis. *Br J Surg* 1958;45:382-7.
11 Brearley R. Treatment of ingrowing toenail. *Lancet* 1958;2:122-5.
12 Dixon GL Jr. Treatment of ingrown toenail. *Foot Ankle* 1983;3:254-60.
13 Heifetz CJ. Ingrown toenail. *Am J Surg* 1937;38:298-315.
14 DeLauro TM. Onychocryptosis. *Clin Podiatr Med Surg* 1995;12:201-13.
15 Lerner LH. Incurvated nail margin with associated osseous pathology. *Curr Podiatr* 1962;11:26-8.
16 Parrinello JF, Japour CJ, Dykyj D. Incurvated nail: does the phalanx determine nail plate shape? *J Am Podiatr Med Assoc* 1995;85:696-8.
17 Zadik FR. Obliteration of the nail bed of the great toe without shortening the terminal phalanx. *J Bone Joint Surg* 1950;32-B:66-7.
18 Winograd AM. A modification in the technique of operation for ingrown toenail. *JAMA* 1929;92:229-30.
19 Bos AM, van Tilburg MW, van Sorge AA, Klinkenbijl JH. Randomized clinical trial of surgical technique and local antibiotics for ingrowing toenail. *Br J Surg* 2007;94:292-6.
20 Espensen EH, Nixon BP, Armstrong DG. Chemical matrixectomy for ingrown toenails: is there an evidence basis to guide therapy? *J Am Podiatr Med Assoc* 2002;92:287-95.
21 Greig JD, Anderson JH, Anderson AJ, Anderson JR. The surgical treatment of ingrowing toenails. *J Bone Joint Surg* 1991;73-B:131-3.
22 Issa MM, Tanner WA. Approach to ingrowing toenails: the wedge resection/segmental phenolization combination treatment. *Br J Surg* 1988;75:181-3.
23 Ross WR. Treatment of the ingrown toenail and a new anesthetic method. *Surg Clin North Am* 1969;49:1499-504.
24 Van der Ham AC, Hackeng CA, Yo TI. The treatment of ingrowing toenails. A randomised comparison of wedge excision and phenol cauterisation. *J Bone Joint Surg Br* 1990;72-B:507-9.

Related links

bmj.com
- Diagnosis and management of primary hyperparathyroidism (BMJ 2012;344:e1013)
- Female genital mutilation: the role of health professionals in prevention, assessment, and management (2012;344:e1361)
- Childhood cough (2012;344:e1177)
- Ductal carcinoma in situ of the breast (2012;344:e797)
- Get Cleveland clinic CME credits for this article

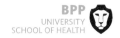

Fungal nail infection: diagnosis and management

Samantha Eisman, dermatologist, Rodney Sinclair, professor of dermatology

¹Sinclair Dermatology, East Melbourne, Vic 3002, Australia

Correspondence to: R Sinclair rodney.sinclair@epworthdermatology.com.au

Cite this as: *BMJ* 2014;348:g1800

DOI: 10.1136/bmj.g1800

http://www.bmj.com/content/348/bmj.g1800

Onychomycosis is the term used for fungal infections of nail. A recent review of population based studies of onychomycosis in Europe and the United States found a mean prevalence of 4.3%.[1] Onychomycosis can be a source of pain and discomfort and can impact on patients' quality of life, with psychosocial and physically detrimental effects.[2] Disease of the fingernails can cause impaired or lost tactile function, whereas disease of the toenails can interfere with walking, exercise, and how shoes fit. Untreated patients can act as source of infection for family members and potentially contaminate communal areas. Infection may be chronic and resistant to treatment, with 16-25% of patients not achieving cure by current treatments.[3] No spontaneous clearing is known to occur. This review provides an evidence based overview of the diagnosis and management of onychmoycosis.

What causes onychomycosis?

Onychomycosis is commonly caused by infection with dermatophytes, a group of three types of fungi that cause skin disease in both animals and humans—namely, *Microsporum, Epidermophyton,* and *Trichophyton.* When nail is affected by dermatophytes, this is referred to as tinea unguium. Around 90% of cases are related to *Trichophyton rubrum*[4] followed by a complex of *Trichophyton interdigitale/ mentagrophytes.* Onychomycosis can also be caused by non-dermatophyte moulds and by yeasts, commonly *Candida albicans.* The distribution of these pathogens is determined by geography, climate, and migration.

Who is at risk?

Onychomycosis is a multifactorial disease. Fungi are ubiquitous and damaged nail increases the risk of infection. Diabetes is an independent risk factor,[5] with one third of patients with diabetes affected. A multicentre survey showed that patients with diabetes are twice as likely as those without diabetes to have onychomycosis.[5] In patients with diabetes, diseased nail can injure surrounding skin, which may go unnoticed because of sensory neuropathy, and this can predispose to osteomyelitis, gangrene, and diabetic ulcers.

Increasing age also poses a risk, and in elderly people (aged >70 years) damaged nail can traumatise the skin and

SOURCES AND SELECTION CRITERIA

We searched Medline, PubMed, the National Institute for Health and Care Excellence website, and the Cochrane Library for systematic reviews, meta-analyses, randomised and non-randomised controlled clinical trials, and case series and reports using the search words "fungal nail disease/infection", "tinea unguium", and "onychomycosis". We also consulted recent guidelines submitted for publication by the British Association of Dermatologists.

provide an entry point for bacteria or other pathogens, causing cellulitis.

Genetics has also been implicated as a risk factor, with *T rubrum* infection showing a familial pattern of autosomal dominant inheritance.[6] Distal lateral onychomycosis caused by *T rubrum* was noted in a familial pattern unrelated to interfamilial transmission.

In a multicentre study, the odds of patients with psoriasis having onychomycosis was 56% greater than in those of the same age and sex without psoriasis, and prevalence of pedal onychomycosis was 13%.[7] In an epidemiological study of 500 participants, the prevalence of onychomycosis in people with HIV was 23.2% and correlated with CD4 counts of $370/mm^3$.[8] In a large series of patients with onychomycosis, 83.3% smoked two or more packets of cigarettes a day compared with 14.8% who were non-smokers,[9] and peripheral arterial disease was another confounding risk factor.

External risk factors reported are increased participation in physical activity, increased exposure to wet work, ill fitting shoes, commercial swimming pools, working with chemicals, walking barefoot, and nail biting.[10] Prevalence rates are also determined by occupation (athletes), climate, living environment, and frequency of travel.

How does it present?

Onychomycosis may involve a single nail or, in exceptional circumstances, all nails. Toenails are seven times more likely to be affected than fingernails. The first and fifth toenails are the most commonly affected, often following an episode of tinea pedis. Fingernail infection is, in contrast, usually associated with tinea corporis or capitis, and is often unilateral. Table 1 lists the different clinical presentations and common infectious agents implicated in onychomycosis.

How is it diagnosed?

Many disorders of nail can mimic onychomycosis (see box for differential diagnoses). It is therefore important to establish a diagnosis microbiologically before starting treatment. The clinical hallmarks of onychomycosis are that nail becomes friable and, owing to the way the fungus invades, characteristic spikes are often visible. They appear as yellow hyperkeratotic bands that progress proximally towards the matrix.

SUMMARY POINTS

- Friable nail plate and nail spikes (yellow hyperkeratotic bands) suggest onychomycosis
- Histopathology of nail clippings can be done easily and quickly and is an economical way to establish a pathogenic role of fungi; specimens can be sent without fixatives or transport medium and results are available in 3-5 days
- Treatment should not be started before confirmation of infection by mycology
- False negative rates for culture are 30%; therefore a negative test result cannot exclude infection and should be repeated if clinical suspicion is high
- Consider non-dermatophyte moulds if onychomycosis is unresponsive to antifungals, and if microscopy provides a positive result but cultures give negative results

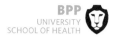

Table 1   Clinical presentations of onychomycoses[11-13]

Type of onychomycosis	Clinical appearance	Cause	Sampling site
Distal and lateral subungual onychomycosis (fig 1)	Hyperkeratosis of undersurface of distal nail plate and bed; onycholysis; dyschromias; one hand-two foot syndrome; tinea pedis often present	*Trichophyton rubrum,Trichophyton mentagrophytes,Trichophyton tonsurans,Epidermophyton floccosum*	Nail bed and underside of nail plate; nail clippings
Superficial white onychomycosis	Crumbling white lesions on nail surface; most common in children	*T mentagrophytes, Aspergillus, Acremonium, Aspergillus, Fusarium*	Surface scrape of white friable area
Proximal (white) subungual onychomycosis	Infection begins in proximal nail fold and distal portion normal; AIDS (gross white discoloration; leukonychia of proximal nail; nail plate surface normal early on	*T rubrum, Trichophyton megnini, Trychophyton schoenleinii, E floccosum*	Curette deeper nail plate and proximal nail bed (pare normal nail plate first); may need biopsy
Endonyx onychomycosis	Milky white discoloration; no subungual hyperkeratosis or onycholysis	*Trychophyton soudanense, Trichophyton violaceum*	Nail clipping
Candida onychomycosis:			
Paronychia	Swollen periungual skin, painful, bacterial superinfection, or nail plate disease	*Candida* species	Proximal and lateral edges; undersurface of nail
Distal nail infection	Onycholysis and subungual hyperkeratosis, fingernails, or vascular abnormality		
Total dystrophic onychomycosis	Gross thickening and hyperkeratosis		
Total dystrophic onychomycosis	Complete destruction of nail plate	Any of above; *Candida* in immunocompromised people	
Mixed	Different patterns in same individual		
Mould	Few specific clinical features; often one nail with previous disease or trauma; toenails; absence of tinea pedis	*Scopulariopsis brevicaulis, Neoscytalidium dimidiatum, Aspergillus, Acremonium, Fusarium, Neoscytalidium hyalinum*	

A recent review suggests carrying out at least two diagnostic investigations to determine the penetration of the nail plate,[14] usually microscopy and culture. Ideally the site should be cleaned with 70% ethanol before sample collection and the sampled material divided into two portions, one for microscopy and the other for culture. For transportation the samples should be stored in commercially available packs, sterile containers, or clean sheets of white paper folded and sealed. The type of onychomycosis will determine the site from which the diagnostic specimen is taken (table 1). Nail clippers can be used to obtain nail clippings of the nail plate (fig 5). Scrapings from subungual hyperkeratosis, nail bed, or nail plate, and surrounding or affected skin, should be taken using a small curette or number 15 scalpel blade. Sampling of the distal nail plate should be avoided because contamination is common. For proximal subungual onychomycosis, the healthy nail plate should be pared away with a number 15 blade and a sharp curette used to remove infected material from the nail bed closest to the lunula.[16] Alternatively, a superficial punch biopsy of the proximal nail plate can be taken from the proximal onycholytic border without anaesthesia. This is a simple procedure that can be performed by a general practitioner.

The specimen can be immediately viewed using direct microscopy by applying potassium hydroxide preparations to small pieces of affected nail on a glass slide. The slide should be warmed over a Bunsen burner flame and a coverslip applied. The specimen can then be examined with ×400 magnification using a normal bright field microscope. The presence of fungal hyphae, spores, or yeast forms should be determined to establish whether fungi are implicated. Direct microscopy is unable to identify particular fungi.

Culture can identify a specific fungus but results take 2-6 weeks to obtain and false negative rates are high (30%).[17] If the clinical suspicion of onychomycosis is high then culture should be repeated. Sections of the nail samples can be directly stained with periodic acid Schiff for histopathological evaluation,[18] which has been shown to be more sensitive (92%) than direct microscopy (80%) and culture (59%).[19]

How and when do you treat topically?

Indications for topical treatment include up to 50% involvement of the distal nail plate with lack of matrix involvement, three or four nails affected, and early distal and lateral subungual onychomycosis and superficial white

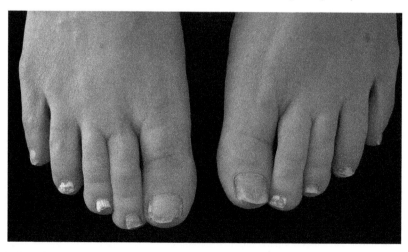

Fig 1 Onycomycosis of toenails showing mixed pattern in same patient—both distal and lateral subungual onychomycosis and superficial white onychomycosis

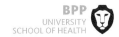

DIFFERENTIAL DIAGNOSIS OF ONYCHOMYCOSIS

Psoriasis (fig 2)

- As in onychomycosis: onycholysis, subungual hyperkeratosis, splinter haemorrhages, leuconychia, dystrophy
- Pitting
- Oil drop sign (a translucent yellow-red discoloration seen in the nail bed)
- Other cutaneous features of psoriasis, family history of psoriasis

Lichen planus

- Cutaneous disease at other sites
- Thin nail plate and ridging
- Dorsal pterygium—scarring at proximal aspect of nail

Trauma

- Nail plate can appear abnormal
- Nail bed should be normal
- Distal onycholysis with repeated trauma
- Single nail affected, shape of nail changed, homogenous alteration of nail colour

Eczema

- Irregular buckled nails with ridging
- Cutaneous signs of eczema

Yellow nail syndrome

- Nail plate is discoloured green-yellow
- Nails are hard with elevated longitudinal curvature
- Nails may be shed, painful
- Associations with bronchiectasis, lymphoedema, and chronic sinusitis

Lamellar onychoschizia (lamellar splitting) (fig 3)

- History of repeated soaking in water
- Usually distal portion of nail

Periungual squamous cell carcinoma/Bowens disease

- Single nail, warty changes of nail fold, ooze from edge of nail

Malignant melanona

- Black discolouration of nail plate or nail bed
- Pigment can extend onto nail fold
- Can get associated bleeding

Myxoid (mucous) cyst

- Cyst at base of nail, groove in nail extending length of nail

Alopecia areata

- Pits, longitudinal ridging, brittleness
- Hair loss

onychomycosis.[20] Other considerations include the patient's age, as children's nails are thin and grow fast, prophylaxis in those at risk of recurrence, and whether oral treatment is contraindicated.

Amorolfine

Amorolfine 5% lacquer has broad spectrum fungicidal and fungistatic activity and has been recommended, according to proposed guidelines, for onychomycosis without matrix involvement and mild cases of distal and lateral disease of up to two affected nails.[20] [21] It is applied once or twice weekly (after nail filing) for six to 12 months. A recent multicentre, randomised, open label, controlled study noted complete cure in 12.7% of patients and mycological cure in 46.5% at 48 weeks.[22]

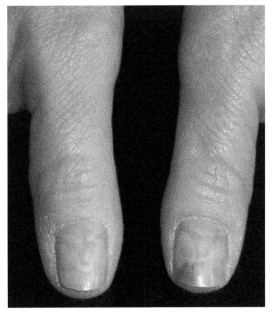

Fig 2 Psoriasis of nails, with irregular proximal border and brown onychodermal band. As with fungal infection, nail surface is not friable

Ciclopirox

Ciclopirox (widely available, but not available in the United Kingdom), which has broad spectrum antifungal activity, is available as an 8% lacquer and is applied once daily for 24 weeks on fingernails and for 48 weeks on toenails. A review of findings from two well designed, double blinded, vehicle controlled, parallel group, multicentre studies showed mycological cure rates of 29% and 36%, compared with complete cure rates of 5.5% and 8.4%.[23] Amorolfine has not been directly compared with ciclopirox but cure rates seem to be lower with ciclopirox. The Cochrane Collaboration[24] suggests that amorolfine might be more effective. A recent multicentre, randomised controlled trial has shown that chemical avulsion of the nail combined with ciclopirox cream and nail lacquer is more effective than amorolfine nail lacquer alone, with clinical cure rates of 53.5% compared with 17% reported in groups receiving amorolfine.[22] Side effects from lacquers include nail fold erythema, burning, and pruritus. These are usually temporary and transient but if severe, treatment should be stopped.

Less commonly used topical treatments

Other topical treatments which may be considered in a specialist setting include tioconazole, available as a 28% solution, which has shown cure rates of up to 22% in an open ended study.[25] Efinaconazole solution 10%, the first triazole antifungal, is applied once daily for 48 weeks. Two identical multicentre, randomised, double blind, vehicle controlled studies conducted in patients with distal lateral subungual onychomycosis showed greater complete cure with efinaconazole (17.8% and 15.2%) compared with vehicle (3.3% and 5.5%).[26] This product has been approved in Canada but is still pending approval in the United States.

What systemic options are available?

Despite the availability of various systemic treatments for onychomycosis (table 2) the search for an ideal agent is ongoing. Even with optimal management, mycological cure rates are about 30% and treatment failure rates are at least 25%.[10] When choosing treatment, consideration needs to be given to the patient's age and health, cost, compliance,

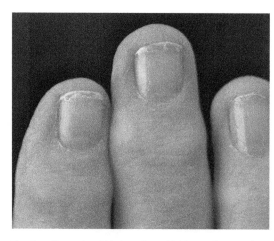

Fig 3 Lamella onychoschizia in patient with history of repeated soaking of hands in water

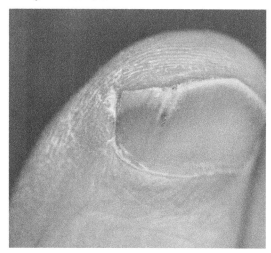

Fig 4 Nail spike showing yellow hyperkeratotic band progressing proximally towards matrix, characteristic of fungal infection of nail, with associated tinea pedis. Cultures confirmed *Trichophyton rubrum*

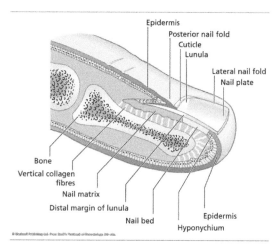

Fig 5 Longitudinal section of nail apparatus. Reproduced from Burns et al,[15] with permission of Wiley-Blackwell

side effects, and drug interactions, and the type and site of infection. Oral treatments are generally more effective than topical ones; however, they have more adverse effects and interactions. Oral treatment is recommended with proximal subungual onychomycosis, when at least 50% of the nail plate is affected, where the nail matrix or multiple nails are involved, and if there has been no response to topical treatment after six months.[21] The two main systemic drugs indicated for the treatment of onychomycosis are terbinafine and itraconazole, but terbinafine should be considered as first line treatment because of lower drug interactions than itraconazole and because it is superior both in vivo and in vitro for dermatophyte onychomycosis. Other systemic therapeutic options include griseofulvin, which remains the only licensed option in children, and fluconazole, used as a third line agent; both are considered below.

Terbinafine

Terbinafine is both fungistatic and fungicidal, with lower activity against *Candida* species. It is given as 250 mg daily for six weeks for fingernails and for 12-16 weeks for toenails. Patients should be re-evaluated three to six months after the start of treatment, the period required for outgrowth of healthy nail. Further treatment should be given if disease persists as the optimal clinical effect is seen some months after mycological cure and cessation of treatment. Trials have investigated pulsed terbinafine 500

mg daily for one week every month for three consecutive months. A large randomised trial has shown mycological cure of 70.9% (continuous) compared with 58.7% (pulsed) at 18 months.[29] Variable success has been shown by other trials studying pulsed or intermittent terbinafine, which would offer a viable option for reducing both the cost and the side effects of treatment. Terbinafine should not be used in patients with chronic or active liver disease. Baseline liver function testing is recommended according to the package insert and periodic monitoring (4-6 weeks) is suggested. Terbinafine should be discontinued immediately in the case of increased liver function.[30]

Itraconazole

Itraconazole is thought to be a fungistatic agent and is active against yeast, dermatophytes, and non-dermatophyte moulds. However, it is less active against dermatophytes than terbinafine. Persistence of itraconazole in the nail plate makes intermittent dosing regimens as effective as daily dosing. In a multicentre randomised trial, intermittent treatment resulted in equal mycological and higher clinical cure compared with continuous treatment.[31] Itraconazole can therefore be given as 200 mg a day (12 weeks for toenails, six weeks for fingernails) or as a monthly pulsed treatment of 400 mg a day for one week of each month (two pulses for fingernails, three pulses for toenails). Itraconazole is contraindicated in those with heart failure or liver abnormalities. Patients receiving continuous treatment for longer than one month should have their liver function tested; however, no monitoring is required for the pulse regimen unless there is a history of hepatic disease, other hepatotoxic drugs, or abnormal liver function at baseline, or if signs or symptoms develop at any time to suggest liver dysfunction.[32]

Several studies have looked at the efficacy rates for terbinafine compared with itraconazole. A multicentre randomised trial showed cure in 55% (continuous terbinafine for 16 weeks) compared with 26% (pulsed itraconazole) at 72 weeks' follow-up.[33] A cumulative meta-analysis of systemic antifungal agents for onychomycosis confirmed these findings.[34] Lower recurrence rates have also been noted with terbinafine in a meta-analysis comparing terbinafine with itraconazole.[35] A recent review reported a synergistic action between itraconazole and terbinafine, and combination treatment may result in better eradication than monotherapy, and may also prevent recurrence of infection.[36]

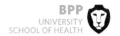

Table 2 Summary of systemic drug treatments in adults[27][28]

Treatment and dose	Contraindications	Cautions/advice	Blood monitoring
First line treatment: itraconazole:			
200 mg/day: 6 weeks for fingernails, 12 weeks for toenails; 400 mg/day for one week a month (pulse): two pulses for fingernails, three pulses for toenails	Chronic and active liver disease; congestive heart failure or ventricular dysfunction; concomitant benzodiazepines, HMG-CoA reductase inhibitors, quinidines, pimozide; pregnancy (category C*); breast feeding	Take with food; numerous drug interactions including hypoglycaemics and antiretrovirals	Liver function test for continuous treatment only and repeat 4-6 weekly; no liver function test for pulsed treatment
First line treatment: terbinafine:			
250 mg/day: 6 weeks for fingernails, 12-16 weeks for toenails	Chronic or active liver disease; breast feeding; pregnancy (category B†)	Stop if AST/ALT increase to 2 normal; if creatinine clearance ‹50 mL/min or creatinine ›300 µmol/L then half normal dose; caution with known autoimmune disorders	Liver function test and full blood count before treatment; monitor with liver function test and full blood count every 4-6 weeks
Fluconazole (unlicensed):			
150 mg/week: 6-9 months for fingernails, 9-18 months for toenails	Renal and hepatic impairment; benzodiazepines (increase sedation); terfenadine, cisapride, astemizole, pimozide, quinidine, or erythromycin; pregnancy (category C*); breast feeding	Many drug interactions; lactose allergen in some preparations; not approved for onychomycosis in United States, Canada, and Australia	Baseline liver function test and full blood count; liver function test if high dosages given, prolonged treatment, concomitant hepatotoxic drugs
Griseofulvin:			
500-1000 mg/day: 6-9 months for fingernails, 12-18 months for toenails	Severe liver impairment; porphyria; lupus erythematosis; pregnancy (category C*); men fathering a child for 6 months after therapy	Take with fatty food; drug interactions (oral contraceptive, anticoagulant, phenobarbital); no longer treatment of choice	Monitor with liver function test regularly if mild hepatic impairment

AST=serum aspartate aminotransferase; ALT=serum alanine aminotransferase.

*Animal reproduction studies have shown an adverse effect on the fetus but there are no adequate and well controlled studies in pregnant women.

†Animal reproduction studies have failed to show a risk to the fetus but there are no adequate and well controlled studies in pregnant women.

Griseofulvin

Griseofulvin has lower efficacy and higher relapse rates than either terbinafine or itraconazole but is the only agent licensed for children. It is indicated when the other drugs are unavailable or contraindicated. Griseofulvin is contraindicated in severe hepatic disease but may be used in mild impairment with regular monitoring of liver function. Doses in adults are 500-1000 mg daily for 6-9 months for fingernails and 12-18 months for toenails.[11]

Fluconazole

Fluconazole, although not licensed for onychomycosis, remains a potential third line treatment. It is cheap, has good compliance rates owing to weekly dosing, and has few drug interactions. It is highly effective against both dermatophytes and *Candida* species. Many studies have evaluated its efficacy in onychomycosis and, based on a systematic review,[37] mycological cure rates between 36% and 100% are reported. A recent meta-analysis recommended a dosage of 150 mg weekly for more than six months for onychomycosis.[38] Fluconazole seems to be less effective (31% cure) than either itraconazole (61%) or terbinafine(75%)[37] but comparative trials are few.[39]

New second generation triazoles include voriconazole, posaconazole, ravuconazole, albaconazole, and pramiconazole. They may play a useful role in immunocompromised hosts, where there is resistance to standard treatment, and in the treatment of non-dermatophyte moulds.[11]

What is the role of nail avulsion and debridement?

Nail avulsion (complete removal) or debridement (partial removal) can be useful in severe onychomycosis, extensive nail thickening, or longitudinal streaks or spikes. These changes can cause a dermatophytoma, representing a granulated nidus of infection, which responds poorly to medical treatment. Avulsion and debridement can help reduce fungal mass and increase the penetration of

antifungal treatment. Chemical avulsion involves dissolving the bond between the nail plate and the nail bed, and softens the nail plate.[40] Agents such as 40% urea or 20% urea with 10% salicylic acid, are recommended for the treatment of single nail disease and are applied with a topical antifungal (1% bifonazole[41] or 1% fluconazole[42]) under occlusion for 1-2 weeks, after which the diseased nail can be removed with a nail elevator or clipper. Surgical avulsion involves separating the nail plate from the nail bed using a nail elevator device. This is an option for disease resistant to topical and systemic antifungals. It is usually followed by a course of systemic antifungals.

Debridement involves partial removal of the nail. In a randomised controlled trial a combination of debridement and 8% ciclopirox lacquer resulted in better (77%) mycological cure than debridement alone (0%).[43]

Is there a role for combination treatments?

Topical ciclopirox, amorolfine, and imidazoles have been used in combination with systemic antifungal agents. In toenail onychomycosis an open randomised trial showed mycological cure rates of 83% for oral itraconazole combined with amorolfine lacquer compared with 41% for itraconazole alone for 12 weeks.[44] Similar benefits were shown with terbinafine.[45] Evidence is sufficient to recommend combination treatment in cases where response to monotherapy may be poor, as is the case in proximal nail disease, treatment failure, or involvement of more than 50% of the nail plate.[20]

What about yeasts and non-dermatophyte moulds?

Candida accounts for 5-10% of all cases of onychomycosis. Itraconazole should be considered as the first line agent for *Candida* species, and fluconazole (although unlicensed) can be used as an alternative. Terbinafine is an effective agent, with cure rates of 70-85% after 48 weeks of treatment with 250 mg daily noted in a series of 65 patients with onychmycosis caused by *C albicans*, *C parasilosis*, or *S*

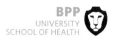

WHEN SHOULD I REFER?[52]

- Patients should be referred if:
- There is coexistent nail disease (psoriasis or lichen planus)
- Onychomycosis is suspected but microscopy and culture give negative results
- Response to treatment is inadequate
- The diagnosis is uncertain
- Disease recurs or there is a relapse
- The nail plate or nail bed shows black discolouration (to exclude nail apparatus melanoma)
- They are children or young people (<18 years)
- The host is immunocompromised

POOR PROGNOSTIC FACTORS[53 54]

These factors may influence treatment type (topical, oral, combination, surgery), length of treatment, duration of treatment, and follow-up:

- Lateral edge involvement
- Area of nail involvement >50%
- Nail thickness >2 mm
- Matrix involvement
- Onycholysis, paronychia, discolouration, dermatophytoma
- Slow nail growth
- Positive culture results at six month follow-up
- Diabetes, peripheral vascular disease, immunosuppression
- The presence of non-responsive organisms, such as *Scytalidium*

NEW TESTS AND TREATMENTS ON THE HORIZON

Diagnosis

- Dermatophyte test strip: visualises mycotic antigens extracted from nail samples by immunochromatography[55]
- Flow cytometry generates distinct profiles for fungi invading the nail plate
- Real time polymerase chain reaction assays can detect and identify dermatophytes in less than two days
- Scanning electron microscopy and confocal microscopy

Treatment

- Techniques to improve topical delivery of antifungals, including phonophoresis, manual and electrical nail abrasion, acid etching, microporation, ultrasonography, laser nail ablation, and iontophoresis
- Technologies to improve drug uptake by fungi: transferosome vesicles (TDT 067), boosted antifungal topical treatment (BATT), and boosted oral antifungal therapy (BOAT)
- Lasers approved for the management of onychomycosis include Nd:YAG short pulse and Q switch 1064 nm and the diode 870, 930, and 980 nm[56] (no randomised controlled trials as yet)
- Photodynamic therapy has been shown in a single centre open trial to achieve cure rates of 44% at 12 months[57]
- Topical germicidal ultraviolet C light[58]

ADDITIONAL EDUCATIONAL RESOURCES

Resources for healthcare professionals

- National Institute for Health and Care Excellence. Fungal nail infection. 2009 (http://cks.nice. org.uk/fungal-nail-infection)—Overview of onychomycosis and extensive review of evidence on treatments
- Cochrane Summaries. 2009 (http://summaries.cochrane.org/CD001434/creams-lotions-and-gels-topical-treatments-for-fungal-infections-of-the-skin-and-nails-of-the-foot)—Discusses creams, lotions, and gels (topical treatments) of fungal infections of the skin and nails of the foot
- *British Journal of Dermatology*. Guidelines for treatment of onychomycosis. 2003 (www.bad.org. uk/Portals/_Bad/Guidelines/Clinical%20Guidelines/Onychomycosis—Detailed guidelines on the management of onychomycosis

Resources for patients

- Dermnet NZ (www.dermnetnz.org/doctors/fungal-infections/tinea-unguium.html)—Provides a summary of causes, diagnosis, clinical appearances, and treatment of onychomycosis
- British Association of Dermatologists (www.bad.org.uk/site/820/Default.aspx)—Overview of fungal nail infection: causes, clinical appearances, diagnosis, and management
- WebMD (www.webmd.com/skin-problems-and-treatments/tc/fungal-nail-infections)—Treatment overview for fungal nail infection

brevicaulis.[46] Non-dermatophyte moulds are difficult to treat. A recent review[47] concluded that the best treatment option may be systemic or topical treatment combined with periodic chemical or surgical debridement or avulsion.

What are the treatment options in children?

The prevalence of onychomycosis in children in the United Kingdom has been reported at 0.2%.[48] Toenails are usually affected and the most common presentation is distal subungual onychomycosis. In children, concomitant tinea capitis and tinea pedis should be excluded, and parents and siblings should be examined to exclude infection. Topical treatment of onychomycosis is often advocated but not licensed in children, and no clinical trials show efficacy in this population.[11] Griseofulvin is licensed for children but is no longer recommended as first line treatment owing to long treatment duration and poor efficacy.[11] Terbinafine is licensed in some countries for use in tinea capitis and can be used in children older than 2 years and with a body weight of more than 12 kg. Children should be referred for specialist review and initiation of treatment. They can, if there are no contraindications, be treated as for adults, using terbinafine, itraconazole, or fluconazole with dose adjusting according to weight and age. None of these treatments are licensed for use in children, but efficacy and safety have been published recently in a systematic review.[49]

Do patients with diabetes or immunosuppression require different treatment?

In patients with diabetes, terbinafine is the treatment of choice and is preferred over itraconazole, which is contraindicated in heart failure. Owing to drug interactions, itraconazole can also induce hypoglycaemia in patients with diabetes. Topical treatments should be considered to avoid the potential for drug interactions with antidiabetic drugs. Terbinafine and fluconazole are the agents of choice in patients with HIV as they interfere least with antiretrovirals.

How do I know if treatment is successful?

Cure of onychomycosis has been defined as the absence of clinical signs or the presence of a negative culture result, with or without negative microscopy results, after an adequate wash-out period of 3-6 months.[50] Even with optimal management 25% to 30% of patients will relapse after initial cure.[51] After three months of treatment, most toenails will still look abnormal after systemic treatment. If normal nail is emerging proximal to the dystrophic nail, a scratch can be made with a scalpel blade at the base of the dystrophy. If the dystrophic nail remains distal to the scratch as it grows out no further treatment is required, but if the dystrophy moves proximal to the scratch then this indicates ongoing infection and further treatment. Serial photography is a helpful additional monitoring tool.

Contributors: SE prepared the manuscript. RS revised and reviewed the manuscript. He is guarantor.

Competing interests: We have read and understood the BMJ Group policy on declaration of interests and declare the following interests: None.

Patient consent: Obtained.

Provenance and peer review: Commissioned; externally peer reviewed.

1 Sigurgeirsson B, Baran R. The prevalence of onychomycosis in the global population—a literature study. *J Eur Acad Dermatol Venereol* 2013; published online 28 Nov.
2 Jesudanam TM, Rao GR, Lakshmi DJ, Kumari GR. Onychomycosis: a significant medical problem. *Indian J Dermatol Venereol Leprol* 2002;68:326-9.

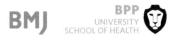

3 Scher RK, Baran R. Onychomycosis in clinical practice: factors contributing to recurrence. *Br J Dermatol* 2003;149(Suppl 65):5-9.

4 Summerbell RC, Kane J, Krajden S. Onychomycosis, tinea pedis and tinea manuum caused by non-dermatophytic filamentous fungi. *Mycoses* 1989;32:609-19.

5 Gupta AK, Konnikov N, MacDonald P, Rich P, Rodger NW, Edmonds MW, et al. Prevalence and epidemiology of toenail onychomycosis in diabetic subjects: a multicentre survey. *Br J Dermatol* 1998;139:665-71.

6 Faergemann J, Correia O, Nowicki R, Ro BI. Genetic predisposition—understanding underlying mechanisms of onychomycosis. *J Eur Acad Dermatol Venereol* 2005;19:17-9.

7 Gupta AK, Lynde CW, Jain HC, Sibbald RG, Elewski BE, Daniel CR 3rd, et al. A higher prevalence of onychomycosis in psoriatics compared with non-psoriatics: a multicentre study. *Br J Dermatol* 1997;136:786-9.

8 Gupta AK, Taborda P, Taborda V, Gilmour J, Rachlis A, Salit I, et al. Epidemiology and prevalence of onychomycosis in HIV-positive individuals. *Int J Dermatol* 2000;39:746-53.

9 Gupta AK, Gupta MA, Summerbell RC, Cooper EA, Konnikov N, Albreski D, et al. The epidemiology of onychomycosis: possible role of smoking and peripheral arterial disease. *J Eur Acad Dermatol Venereol* 2000;14:466-9.

10 Hay RJ. The future of onychomycosis therapy may involve a combination of approaches. *Br J Dermatol* 2001;145(Suppl 60):3-8.

11 Ameen M, Lear JT, Madan V, Mohd Mustapa MF, Richardson M. British Association of Dermatologists' guidelines for the management of onychomycosis 2013; (in press).

12 Singal A, Khanna D. Onychomycosis: diagnosis and management. *Indian J Dermatol Venereol Leprol* 2011;77:358-75.

13 Hay RJ, Baran R. Onychomycosis: a proposed revision of the clinical classification. *JAAD* 2011;65: 1219-27.

14 Gupta AK, Simpson FC. Diagnosing onychomycosis. *Clin Dermatol* 2013;31:540-3

15 Burns T, Breathnach S, Cox N, Griffiths C, eds. Rook's textbook of dermatology, 8th edn. Wiley-Blackwell, 2010.

16 Rodgers P, Bassler M. Treating onychomycosis. *Am Fam Physician* 2001;63:663-73.

17 Hay R. Literature review. Onychomycosis. *J Eur Acad Dermatol Venereol* 2005;19(Suppl 1):1-7.

18 Barak O, Asarch A, Horn T. PAS is optimal for diagnosing onychomycosis. *J Cutan Pathol* 2010;37:1038-40.

19 Weinberg JM, Koestenblatt EK, Tutrone WD, Tishler HR, Najarian L. Comparison of diagnostic methods in the evaluation of onychomycosis. *J Am Acad Dermatol* 2003;49:193-7.

20 Lecha M, Effendy 'I, Feuilhade de Chauvin M, Di Chiacchio N, Baran R. Taskforce on onychomycosis education. Treatment options-development of consensus guidelines. *J Eur Acad Dermatol Venereol* 2005;19(Suppl 1):25-33.

21 Gupta AK, Paquet M, Simpson FC. Therapies for the treatment of onychomycosis. *Clin Dermatol* 2013;31:544-54.

22 Paul C, Coustou D, Lahfa M, Bulai-Livideanu C, Doss N, Mokthar I, et al. A multicenter, randomized, open-label, controlled study comparing the efficacy, safety and cost-effectiveness of a sequential therapy with RV4104A ointment, ciclopiroxolamine cream and ciclopirox film-forming solution with amorolfine nail lacquer alone in dermatophytic onychomycosis. *Dermatology* 2013;227:157-64.

23 Gupta AK, Baran R. Ciclopirox nail lacquer solution 8% in the 21st century. *J Am Acad Dermatol* 2000;43(Suppl):S96-102.

24 Crawford F, Hollis S. Topical treatments for fungal infections of the skin and nails of the foot. *Cochrane Database Syst Rev* 2007;3:CD001434.

25 Hay RJ, Mackie RM, Clayton YM. Tioconazole nail solution—an open study of its efficacy in onychomycosis. *Clin Exp Dermatol* 1985;10:111-5.

26 Elewski BE, Rich P, Pollak R, Pariser DM, Watanabe S, Senda H, et al. Efinaconazole 10% solution in the treatment of toenail onychomycosis: two phase III multicenter, randomized, double-blind studies. *J Am Acad Dermatol* 2013;68:600-8.

27 Sotiriou E, Koussidou-Eremonti T, Chaidemenos G, Apalla Z, Ioannides D. Photodynamic therapy for distal and lateral subungual toenail onychomycosis caused by Trichophyton rubrum: preliminary results of a single-centre open trial. *Acta Derm Venereol* 2010;90:216-7.

28 Dai T, Tegos GP, Rolz-Cruz G, Cumbie WE, Hamblin MR. Ultraviolet C inactivation of dermatophytes: implications for treatment of onychomycosis. *Br J Dermatol* 2008;158:1239-46.

29 Warshaw EM, Fett DD, Bloomfield HE, Grill JP, Nelson DB, Quintero V, et al. Pulse versus continuous terbinafine for onychomycosis: a randomized double-blind, controlled trial. *J Am Acad Dermatol* 2005;53:578-84.

30 Electronic Medicines Compendium. Lamisil tablets 250mg. www.medicines.org.uk/emc/medicine/1290/SPC/Lamisil+Tablets+250mg/.

31 Havu V, Brandt H, Heikkilä H, Hollmen A, Oksman R, Rantanen T, et al. A double-blind, randomized study comparing itraconazole pulse therapy with continuous dosing for the treatment of toe-nail onychomycosis. *Br J Dermatol* 1997;136:230-4.

32 Gupta AK, Chwetzoff E, Del Rosso J, Baran R. Hepatic safety of itraconazole. *J Cutan Med Surg* 2002;6:210-3.

33 Evans EG, Sigurgeirsson B. Double blind, randomised study of continuous terbinafine compared with intermittent itraconazole in treatment of toenail onychomycosis. The LION Study Group. *BMJ* 1999;318:1031-5.

34 Gupta AK, Ryder JE, Johnson AM. Cumulative meta-analysis of systemic antifungal agents for the treatment of onychomycosis. *Br J Dermatol* 2004;150:537-44.

35 Yin Z, Xu J, Luo D. A meta-analysis comparing long-term recurrences of toenail onychomycosis after successful treatment with terbinafine versus itraconazole. *J Dermatolog Treat* 2012;23:449-52.

36 Gupta AK, Paquet M. Improved efficacy in onychomycosis therapy. *Clin Dermatol* 2013;31:555-63.

37 Brown SJ. Efficacy of fluconazole for the treatment of onychomycosis. *Ann Pharmacother* 2009;43:1684-91.

38 Gupta AK, Drummond-Main C, Paquet M. Evidence-based optimal fluconazole dosing regimen for onychomycosis treatment. *J Dermatolog Treat* 2013;24:75-80.

39 Havu V, Heikkilä H, Kuokkanen K, Nuutinen M, Rantanen T, Saari S, et al. A double-blind, randomized study to compare the efficacy and safety of terbinafine (Lamisil) with fluconazole (Diflucan) in the treatment of onychomycosis. *Br J Dermatol* 2000;142:97-102.

40 Pandhi D, Verma P. Nail avulsion: indications and methods (surgical nail avulsion). *Indian J Dermatol Venereol Leprol* 2012;78:299-308.

41 Lahfa M, Bulai-Livideanu C, Baran R, Ortonne JP, Richert B, Tosti A, et al. Efficacy, safety and tolerability of an optimized avulsion technique with onyster® (40% urea ointment with plastic dressing) ointment compared to bifonazole-urea ointment for removal of the clinically infected nail in toenail onychomycosis: a randomized evaluator-blinded controlled study. *Dermatology* 2013;226:5-12.

42 Baran R, Coquard F. Combination of fluconazole and urea in a nail lacquer for treating onychomycosis. *J Dermatolog Treat* 2005;16:52-5.

43 Malay DS, Yi S, Borowsky P, Downey MS, Mlodzienski AJ. Efficacy of debridement alone versus debridement combined with topical antifungal nail lacquer for the treatment of pedal onychomycosis: a randomized, controlled trial. *J Foot Ankle Surg* 2009;48:294-308.

44 Lecha M. Amorolfine and itraconazole combination for severe toenail onychomycosis; results of an open randomized trial in Spain. *Br J Dermatol* 2001;145(Suppl 60):21-6.

45 Baran R, Feuilhade M, Combernale P, Datry A, Goettmann S, Pietrini P, et al. A randomized trial of amorolfine 5% solution nail lacquer combined with oral terbinafine compared with terbinafine alone in the treatment of dermatophytic toenail onychomycoses affecting the matrix region. *Br J Dermatol* 2000;142:1177-83.

46 Nolting S, Brautigam M, Weidinger G. Terbinafine in onychomycosis with involvement by non-dermatophytic fungi. *Br J Dermatol* 1994;130(Suppl 43):16-21.

47 Gupta AK, Drummond-Main C, Cooper EA, Brintnell W, Piraccini BM, Tosti A. Systematic review of nondermatophyte mold onychomycosis: diagnosis, clinical types, epidemiology, and treatment. *J Am Acad Dermatol* 2012;66:494-502.

48 Philpot CM, Shuttleworth D. Dermatophyte onychomycosis in children. *Clin Exp Dermatol* 1989;14:203-5.

49 Gupta AK, Paquet M. Systemic antifungals to treat onychomycosis in children: a systematic review. *Pediatr Dermatol* 2013;30:294-302.

50 Ghannoum M, Isham N, Catalano VA. Second look at efficacy criteria for onychomycosis: clinical and mycological cure. *Br J Dermatol* 2014;170:182-7.

51 De Berker D. Clinical practice. Fungal nail disease. *N Engl J Med* 2009;14:2108-16.

52 National Institute for Health and Care Excellence. Fungal nail infection—summary. 2013. http://cks.nice.org.uk/fungal-nail-infection#!topicsummary.

53 Scher RK, Baran R. Onychomycosis in clinical practice: factors contributing to recurrence. *Br J Dermatol* 2003;149(Suppl 65):5-9.

54 Sigurgeirsson B. Prognostic factors for cure following treatment of onychomycosis. *J Eur Acad Dermatol Venereol* 2010;24:679-84.

55 Tsunemi Y, Takehara K, Miura Y, Nakagami G, Sanada H, Kawashima M. Screening for Tinea unguium by Dermatophyte Test Strip. *Br J Dermatol* 2014;170:328-31.

56 Gupta A, Simpson F. Device-based therapies for onychomycosis treatment. *Skin Therapy Lett* 2012;17:4-9.

57 Katz HI, Gupta AK. Oral antifungal drug interactions. *Dermatol Clin* 1997;15:535-44.

58 Gupta AK, Lynde CW, Lauzon GJ, Mehlmauer MA, Braddock SW, Miller CA, et al. Cutaneous adverse effects associated with terbinafine therapy: 10 case reports and a review of the literature. *Br J Dermatol* 1998;138:529-32.

Related links

bmj.com/archive

- Management of sickle cell disease in the community (*BMJ* 2014;348:g1765)
- Coeliac disease (*BMJ* 2014;348:g1561)
- Fibromyalgia (*BMJ* 2014;348:g1224)
- Trigeminal neuralgia (*BMJ* 2014;348:g474)

bmj.com

- Get Cleveland Clinic CME credits for this article

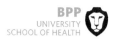

Evaluation of oral ulceration in primary care

Vinidh Paleri, consultant head and neck and thyroid surgeon[1],
Konrad Staines, consultant in oral medicine[1], Philip Sloan, professor of pathology[1],
Adam Douglas, general practitioner[2],
Janet Wilson, professor of otolaryngology-head and neck surgery[1]

[1]Newcastle upon Tyne Hospitals NHS Foundation Trust, High Heaton, Newcastle upon Tyne NE7 7DN

[2]Cestria Health Centre, County Durham DH2 3DJ

Correspondence to: V Paleri vinidh.paleri@ncl.ac.uk

Cite this as: BMJ 2010;340:c2639

DOI: 10.1136/bmj.c2639

http://www.bmj.com/content/340/bmj.c2639

Introduction

Oral ulcers are common, with an estimated point prevalence of 4% in the United States.[1] Aphthous ulcers may affect as many as 25% of the population worldwide. Patients with an oral ulcer may present initially to a general practitioner or a dental practitioner. Most ulcers are benign and resolve spontaneously but a small proportion of them are malignant. The incidence and prevalence of oral cancers varies across the world. The five year prevalence of oral cavity cancer in developed countries is 275 373 cases and in less developed countries 464 756 cases.[2] Some of the highest incidences are seen in the Indian subcontinent, southern France, and South America. Importantly, the incidence of oral cancer is rising in most populations, particularly in young women. In the United Kingdom, around 2500 cases of oral cavity cancers are seen every year.

A community based, cluster randomised intervention trial has shown that early detection of an oral squamous cell malignancy reduces mortality. According to the UK Department of Health's national referral guidelines for suspected cancer, a generalist may refer an oral ulcer that persists for more than three weeks to a specialist to be seen within two weeks of referral.[3] An audit of 1079 such referrals, which showed that only 18% of patients referred had a malignancy, highlighted the difficulties encountered by health care practitioners in differentiating potentially malignant ulcers from benign ones.[4] A recent study used a validated theoretical framework to evaluate general medical practitioners' attitudes towards oral examination and found that lack of confidence, knowledge, and training contributed to difficulties in differentiation.[5] The aim of this review is to provide a clinically oriented overview of the common causes of acute oral ulcers and to present a structured clinical assessment to assist in distinguishing malignant ulcers from non-malignant ones.

SOURCES AND SELECTION CRITERIA

We searched for papers published between 1990 and 2009 using key index terms (oral ulcer, mouth ulcer) on PubMed (Medline and life science journals), Cochrane systematic reviews, and BMJ Clinical Evidence. We searched national and international clinical trial databases. This search was supplemented by published reviews known to us and our own clinical practice.

SUMMARY POINTS

- Oral ulceration is common and mostly benign
- Some oral ulcers may be associated with systemic disease or particular drugs
- A systematic approach to examination of the oral cavity with good lighting and retraction of mobile tissues is critical
- A substantial minority of oral ulcers are malignant
- Patients with an ulcer that persists for more than three weeks should be referred; suspected malignancy requires urgent referral to a specialist
- Non-malignant oral ulceration may be investigated and treated in primary care or referred
- If a patient with a benign ulcer is not referred re-evaluate the lesion to ensure that healing has occurred.

What causes oral ulcers?

Oral ulcers may have a great many causes, although in some no cause is identified. Oral ulcers are termed "acute" if they persist for less than three weeks duration and "chronic" if they persist for longer than three weeks. They may be recurrent.

Non-neoplastic causes of acute oral mucosal ulcers

Trauma, minor aphthous ulcers, drugs, and infections are responsible for most acute, self limiting oral ulcers. Traumatic injury to the oral mucosa may be caused by a sharp tooth margin, an overextended denture flange, or cheek biting (fig 1A). Chemical and thermal trauma can also cause oral ulceration (fig 1B). Traumatic ulceration may mask or mimic more serious causes. The cause of trauma should be identified and removed with follow up to ensure that healing has occurred.

Minor aphthous ulcers are painful, discrete, and round, measuring less than 1 cm in diameter with a greyish base and a red halo (fig 1C). As many as six may occur at a time on multiple oral mucosal sites. The cause is unknown in most patients, although predisposing factors such as familial tendency, local trauma, and stress are often cited. Such ulcers most commonly involve non keratinised oral mucosa. They typically heal spontaneously within 10 days, although more severe forms may persist, and recurrence is common. The majority of patients presenting with aphthous ulcers do not have an associated underlying systemic disease, but aphthous-like ulcers may occur in association with systemic disease such as inflammatory bowel disease, or use of medication such as non-steroidal anti-inflammatory drugs.

Various infectious agents can cause acute oral ulceration (box 1). The most common infective causes are the herpesviridae. Herpetic ulcers are usually ragged and well delineated and occur within a precise sensory nerve distribution (fig 1D). They may resolve within three weeks but can persist for longer, especially in immunocompromised patients.

Non-neoplastic causes of chronic oral mucosal ulcers

The majority of chronic oral ulcers are accounted for by major aphthous ulcers, traumatic ulceration with persistent irritation (for example, from a sharp tooth, denture flange, or in rare cases deliberate self harm), oral lichen planus, drugs, and chronic infections. Major aphthous ulcers tend to be larger than minor ones and may involve the keratinised oral mucosa such as the hard palate. Large ulcers may take longer than three weeks to resolve and often leave a scar. Their clinical appearance may suggest malignancy (fig 2A). Herpetiform aphthous ulcers are characterised by small, numerous, 1-3 mm lesions that are clustered and appear in crops. They typically heal in less than a month without scarring. They can be mistaken for infective ulcers caused by herpesviridae but are never preceded by vesicles.

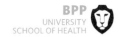

Chronic traumatic ulcers are painful and soft on palpation and may have rolled margins with whitish surrounding mucosa. Lichen planus is an autoimmune skin condition that may have oral and genital involvement. Oral lichen planus may occur as an isolated entity. The ulceration is typically superficial, often described as erosion, and blends with surrounding inflamed tissue (fig 2B and C). Fine white striae represent keratosis. The ulcer may be associated with desquamative full thickness gingivitis. The differential diagnosis for such widespread ulceration includes rarer causes such as systemic lupus erythematosus, graft versus host disease, and immunobullous disorders (mucous membrane pemphigoid and pemphigus vulgaris).

Drug related chronic ulcers may mimic aphthous ulcers (aphthous like ulceration) or oral lichenoid lesions (fig 2D). Solitary fixed eruptions, pemphigus, and mucous membrane pemphigoid induced by drugs may rarely involve the oral mucous membrane; bullae form and subsequently ulcerate. Drug related lesions may be associated with other mucocutaneous lesions.

Many infectious agents can cause chronic oral ulceration. In patients with HIV infection, causes can range from severe and chronic aphthous type ulceration to lymphoma. Immunocompromised patients may have mouth infections such as recurrent intraoral herpes. Secondary syphilis should be considered, even though associated oral ulcers often resolve spontaneously, since the patient may go on to develop complications of tertiary syphilis if left untreated. Chronic periapical dental infections can present with a draining dental sinus in the gingival tissue or the palate.

Neoplastic causes of oral mucosal ulcers

Many patients who present with an oral ulcer as the initial sign of malignancy will have had symptoms for more than three weeks. Box 2 lists malignant causes of oral ulcers. Oral squamous cell carcinoma is the most common epithelial malignancy within the oral cavity. Other cancers, such as minor salivary gland tumours and lymphomas, more commonly present as masses but can also present as an ulcer.

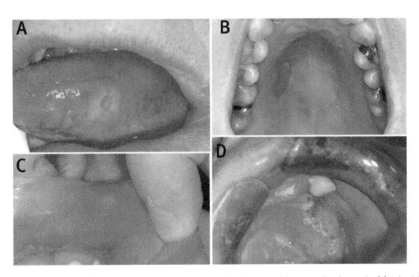

Fig 1 Acute non-neoplastic oral ulcers. (A) Traumatic ulcer of the lateral border of tongue with surrounding keratosis. (B) Palatal burn caused by aspirin. (C) Minor aphthous ulcer. (D) Herpes zoster of the palate showing distribution of ulcers along the course of the greater palatine nerve

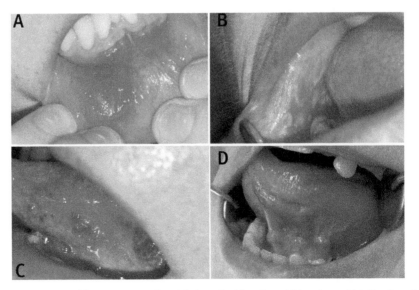

Fig 2 Chronic non-neoplastic ulcers. (A) Major aphthous ulcer of the lower lip. (B) Erosive oral lichen planus with bullous formation and ulceration of left cheek mucosa. (C) Oral ulceration secondary to oral lichen planus healing with granulation tissue visible at ulcer base. (D) Ulcer on lateral tongue caused by nicorandil

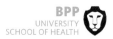

BOX 1 INFECTIONS CAUSING ORAL ULCERS

Common
- Primary herpetic stomatitis (herpes simplex virus 1)
- Recurrent intraoral herpes (herpes simplex virus 1)
- Herpes zoster intraoral ulceration (varicella zoster virus)

Uncommon
- Actinomycosis
- Tuberculosis
- Syphilis
- HIV

BOX 2 MALIGNANT CAUSES OF ORAL ULCERS
- Oral squamous cell carcinoma (most common)
- Lymphoma
- Minor salivary gland tumours
- Tumour extension from maxillary sinus
- Odontogenic tumours
- Metastatic neoplasms
- Neoplasms of bone
- Neoplasms of connective tissue
- Neoplasms of melanocytes
- Vascular neoplasms

BOX 3 CLINICAL FEATURES OF MALIGNANT ORAL ULCER

Features that should raise suspicion
- Non-healing painless ulcer present for >3 weeks
- Induration and lack of inflammation surrounding ulcer
- Ulcer with rolled thickened edge
- Smoking and alcohol use
- Age (85% of cases at age >50 years)
- Male sex (2:1)
- Previously diagnosed premalignant lesion in the area
- No history of previous ulceration
- No local factors that could potentially cause ulceration
- No systemic factors that could potentially cause ulceration
- History of oral squamous cell carcinoma

Features that may reduce suspicion
- Recurrent ulceration that heals in between episodes
- Multiple ulcers that occur synchronously
- Clustering of ulcers
- Occurrence in association with systemic diseases, especially autoimmune
- Blister formation
- Associated sore and bleeding gums
- Identifiable local causes (for example, sharp tooth)

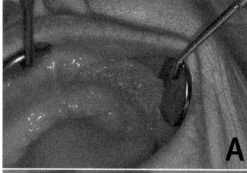
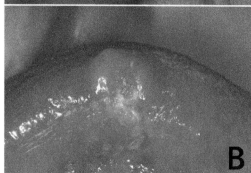

Fig 3 Squamous cell cancer of (A) upper maxillary alveolus with an area of denture hyperplasia and (B) lateral border of tongue

What features increase suspicion of a malignant ulcer?

Who gets oral squamous cell carcinoma?

Oral squamous cell carcinoma characteristically affects older men but the incidence in women and in younger adults is increasing.[6] The main risk factors for its development worldwide are the habitual use of tobacco[7] and alcohol,[8] which have a synergistic effect. Cultural habits such as betel quid or nut chewing also increase risk in some populations. The main risk factor for cancer of the lip is exposure to ultraviolet light.[9] There is increasing evidence of a causative role for high risk human papillomaviruses (HPVs) in oropharyngeal cancer[10] and HPV 16 DNA has been shown to be present in over 70% of such cancers. Although HPV DNA has been detected in oral cancer, a cause-effect relation is yet to be proven.[11] Other risk factors include the presence of premalignant lesions of the oral mucosa, such as leukoplakia and erythroplakia (white and red patches that cannot be characterised clinically or pathologically as any other disease), and various general mucosal disorders in which mucosal atrophy occurs.[12]

Clinical characteristics of oral squamous cell carcinoma

Clinical features of a malignant oral ulcer are listed in box 3. Oral squamous cell carcinoma typically presents as a non-healing painless ulcer. Varying presentation in the early stages can lead to misdiagnosis. Carcinoma may develop in clinically normal mucosa or in an area of clinically altered oral mucosa such as leukoplakia or erythroplakia.[12]

A non-healing ulcer that persists for more than three weeks is the most frequent presentation of early stage oral squamous cell carcinoma. Several clinical clues may differentiate such an ulcer from other causes (box 3). Induration, lack of surrounding inflammation, and rolled thickened margins in an ulcer that has been present for three weeks when other causes have been excluded suggest a malignant process (fig 3). Other causes, such as traumatic ulcers, can have a similar and chronic presentation, which can hinder recognition of malignant ulcers.

In advanced cases, infiltration of the malignant growth beneath the oral mucosa results in palpable induration around the ulcer or a mass that may ulcerate through the skin or cause fixation of mobile oral tissues. A fungating mass may become apparent after dental extraction. Involvement of nerves may cause pain and paraesthesia. Presenting symptoms may also include referred earache, trismus, dysphagia, halitosis, and enlarged cervical nodes.

The most common site for oral squamous cell carcinoma is the lateral border of the tongue, followed by the floor of the mouth. Squamous cell carcinomas of the gums tend to occur in the molar and premolar regions of the lower jaw. Lymph node enlargement may be seen early in the course of the disease. Involvement of the lymph nodes is dictated by several tumour and host factors.

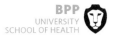

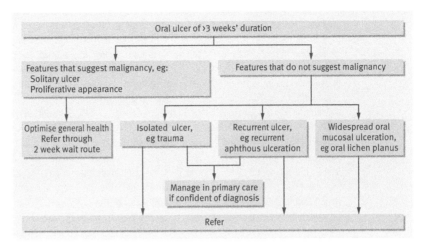

Fig 4 Suggested clinical algorithm for chronic oral ulcers

What is the best way to approach clinical evaluation of a patient with oral ulcer?

We suggest that general medical practitioners should focus initially on identifying features that suggest a malignant process (box 3), which would trigger an urgent referral to secondary care. If malignancy has been excluded or is extremely unlikely other diagnoses may be considered. Figure 4 presents an algorithm to guide the general practitioner through differential diagnoses and appropriate management for chronic oral ulcers.

History

Attention to detail in the history is vital. For example, a patient could perceive recurrent spontaneously healing ulcers in different sites as a single chronic ulcer. Remember to ask about dental procedures such as tooth restorations before the emergence of the ulcer, and about problems with dental prostheses.

Ask about current use of drugs and history of tobacco and alcohol use. NSAIDS and antihypertensives are examples of drugs that have been associated with oral ulceration. Bisphosphonates may cause oral ulceration directly or through osteonecrosis of the jaw; oral ulceration may develop in mucosa directly overlying an area of necrosis, or in an adjacent area such as the tongue after frictional trauma from exposed bone. Nicorandil can cause one or more large (0.5-3 cm) chronic painful ulcers that are usually localised on the inner aspect of the cheeks or on the tongue. Healing should occur with dose reduction or complete cessation of the drug.

Enquiry about any possible co-existing diseases, such as those listed below, may help to differentiate between malignant and non-malignant cases.

- Autoimmune diseases: systemic lupus erythematosus and Behçet's syndrome
- Dermatological diseases: lichen planus, erythema multiforme, and mucous membrane pemphigoid can involve oral mucosa without any extraoral involvement or may be associated with skin and extraoral involvement. They can be difficult to distinguish intraorally because they can all cause widespread erosions, blisters, and full thickness gingivitis (desquamative gingivitis).
- Gastrointestinal disease: inflammatory bowel disease (Crohn's disease and ulcerative colitis) may be associated with aphthous like ulcers or with snail track ulceration involving the oral mucosa and gingival tissue or pustular

patches (pyostomatitis vegetans). Coeliac disease is associated with recurrent aphthous like ulcers.
- Haematological disease: history of anaemia or myeloproliferative disorder may be associated with ulceration. Chemotherapy can cause mucositis and oral ulceration.
- Psychosocial factors: repeated intended or inadvertent self inflicted trauma.

Examination

A thorough intraoral examination to assess the mucosa of the oral cavity requires a good light source and preferably two dental mirrors (see supplemental video). Alternatively, tissues can be held back with tongue depressors to maximise visualisation of the mucosa. If patients open the mouth completely, retraction of taut cheeks makes effective examination difficult, so they should only partly open their mouths.

Seven regions in the oral cavity must be examined systematically to avoid missing a lesion—the lips, cheek mucosa, floor of mouth (particularly the posterior floor of mouth between the tongue and the mandible), teeth and gums, hard palate, oral tongue, and the retromolar trigone.

If an ulcer is present assess whether it is localised or part of widespread ulceration and whether the surrounding areas seem inflamed. Note the shape and margins of the ulcer. Feel for induration of the ulcer and surrounding tissue and ensure that there is no fixation of mobile tissues such as the tongue. Note the relation of any prosthesis, sharp teeth, or dental restorations to an ulcer if present. Extraoral examination to look for swelling or lymphadenopathy in the head and neck region should always be performed.

What can primary care doctors do before referral?

Patients often need symptom relief even before a diagnosis is established. The options include saline mouthwash, topical analgesic or anti-inflammatory preparations (such as benzydamine, available as mouthwash or spray), antimicrobial agents (such as chlorhexidine, available as mouthwash, spray, or gel), barrier paste (such as carmellose gelatine), topical anaesthetics (such as lidocaine, available as spray or ointment), and systemic analgesics.

Conditions that predispose to oral ulceration, such as iron deficiency anaemia, vitamin B12 deficiency, and folate deficiency can be excluded in primary care. If the diagnostic process should include histopathological analysis then referral at an earlier stage is indicated.

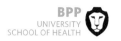

More than 60% of patients with head and neck cancer have a comorbid disease, usually of the cardiovascular or respiratory system. Treatment for such tumours can be intensive and optimisation of general health is important to avoid delays in treatment delivery. Advice from a primary care practitioner to reduce or stop tobacco and alcohol consumption and support in doing so is important.

Where should a patient with chronic oral ulceration be referred?

In the United Kingdom, when a general practitioner suspects oral malignancy, guidelines from the National Institute for Health and Clinical Excellence (NICE) recommend referral to be seen within two weeks at a local head and neck cancer unit.[13]

ONGOING RESEARCH

- Several trials are in progress to evaluate rapid diagnosis and techniques to predict likelihood of transformation of oral premalignant lesions. Diagnostic aids being evaluated include brush cytology, autofluorescence, and tissue reflectance. A National Institute for Health Research portfolio study is evaluating dielectrophoresis, a non-invasive method of determining electrophysiological parameters of cellular cytoplasm, for diagnosing oral cancer
- An ongoing National Institute for Health Research portfolio trial is studying the efficacy of oral topical cyclo-oxygenase 2 inhibitors mouthwash for treatment of oral dysplasia

---

USEFUL ONLINE RESOURCES (NO REGISTRATION REQUIRED)

Resources for non-specialist healthcare professionals

- Referral Guidelines for Suspected Cancer (www.nice.org.uk/nicemedia/pdf/CG027quickrefguide.pdf)—This quick reference guide from the NICE summarises the current referral guidance for all cancer types; pages 19 and 20 relate to head and neck.
- Problems in the mouth (www.patient.co.uk/doctor/problems-in-the-mouth.htm)—This article from Patient UK provides a general overview of different types of intraoral pathology, with links to other resources allowing further enquiry.
- Mouth problems (www.dermnet.org.nz/site-age-specific/mouth.html)—From the website of The New Zealand Dermatological Society, provides links to vignettes of several oral diseases, with accompanying pictures.
- Oral cancer: prevention and detection (www.gla.ac.uk/departments/dentalschool/oralcancer)—From the website of University of Glasgow Dental School.

Resources for patients

- Mouth cancer foundation (www.rdoc.org.uk)—Professional support organisation solely dedicated to supporting people with mouth, throat, and other head and neck cancer.
- Mouth problems (http://familydoctor.org/online/famdocen/home/tools/symptom/509.html)—Self help flow chart of mouth symptoms and possible diagnoses, from the American Academy of Family Physicians.
- Mouth Cancer (www.nhs.uk/conditions/cancer-of-the-mouth/pages/introduction.aspx)—This web page from NHS Choices gives an overview of prevention, diagnosis and management of oral cancer.
- Patient UK patient information leaflets—mouth ulcers (www.patient.co.uk/health/Mouth-Ulcers-(Minor-Aphthous-Type).htm), cancer of the mouth (www.patient.co.uk/health/Cancer-of-the-Mouth.htm)

ADDITIONAL EDUCATIONAL RESOURCES

- Bruce AJ, Rogers RS 3rd. Acute oral ulcers. *Dermatol Clin* 2003;21:1-15.
- Scully C, Bagan JV, Hopper C, Epstein JB. Oral cancer: current and future diagnostic techniques. *Am J Dent* 2008;21:199-209.
- Muñoz-Corcuera M, Esparza-Gómez G, González-Moles MA, Bascones-Martínez A. Oral ulcers: clinical aspects. A tool for dermatologists. Part I Acute ulcers. *Clin Exp Dermatol* 2009;34:289-94.
- Muñoz-Corcuera M, Esparza-Gómez G, González-Moles MA, Bascones-Martínez A. Oral ulcers: clinical aspects. A tool for dermatologists. Part II Chronic ulcers. *Clin Exp Dermatol* 2009;34:456-61.
- Clinical knowledge summaries. Oral health. www.cks.nhs.uk/clinical_topics/by_clinical_specialty/oral_health.
- Oral lichen planus. www.dermnetnz.org/scaly/oral-lichen-planus.html.

In cases where a malignant cause is unlikely or has been excluded but the ulcer is chronic or troublesome, referral to a local oral medicine specialist unit is appropriate. Where such a service is not available, referrals can be directed to an oral and maxillofacial or otolaryngology unit.

Should we screen for oral malignancy?

Oral precancers and cancers have distinctive appearances and are suitable for screening by visual inspection of the oral cavity. A cluster randomised controlled study of more than 180 000 patients in a South Indian area with a high burden of the disease showed that screening significantly increased the number of early cancers identified and led to decreased mortality.[14] A Cochrane systematic review concluded that evidence was insufficient to support or refute the use of visual examination to screen for oral cancer in the general population.[15] A decision analysis model informed by published costs, systematic reviews, and expert opinion suggested that opportunistic screening of high risk groups (men older than 40 years who smoke and drink) by general medical or dental practitioners may be cost effective.[16]

A PATIENT'S PERSPECTIVE

At the beginning I felt as if the roof of my mouth was like a fur lined carpet. After a few days I coughed up a big chunk of skin from the roof of my mouth. This prompted me to see the GP as I found it difficult to see what was on the roof of my mouth even when I tipped my head back. The GP said she had never seen anything like this and asked if she could show a colleague. They both decided I should be referred to the Freeman hospital to be seen within two weeks. At this point I thought I had cancer.

Mr Paleri told me he had seen very few conditions with rapid progression like this; he took some photographs and was concerned that this might be cancer. The ulcer was biopsied at the same visit and I had to return a week or two later to see him for the results. When I returned home I needed to see the GP for painkillers as the ulcer was painful, especially when eating and swallowing. I am a paramedic and my GP asked me if I realised what the likely diagnosis was. He said cancer was a possibility. I didn't know what they could do about cancer on the roof of my mouth; I started to put my affairs in order and thought about what was going to happen to my children.

When I went back to get the results, Mr Paleri said that this was some form of ulcer with an unpronounceable name, and that it could be treated and probably would heal itself. The relief was absolutely fantastic, it felt like a bus had been lifted from my shoulders. I can't remember what the treatment was but things started to heal spontaneously. It did however cause some problems while it healed, especially with medication and food getting stuck in the ulcer. Occasionally this can still be a problem, but it is looking good now.

While this was a frightening thing at that time, I now understand the need to exclude serious disease. I hope everyone reading this article appreciates that they will need to seek prompt medical advice rather than being worried about what the problem may or may not be.

David Page, Ashington

Necrotising sialometaplasia is an uncommon, self resolving cause of oral ulcer. This is clearly a rapid, yet worrying presentation and the priority is to rule out malignancy. The clinician's concern has understandably caused a great deal of emotional distress, but the biopsy results were unequivocal and reassuring. This case exemplifies the varied nature of mouth ulcers and the need to achieve clinical diagnosis supplemented by a tissue diagnosis when needed. Vinidh Paleri

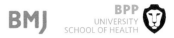

Competing interests: All authors have completed the Unified Competing Interest form at www.icmje.org/coi_disclosure.pdf (available on request from the corresponding author) and declare (1) no support from companies for the submitted work; (2) no relationships with companies that might have an interest in the submitted work in the previous 3 years; (3) no spouses, partners, or children with financial relationships that may be relevant to the submitted work; and (4) no non-financial interests that may be relevant to the submitted work.

Provenance and peer review: Not commissioned, externally peer reviewed.

Patient consent obtained.

1. Shulman JD, Beach MM, Rivera-Hidalgo F. The prevalence of oral mucosal lesions in US adults: data from the third national health and nutrition examination survey, 1988-1994. *J Am Dent Assoc* 2004;135:1279-86.
2. Ferlay J, Bray F, Pisani P, Parkin DM. GLOBOCAN 2002: cancer incidence, mortality and prevalence worldwide. IARCPress, 2004.
3. Department of Health. Referral guidelines for suspected cancer. Department of Health, 2000; 39-41.
4. McKie C, Ahmad UA, Fellows S, Meikle D, Stafford FW, Thomson PJ, et al. The 2-week rule for suspected head and neck cancer in the United Kingdom: referral patterns, diagnostic efficacy of the guidelines and compliance. *Oral Oncol* 2008;44:851-6.
5. Wade J, Smith H, Hankins M, Llewellyn C. Conducting oral examinations for cancer in general practice: what are the barriers? *Fam Pract* 2010;27:77-84.
6. Curado MP, Hashibe M. Recent changes in the epidemiology of head and neck cancer. *Curr Opin Oncol* 2009;21:194-200.
7. Gandini S, Botteri E, Iodice S, Boniol M, Lowenfels AB, Maisonneuve P, et al. Tobacco smoking and cancer: a meta-analysis. *Int J Cancer* 2008;122:155-64.
8. Bagnardi V, Blangiardo M, La Vecchia C, Corrao G. A meta-analysis of alcohol drinking and cancer risk. *Br J Cancer* 2001;85:1700-5.
9. Perea-Milla Lopez E, Minarro-Del Moral RM, Martinez-Garcia C, Zanetti R, Rosso S, Serrano S, et al. Lifestyles, environmental and phenotypic factors associated with lip cancer: a case-control study in southern Spain. *Br J Cancer* 2003;88:1702-7.
10. D'Souza G, Kreimer AR, Viscidi R, Pawlita M, Fakhry C, Koch WM, et al. Case-control study of human papillomavirus and oropharyngeal cancer. *N Engl J Med* 2007;356:1944-56.
11. Robinson CM, Sloan P, Shaw R. Refining the diagnosis of oropharyngeal squamous cell carcinoma using human papillomavirus testing. *Oral Oncology* (forthcoming).
12. van der Waal I. Potentially malignant disorders of the oral and oropharyngeal mucosa; terminology, classification and present concepts of management. *Oral Oncol* 2009;45:317-23.
13. National Institute for Health and Clinical Excellence. Referral guidelines for suspected cancer. 2005. www.nice.org.uk/CG027.
14. Sankaranarayanan R, Ramadas K, Thomas G, Muwonge R, Thara S, Mathew B, et al. Effect of screening on oral cancer mortality in Kerala, India: a cluster-randomised controlled trial. *Lancet* 2005;365:1927-33.
15. Kujan O, Glenny AM, Oliver RJ, Thakker N, Sloan P. Screening programmes for the early detection and prevention of oral cancer. *Cochrane Database Syst Rev* 2006;3:CD004150.
16. Speight PM, Palmer S, Moles DR, Downer MC, Smith DH, Henriksson M, et al. The cost-effectiveness of screening for oral cancer in primary care. *Health Technol Assess* 2006;10:1-144, iii-iv.

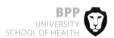

Improving healthcare access for people with visual impairment and blindness

M E Cupples, clinical reader[1], P M Hart, consultant ophthalmologist[2], A Johnston, care co-ordinator[3], A J Jackson, head of optometry[2], head of clinical services[4]

[1]Department of General Practice, Queen's University, Belfast BT9 7HR, UK

[2]Belfast Health and Social Care Trust, Belfast

[3]Royal National Institute for the Blind, Belfast

[4]Australian College of Optometry, Melbourne, Australia

Correspondence to: Margaret E Cupples m.cupples@qub.ac.uk

Cite this as: *BMJ* 2012;344:e542

DOI: 10.1136/bmj.e542

http://www.bmj.com/content/344/bmj.e542

Worldwide, visual impairment is increasing in prevalence: current data indicate that 284 million people have impaired vision,[1] 10% of whom live in the developed world. In the UK sight loss affects about two million people,[2] including an estimated 80 000 of working age and 25 000 children. The prevalence of visual impairment is higher among those with multiple disability and older people.[3] According to estimates from the UK's Royal National Institute for the Blind (RNIB) one in 30 people of any age, one in five aged 75 or over, and half of those over age 90 years in the UK are living with sight loss.[4] Older people with vision impairment report greater difficulty performing activities of everyday living than those with other or no sensory impairments.[5] Individuals with impaired vision may have great difficulty in accessing and negotiating healthcare services. We discuss the difficulties that visually impaired patients encounter in the healthcare environment and ways in which problems may be overcome.

What is the range of visual impairment?

People who are registered as severely sight impaired (previously known as blind registration) are defined as having central visual acuity of less than 3/60 with normal fields of vision, or gross visual field restriction. They cannot see at 3 m what the normally sighted person sees at 60 m. Those registered as sight impaired (previously known as partially sighted) can see at 3 m, but not at 6 m, what the normally sighted person sees at 60 m. Less severe visual impairment is not captured by registration data, and its prevalence is difficult to quantify. People classified as having low vision have a visual acuity of less than 6/18 but more than 3/60. They are not eligible to drive and may have difficulty recognising faces across a street, watching television, or choosing clean, unstained, co-ordinated clothing.

What effect does visual impairment have on the individual?

If loss of vision is gradual, individuals may adapt better to changed circumstances than if it is sudden. However, regardless of the mode of onset, many who experience loss of vision withdraw from social contact,[6] perhaps partly

SOURCES AND SELECTION CRITERIA

The material for this article was based on discussion between an optometrist, an ophthalmologist, and a general practitioner, who were engaged in research exploring the needs of people with visual impairment in achieving medication compliance. This work resulted in a personal archive of references reflecting needs of people with impaired vision in accessing healthcare. To ensure applicability of the article to this population we consulted the regional base of the Royal National Institute for the Blind (RNIB) and asked its eye care co-ordinator to ask members of the lay public to share their recent experiences of healthcare services and to identify the best advice to improve care provision in practice.

because they lose awareness of the nuances of body language that are part of social interactions. A patient's fear of experiencing "total darkness" may be associated with profound psychological distress. For older patients, losing physical mobility and other senses such as hearing and touch adds to a sense of difficulty and isolation and may lead to poor mental health, which in turn may affect families.[7] An increased risk of depression,[8] suicide,[9] falls,[10] and cognitive decline[11] may be exacerbated if healthcare providers do not recognise the particular problems of people with visual impairment. Previously identified problems[12] include receiving written information in inaccessible formats, difficulties communicating with practitioners and staff, doctors failing to respect people's ability to participate in their own care, and physical difficulties with getting around healthcare facilities. Challenges in obtaining safe, effective, and timely care have been reported; common courtesy and an approach to communication tailored to the individual could improve patients' experiences.[12]

People who lose their vision, especially in later life, may attempt to conceal it, although their ability to do so may vary. They may develop good social support networks, with family members or friends on whom they depend as a confidante for information, directions, and treatment details. The impact of loss of vision is related to the extent to which resolution (relevant to reading, television viewing), panoramic vision (mobility, safe travel) and contrast detection (face recognition, identifying objects in low light) are affected. Those with severe central vision loss, as in macular degeneration, may still move around confidently, especially in familiar surroundings. Their inability to see facial details or to read may go unnoticed. People with glaucoma, who lose their peripheral vision and experience impaired contrast detection, may find it more difficult to function even in familiar environments.

Vivid, recurrent visual hallucinations (Charles Bonnet Syndrome) are an increasingly recognised feature of visual loss, which may result from impaired visual signals being transmitted to the brain. In one recent study[13] a third of people with low vision had experienced such hallucinations; some had not reported them and others had received inadequate explanations. Warning about the possibility of this phenomenon would help alleviate distress.

SUMMARY POINTS

- Visual impairment can have adverse consequences for health and wellbeing, and its prevalence is increasing, especially among older people
- People with visual impairment are likely to have limited access to information and healthcare facilities, and to receive sub-optimal treatment because staff are unaware of specific needs related to vision
- Being aware that people may have problems with vision is an important pre-requisite for good healthcare
- Taking time to communicate effectively about access, facilities, diagnosis, and management plans is necessary; communications, in visual or audio format, should be tailored to individuals' needs
- Checking that personal resources are in place to facilitate compliance with treatment plans is essential for good clinical care

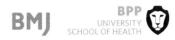

How might we recognise that someone has impaired vision in the clinical environment?

Unlike physical impairment, visual impairment is rarely obvious to a casual observer. A few patients with visual impairment will have a guide dog, some a white cane, and even fewer use electronic navigation aids. Those registered as sight impaired or severely sight impaired should have this documented in their medical records but it may not be readily apparent.

Some people have sufficient confidence and insight to inform those involved in their healthcare about their difficulties but many, especially older individuals, are embarrassed that they can no longer see well. Some may assume that professionals working with them will be aware of their problems. Many will take proffered leaflets politely and sign on dotted lines without understanding what is being agreed to, rather than ask questions. In new situations people may become timid and hesitant. Older people may become confused easily and appear angry or demanding. An individual's behaviour may be perceived as strange and misunderstood without awareness of their impairment.

Health professionals need to be alert to the subtle signs that a patient may be visually impaired. Patients with severe impairment may have difficulty in finding a chair or negotiating furniture, may not make eye contact when conversing, or may not respond when something is handed to them.

How might contact with healthcare services be optimised for patients with visual impairment?

People with visual impairment may encounter difficulties at any point in their interaction with healthcare services, from identification of a potential problem to the ongoing management of diagnosed illness. Effective communication and anticipation of difficulties are key to avoiding and resolving problems.

Improving delivery of information about appointments and treatment

Example 1

The daughter of an 87 year old patient with age related macular degeneration highlights how not being able to read printed information may be a problem: "At the ophthalmology clinic my father was told he had 'wet ARMD' and nothing could be done because he did not attend two appointments and had missed his 'window of opportunity'. The doctor said that all she could do was register him as blind. I told the staff that we had never received previous appointments, but I don't think they believed me. My father keeps asking if I know where the two appointments went, and this upsets me. I feel guilty—if we had attended sooner my father's sight loss might have been avoided. I feel that he thinks this too and blames me."

A review published by the RNIB[14] noted that "Receiving inaccessible health information has serious consequences for blind and partially sighted people"—such as the loss of privacy and independence (someone else must read the information for them), potential risks to personal safety (regarding medication), and a loss of ability to make informed choices about healthcare. The example above illustrates the serious consequences of a delayed consultation, which might have occurred because the patient could not read appointment letters. Many people do not admit to friends or family that they have problems with their health or eyesight. It may not be easy to ask

for help to find telephone numbers to make appointments, arrange transport to the surgery or hospital, and navigate the process of attendance. People may miss information that is presented in leaflets or posters.

When dealing with patients with visual impairment consider carefully how to share information appropriately with the patient, family, and points of referral. Depending on the patient's level of disability appropriate communication might comprise sending letters in large print, with different font styles, or with background contrast, or offering information in audio format, by telephone, or electronically (email or compact disc), rather than letter. For a very few profoundly affected individuals, Braille letters or information could be needed. Patients should be asked about their supporting network of family or friends and how this can be employed in assisting with their healthcare needs.

Perhaps the primary focus of information provision should be to ensure that information about access to general practitioners' surgeries and clinics is offered in various formats, both visual and audio, including large print and computer or web based versions.

Helping patients to navigate unfamiliar environments

Example 2

A 50 year old man, registered as severely sight impaired, reports how modern technologies have made things more difficult for him: "Electronic systems have reduced my independence. Signing in on the computer installed at my GP's surgery is not possible and saying that I need help is difficult. It's hard to know if anyone's at the reception desk. Before this someone always greeted me as soon as I went through the door. And then, when I was at accident and emergency, I didn't see the button to open the door. The staff shouted at me to press the button but I couldn't see it."

An initial greeting to everyone entering healthcare premises should include a verbal offer of help. People with visual impairment may require simple clear instructions or personal physical guidance to find their way around. Key points to be aware of when guiding people are shown in box 1. Furniture placement and style, lighting levels, glare reduction, use of contrasting colours, and tactile and dual audio and visual signage are important considerations in improving access.

If patients cannot read signs or observe others they may have difficulty finding their way around healthcare premises. They might not be able to communicate effectively with staff because they cannot see visual cues, gestures, or facial expressions. As clinics and surgeries adopt electronic systems to summon patients, visually impaired patients may find that they miss their slots because they are not "called". Healthcare staff should be alert to recognise those for whom electronic systems, particularly those with visual instructions only, pose problems.

In a clinic situation, come out to the waiting room to call the patient and guide them to the consulting room if necessary. Use accurate and specific language when giving directions or explaining the layout of a room. For example, "the door is on your left", rather than "the door is over there". Remember that the person is unlikely to see non-verbal cues and gestures or information. Take time to explain the layout of a room and describe where things are placed if a patient is obliged to stay in an unfamiliar setting. An example of a consequence of not describing the layout of a bathroom to a blind patient was that he fell, hit his

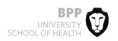

BOX 1: KEY POINTS FOR BASIC GUIDING TECHNIQUES

- If the patient is not familiar with the surroundings, ask politely if they would like to be guided; do not be offended if your offer is not accepted
- Offer your arm for the person to grip just above the elbow (they may prefer to grip your shoulder)
- When guiding someone with sight problems, walk slightly in front, making sure that the pace is not too fast or too slow
- If steps or stairs are involved always state whether they go up or down and give warning of approaching ground level
- Explain changes in ground surface, such as moving from a tiled floor to carpet
- Never guide someone into a seat backwards: instead, describe the chair, place your hand on the back of the chair, and enable the person to orientate themselves into the seat independently

BOX 2 TIPS TO IMPROVE HEALTHCARE FOR PATIENTS WITH VISUAL IMPAIRMENT

Communicating effectively with people who are blind or vision impaired

- Identify yourself—do not assume someone will recognise you by your voice; use your full name and indicate your role in their care
- Face the person directly and use their name when introducing yourself or directing conversation to them in a group
- Speak naturally and clearly: loss of eyesight does not mean loss of hearing
- Do not expect eye contact or assume that lack of eye contact means lack of attention to what you are saying
- Never channel conversation through a third person
- In a group setting, introduce the other people present
- Never leave a conversation without saying so
- Try to avoid situations where competing background noise may be a problem
- Ask the patient to describe their level of vision and if they require any help; remember, not all vision impaired patients wear dark glasses or use a guide dog or cane
- Continue to use non-verbal body language; this will affect the tone of your voice and adds useful information to someone who is vision impaired
- Use everyday language—do not avoid words like "see" or "look" or talking about activities such as watching television
- During a consultation, if an examination is needed, explain that physical contact may be required (or that eye drops may be used)
- If an interpreter or support worker is involved, ensure the patient is happy with their presence at each stage of the consultation
- Ensure the patient knows who is in the consulting room; for example, medical students or nurses—ask them to introduce themselves, indicate their role, and gain consent to remain
- Use accurate and specific language when giving directions. For example, "the door is on your left", rather than "the door is over there"; remember the person is unlikely to see non-verbal cues and gestures or information
- Always ask whether help is needed, for example, to be guided to another department
- Be aware that changing light levels can affect vision: bright sunlight may be a greater problem than dark corridors
- Explain where things are placed; for example, "your cup of tea is on the table directly in front of you"—or use the "clockface" method; for example, "it's on the plate at 3 o'clock"
- Offer to read any written materials aloud; identify exactly where signatures are required
- If providing information for later reference, ensure it is in an accessible format and ask about preferred format; for example, large print, audio, or electronic

Points to consider

- Clarify plans for follow-up—discuss format of information, to whom a letter should be addressed, appropriate telephone numbers, transport requirements, support worker, interpreter. If potentially sensitive information to be conveyed, should the patient return to the surgery to be informed verbally by the doctor?
- When visual impairment is diagnosed, share information with other health professionals who are involved in the patient's healthcare provision. "Flag" medical records to alert others to their needs and include the information in referral letters
- Be patient and recognise that extra time may be required for consultations

head on the toilet, and incurred a head injury. He was also embarrassed and commented "Never will I forget what I had to go through"; he blamed a lack of staff awareness for his unpleasant experience.

Communication and consultation skills

Example 3

A 27 year old woman with visual impairment secondary to congenital glaucoma describes her experience of consultation with healthcare practitioners: "I was so frustrated at the lack of awareness of staff of the basics of interacting with a person who's blind. Sometimes they would talk to members of my family rather than me. Also, they'd create such a drama over having to guide me somewhere. I just think that with some basic training, this could've been a non-issue. I can understand blind or partially sighted people dreading dealing with health services. I have, myself, missed appointments because I couldn't read the appointment letter or simply didn't know it had come until someone with eyesight happened to visit my house."

Pointers for communicating effectively with people who have visual impairment are provided in box 2. Asking routinely, "Do you have any problems with vision that I should know about?" could make life easier for many who find it difficult to admit spontaneously to their disability. Do not assume that those with a visual disability have a lesser level of understanding or autonomy than those who can see. Even if patients do not make eye contact, face them and talk to them directly, not through a third person. Introduce yourself and all people present in the consulting room. Explain what you are doing and what you plan to do. Tell the patient if you plan to leave the room. If you are moving from one location to another, offer to guide the person, but also offer a description of the environment so that the patient can choose which he or she would prefer. Extra time may be needed for consultations in order to explain things that might otherwise be communicated in writing, to make a plan for appropriate follow-up and delivery of test results, or to allow the patient to ask questions.

Providing an escort to the location for investigations, making an agreed plan for communication of results, writing clear information in referrals about needs relating to vision, and flagging records for future visits facilitates access to good quality care. Good communication empowers patients and enhances their contribution to concordant management plans.

Example 4

A 54 year old woman with visual impairment describes a clinic visit that went smoothly: "At a recent clinic visit the registrar met me in the waiting room, walked with me to the consulting room, explained the examination I would have and the tests I'd have done, and checked I understood the plan for getting results. He was great—I found out that he had recently received visual awareness training."

Consider the huge impact of loss of vision and refer to services as appropriate. Be aware that some patients may require increased self confidence to alert staff to their limitations related to vision and offer referral to counselling or assertiveness classes. Also, be prepared to offer referral to a low vision clinic; evidence shows clearly that even after one appointment, difficulty in daily visual tasks decreases.[15]

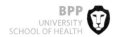

Example 5

A 37 year old woman describes her experience with her general practitioner after suddenly losing her vision: "After being registered blind and sent home from hospital without any information I went to see my GP for advice. I was aged 37, had lost my job, my [driving] licence, and most of all my confidence. Even though I was really upset, rather than listening to me, the GP opened a copy of the yellow pages. She told me she was looking for the address of a local sensory support team but that she had no idea what they could offer me, nor how long it would take them to contact me. When they did phone me months later it emerged that the GP had not considered the referral urgent. However, my mental health had deteriorated so much that I was referred urgently to the mental health team—I blame my GP and her lack of awareness for this."

The "Additional educational resources" box lists useful sources of information for healthcare practitioners treating patients with visual impairment or blindness. In most countries advice is available from charities and from professional bodies. Within the UK such sources include the Royal College of Ophthalmologists, the College of Optometrists, the British and Irish Orthoptists Society, and specific support groups such as the Albinism Fellowship, British Retinitis Pigmentosa Society, International Glaucoma Association, and Macular Disease Society.

Various sources of support are available for people with visual impairment. For example, a visit to the surgery or hospital could be less daunting if accompanied by a voluntary support worker. The concept of an eye care liaison officer is relatively recent. Where medication is needed, healthcare professionals should check that the patient is able to adhere to prescribed treatment. Request that pharmacists offer information in large print or audio format and offer compliance packs that can assist self administration of medication. Visually impaired patients may encounter difficulties with opening certain packaging, distinguishing different packaging and tablets from each other, and measuring liquids. Using eye drops and administering injections are not easy without good vision. Commercial systems of support can be accessed, including "talking labels" (simple electronic devices providing short pre-recorded audio messages attached to the medication package) and "pen friends" (pen-like devices that scan minute barcodes and convert information to audio format).

Conclusion

Doctors might consider journeying from home to the consulting room while blindfolded or wearing spectacles with semi-opaque lenses, to help them imagine the emotional background against which people with impaired vision present to healthcare services. If healthcare professionals do not recognise the unique needs of patients with impaired vision, access to good quality healthcare for this group of patients is impeded, whereas anticipation of their needs promotes wellbeing and limits disability.

ADDITIONAL EDUCATIONAL RESOURCES

- World Blind Union (Union Mondiale des Aveugles) (www.worldblindunion.org)—International non-governmental coalition of representatives from associations of blind people and agencies providing services to them. Members are grouped into seven geographical unions: Africa, Asia, Europe, East Asia/Pacific, Latin America, Middle East, and North America/Caribbean, and provide an international forum for the exchange of knowledge and experience in the field of blindness and vision impairment
- Royal National Institute of Blind People (RNIB) (www.rnib.org.uk)—Information, support and advice to people with sight loss
- Action for Blind People (www.actionforblindpeople.org.uk)—Practical help and support for blind and partially sighted people of all ages
- SeeAbility (www.seeability.org)—Supports adults who are visually impaired with multiple disabilities (learning, physical, or mental health)
- Guide Dogs for the Blind Association (www.guidedogs.org.uk/aboutus/whatwedo)—Provides mobility for blind and partially sighted people, educates, funds research
- Calibre Audio Library (www.calibre.org.uk)—Free postal service of audio books for adults and children with sight problems, dyslexia, or other disabilities
- National Talking Newspapers and Magazines (www.tnauk.org.uk)—Provides newspapers and magazines in audio and digital format
- StyleAble (www.styleable.co.uk/about)—Lifestyle resource for blind and partially sighted people, who want to create their own image and personal style and feel confident
- The Accessible Friends Network (www.tafn.org.uk)—Worldwide internet based computer support for people with blindness and partial sight
- St Dunstans (www.st-dunstans.org.uk/about_us/index.html)—Physical and emotional support for blind and visually impaired ex-service men and women
- VISION 2020 UK (www.vision2020uk.org.uk)—Facilitates collaboration between national, regional, and international organisations in the UK that focus on vision impairment
- Thomas Pocklington Trust (www.pocklington-trust.org.uk)—Housing, care, and support services for people with sight loss in the UK
- The Torch Trust (www.torchtrust.org)—A Christian organisation with a worldwide vision for people with sight loss
- The National Blind Children's Society (www.nbcs.org.uk/aboutus/Our-Work/195)—Provides services such as educational advocacy advice and support and information for families

See also www.ehow.co.uk/list_5886520_list-charities-blind.html

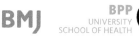

AJ is employed by RNIB. MEC is partly funded by the Centre of Excellence for Public Health (Northern Ireland), a UKCRC Public Health Research Centre of Excellence. We thank the British Heart Foundation, Cancer Research UK, Economic and Social Research Council, Medical Research Council, Research and Development Office for the Northern Ireland Health and Social Services, and the Wellcome Trust, under the auspices of the UK Clinical Research Collaboration for funding.

Contributors: MEC, AJJ, and PMH contributed to the conception and design of the article. MEC wrote the first draft of the paper. All authors contributed to the literature search and re-drafting of the paper, revising it critically for important intellectual content and approving the final version to be published. MEC is the guarantor.

Competing interests: All authors have completed the Unified Competing Interest form at http://www.icmje.org/coi_disclosure. pdf (available on request from the corresponding author) and declare: no support from any organisation for the submitted work; no financial relationships with any organisations that might have an interest in the submitted work in the previous three years; no other relationships or activities that could appear to have influenced the submitted work.

Provenance and peer review: Not commissioned; externally peer reviewed.

Patient consent obtained.

1   World Health Organization. Visual impairment and blindness. Fact sheet. WHO, 2011: 282.
2   Bosanquet N, Mehta P. Evidence base to support the UK Vision Strategy. RNIB and The Guide Dogs for the Blind Association. www.vision2020uk.org.uk/ukvisionstrategy/core/core_picker/download.asp?id=16.
3   van den Broek EG, Janssen CG, van Ramshorst T, Deen L Visual impairments in people with severe and profound multiple disabilities: an inventory of visual functioning. *J Intellect Disabil Res* 2006;50:470-5
4   Royal National Institute for the Blind. Key information and statistics. www.rnib.org.uk/aboutus/Research/statistics/Pages/statistics.aspx.
5   Crews JE, Campbell VA. Vision Impairment and hearing loss among community-dwelling older Americans: implications for health and functioning. *Am J Pub Health* 2004;94:823-9.
6   Thurston M, Thurston A, McLeod J. Socio-emotional effects of the transition from sight to blindness. *B J Visual Impair* 2010;28:90-112.
7   Silverstone B. Aging, vision rehabilitation, and the family. In: Crews JE, Whittington FJ, eds. Vision loss in an aging society: a multidisciplinary perspective. AFB Press, 2000.
8   Rovner BW, Ganguli M. Depression and disability associated with impaired vision: the MoVies Project. *J Am Geriatr Soc* 1998;46:617-9.
9   Waern M, Rubenowitz E, Runeson B, Skoog I, Wilhelmson K, Allebeck P. Burden of illness and suicide in elderly people: casecontrol study. *BMJ* 2002;324:1355-7.
10   Ivers RQ, Cumming RG, Mitchell P and Attebo K. Visual impairment and falls in older adults: The Blue Mountain Study. *J Am Geriat Soc* 1998;46:58-64.
11   Lin MY, Gutierrez PR, Stone KL, Yaffe K, Ensrud KE, Fink HA, et al. Vision impairment and combined vision and hearing impairment predict cognitive and functional decline in older women. *J Am Geriatr Soc* 2004;52:1996-2002.
12   O'Day BL, Killeen M, Iezzoni LI. Improving health care experiences of persons who are blind or have low vision: suggestions from focus groups. *Am J Med Qual* 2004;19:193-200.
13   Gilmour G, Schreiber C, Ewing C. An examination of the relationship between low vision and Charles Bonnet Syndrome. *Can J Ophthalmol* 2009;44:49-52.
14   Sibley E, Alexandrou B. Towards an inclusive health service: a research report into the availability of information for blind and partially sighted people. www.rnib.org.uk/aboutus/Research/reports/2009andearlier/Access_Health.pdf.
15   Pearce E, Crossland MD, Rubin GS. The efficacy of low vision device training in a hospital-based low vision clinic. *Br J Ophthalmol* 2011;95:105-8.

Related links

bmj.com/archive
Previous articles in this series

bmj.com
- Get Cleveland Clinic CME credits for this article

BMJ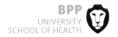

Care of the dying patient in the community

Emily Collis, consultant in palliative medicine[1],
R Al-Qurainy, community consultant in palliative medicine[1]

[1]Pembridge Palliative Care Centre, Central London Community Healthcare Trust, St Charles Centre for Health and Wellbeing, London W10 6DZ, UK

Correspondence to: E Collis emily.collis@clch.nhs.uk

Cite this as: BMJ 2013;347:f4085

DOI: 10.1136/bmj.f4085

http://www.bmj.com/content/347/bmj.f4085

The consensus from international studies of patient preferences is that, given adequate support, most people would prefer to die at home.[1 2 3] However, more than half of all deaths in the United Kingdom occur in hospital, with only 18% of people dying in their own home.[4] Suggested reasons for this include a lack of anticipatory care planning, poor coordination between healthcare agencies, and insufficient community resources. National and local policies now focus on facilitating home deaths, and recently there has been a small increase in the proportion and absolute number of people dying at home.[5]

The demographics of deaths across Europe are changing with the ageing population, with deaths from dementia, cancer, and chronic diseases becoming more common.[6 7] Caring for such patients in hospital will probably become unsustainable in terms of capacity, cost, and patient satisfaction. The focus of end of life care is therefore shifting to the community—to homes and care homes—where the role of the general practitioner, with support from the community palliative care team, is key. The onus is on all health and social care professionals to work collaboratively across settings to enable patients to receive high quality end of life care in the place of their choice.

Where do people want to die?

The English national end of life care strategy states that, whenever possible, people should be able to spend their last days in the place of their choosing.[1] In Europe and the United States, more than half of patients express a wish to be cared for and to die at home.[1 2 8] Wherever their final place of death, most people spend most of their last year of life at home. Younger patients have a higher preference for home death, whereas older patients tend to prefer home or hospice.[9] Patients' preferences should be interpreted with the caveat that they usually come from surveys of well people. A recent systematic review reported that around a fifth of patients changed preference as their

illness progressed.[10] This highlights the importance of ongoing discussions with patients and carers over time and of providing rapidly accessible high quality end of life care across settings.

Where do people die?

Demographic data from 2010 show that over half of all deaths in England occurred in hospital, with 18% in care homes and 5% in hospices.[9] The proportion of deaths at home increased slowly but steadily—from 18.3% in 2004 to 20.8% in 2010.[5] This is a welcome reversal of the previous trend towards a decrease in home deaths, which in 2008 had been predicted to fall to 10% by 2030.[11] This latest trend mirrors that reported in the US, where hospital deaths have decreased to 36%.[12]

What factors are associated with achieving preferred place of death?

Comparison between preferred and actual place of death shows a gap of at least 39% (table).[9] Systematic review has identified several factors associated with achieving home death, including younger age and a diagnosis of cancer.[9] A recent UK population based study found that home deaths for patients with cancer have increased to 24.5%,[13] compared with 12% for respiratory or neurological diseases and 6% for dementia.[14] Other factors associated with home deaths are living with relatives, patients' low functional status, and support from extended family or home care services.[15] Patients receiving specialist end of life care community services (such as "hospice at home") are significantly more likely to die at home than those receiving usual care.[16 17] For many patients, care homes are home. More than half of deaths from dementia across five European countries occur in care homes.[7 14]

Although many patients express a wish to die at home they also recognise "the practical and emotional difficulties of exercising this choice."[16] Social trends have seen changes in family structure, with many more people living alone with a low level of informal support. Patients express concern about being a "burden." They also worry about their families seeing them in distress or having to help with intimate aspects of care.[18] The preference to be cared for at home ranks higher among patients than among family and carers.[10] Carers can become overwhelmed by the enormity of the task they have committed themselves to and if inadequately supported may seek hospice or hospital care as an alternative.

How can we facilitate home deaths for patients who want this?

Step 1: Identification of patients in the last year of life
Patients need to be identified in advance to discuss and plan care, anticipate the physical and psychosocial problems that are likely to arise, and enable patients to make informed decisions about all aspects of care, including ceilings of management and preferred place of care.

SOURCES AND SELECTION CRITERIA

We searched the *Cochrane Database of Systematic Reviews*, Medline, Embase, and Clinical Evidence online. Search terms included "death or dying" and "home or community". Studies were limited to those conducted in adults that were written in English. They included recent systematic reviews, meta-analyses, randomised controlled trials, and high quality prospective or retrospective audits. We also consulted relevant reports and national guidelines, including those published by the National Institute for Health and Care Excellence.

SUMMARY POINTS

- Most people report a preference to die at home
- To support this preference, doctors in all settings need to identify relevant patients early
- Anticipatory care planning should include discussion and documentation of patient preferences, anticipatory prescribing, and completion of a do not attempt cardiopulmonary resuscitation order
- General practitioners have a key role, in both homes and care homes, before and after death
- Good communication and effective coordination of care 24 hours a day are essential to prevent unwanted and unnecessary hospital admissions towards the end of life

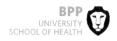

Place of death	Age group (years)					
	45-64		65-74		≥75	
	Preferred (%)	Actual (%)	Preferred (%)	Actual (%)	Preferred (%)	Actual (%)
Home	63	32	56	28	45	17
Hospice	32	11	37	9	41	3
Hospital	1	50	4	54	6	54
Care home	1	3	1	7	5	25

Preferred versus actual place of death by age group (England, 2010)[9]

The 3 selected age groups represented 96% of all deaths in 2010 (45-64 years made up 13%, 65-74 years 16%, ≥75 years 67%).

It can be difficult to identify these patients, especially those with non-malignant disease who may experience a slower and more fluctuating deterioration than those with cancer. Systematic review found that the lack of a clearly predictable disease course in chronic heart failure and chronic obstructive pulmonary disease had a marked impact on the patient's level of awareness of deterioration and on engagement with advance care planning.[14] By contrast, those with long term neurological conditions had a heightened awareness of their deteriorating condition and often planned ahead.[14]

Several initiatives can help identify patients in their last year of life. The "find your 1%" campaign in the UK refers to the identification of the 1% of the population who die each year. GPs in the UK see on around 20 deaths a year, most of which are predictable.[19] Only about five of these deaths are from cancer. Although no direct evidence exists to support the campaign, there is evidence that early engagement in end of life care can increase home deaths and patient satisfaction.[20]

The question "would you be surprised if this patient were to die in the next year?" is a useful starting point to aid identification.[1] The supportive and palliative care indicators tool (SPICT) provides a more detailed algorithmic approach, using a combination of specified general clinical and disease specific indicators of deterioration.[21] [22] Clinical indicators include poor performance status, increasing care requirements, progressive weight loss, and multiple unplanned hospital admissions. Disease specific clinical indicators are more detailed for each category of disease—for example, urinary and faecal incontinence in dementia and cardiac cachexia in cardiac disease. Similar tools are being developed in Holland, the US, and Spain.[23] [24] [25] Despite the implementation of directives advocating early intervention, most patients with advanced chronic illness are not identified before they die, so further work is needed.[26]

Step 2: Assessment

After identification, the next step is to gently explore the patient's insight into his or her condition and complete a holistic assessment of the full range of physical, psychological, social, spiritual, and cultural needs. An assessment of carers' needs should also be completed.[1] Patients with symptom control needs, complex psychosocial needs, or terminal care needs benefit from referral to the local community palliative care service. Consider referral to other health and social care professionals with expertise in all aspects of the patient and carer's holistic care to help meet identified areas of unmet need (box 1). These include help with applications for appropriate benefits and early support from social workers if young children are involved or complicated bereavement is anticipated. The evidence basis for spiritual support may be lacking,[27] but many patients value an opportunity to raise existential issues, and guidance for this is available.[28]

Step 3: Anticipatory care planning

Retrospective studies have shown a positive association between having an advanced care plan and meeting patient preferences,[29] whereas failure to implement a timely end of life care plan has been identified as a key obstacle to high quality end of life care.[30] Give patients the opportunity to have early anticipatory care planning discussions. This should be done in a sensitive way so that damaging communication is not imposed at the wrong time or on patients who will never cope with this kind of thinking. Barriers to advance care planning in primary care have been identified and include prognostic uncertainty, desire to maintain hope, and resistance to a "tick box" approach.[31]

The principle is to give patients control of the information flow, within a wider context of open communication with family and carers. For example, if a parenteral feeding tube is an option—as in motor neurone disease or head and neck cancers—elicit and document patient preferences in advance, while the patient is well enough for the procedure. The subject may be best broached with open questions, such as: "Do you like to plan ahead with regard to your health?," progressing to more specific questions as guided by patient cues. "Some specific interventions are useful to plan in advance. Have you thought about whether you would consider a feeding tube if you aren't able to swallow safely? If so, it's often better to have the tube placed sooner, so it's ready for when you need it. The procedure itself can be risky if you're not well enough."

Information giving is a continuous process. At each stage, check what patients or carers already understand and whether they have any particular concerns, perhaps around practicalities or what to expect during the dying process. Inform patients and carers about what to expect so that, as far as possible, there are no surprises. Adjust how much information you give, and how and when you give it, to the individual circumstances. A recent European survey of patient preferences found that 73.9% wanted to be fully informed of poor prognosis.[32] A large minority of patients therefore prefer not to be fully informed. It is a doctor's duty to distinguish between these patients and communicate accordingly.

Regular review allows professionals to provide information and manage any deterioration in the patient's condition. Medication review is recommended to rationalise oral drugs. This should be tailored to the individual but may include stopping drugs with mostly long term benefit (such as statins) or those with intolerable side effects, such as constipation from ferrous sulphate. As patients become less well and lose weight, blood pressure and blood glucose monitoring should guide appropriate reduction in antihypertensive and hypoglycaemic drugs.

Agree and document a plan for managing predictable complications such as a bleed, seizure, or infection. Share a copy of the current care plan and contact numbers (including out of hours) with the patient and the family or carers. The overall aim is to avoid crises and to ensure the right care is given at the right time and in the right place.

Coordination of care

A coordinated team approach results in better outcomes for patient experience, quality of care, and family or carer satisfaction than when professionals work in silo. Patients in their last year of life have a high frequency of hospital admissions (average 3.5; varies from 2.3 for patients with

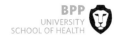

stroke to 5.1 for cancer).[33] Discharge planning for end of life care is a multidisciplinary process. An integrated model of care across settings, with effective communication between hospital and primary healthcare teams, is essential to avoid recurrent unnecessary and unwanted hospital admissions.

The gold standards framework provides a systematic approach to formalising best practice in end of life care in the community, starting with a register of patients in their last year of life and regular multidisciplinary meetings (level one). Level two helps to structure symptom assessment and level three focuses on carer support.[34] Introduction of the framework into primary care has improved end of life care (as reported by the practices involved).[35] [36] The framework has since been introduced into care homes and more recently to some hospitals, where identification using a systematic approach may be useful.[37] An evaluation of national uptake and further research into clinical outcomes is needed.[38]

Recent international initiatives include the implementation of electronic palliative care coordination systems (or EPaCCS), such as electronic medical orders for life sustaining treatment (eMOLST) in New York and coordinate my care (CMC) in London.[38] [39] EPaCCS share the care plan electronically. The aim is to ensure effective handover of information between professionals (without duplication), improve continuity of care, and prevent hospital admissions. Provisional reports suggest that use of an EPaCC increases the number of patients dying in their preferred place of care.[39] However, only a small proportion of the target population is covered by EPaCC projects and any improvements probably have a multitude of causes.

How can the dying phase be managed in the community?

Most, but not all, patients have an identifiable dying phase that lasts hours or days, and occasionally up to a week or so. Box 2 provides help in identifying transition to the dying phase.[22] Diagnosis of dying should prompt a further holistic needs assessment to guide anticipatory care and access to appropriate 24 hour support. If possible, discuss spiritual care needs with the patient or carers to enable practices in keeping with the patient's religious beliefs to be observed before and after death.

Use of an integrated pathway

Integrated pathways for end of life care, such as the Liverpool care pathway, have been introduced into the community setting with the aim of translating the gold standard of hospice end of life care to home and care homes. Such pathways may act as a prompt for improved communication and regular reviews of symptom control. Owing to the adverse media attention regarding the use of the Liverpool care pathway in the acute setting in the UK, it is the subject of an independent review by the Department of Health, with results due to be published later this year.[40]

Physical symptoms

Whatever the cause of death, patients may experience pain, shortness of breath, agitation, secretions, or nausea. Drugs should be prescribed pre-emptively for these common symptoms and be available at the patient's home or care home.[41] A community drug prescription chart should be completed. If a patient requires two or more injections for symptom control within 24 hours, or is taking essential drugs that can no longer be given orally (such

---

BOX 1 KEY AGENCIES IN END OF LIFE CARE IN THE UK

- General practitioners
- Specialist palliative care services: community teams, hospital support teams, outpatient clinics, hospices
- District nursing teams
- Social services
- GP out of hours service
- Hospice at home service
- Marie Curie nursing service
- Hospital specialists
- Ambulance service
- Allied health professionals: physiotherapists, occupational therapists, speech and language therapists
- Clinical nurse specialists: heart failure, respiratory, diabetes, oncology
- Tissue viability nurses
- Social workers
- Chaplains

BOX 2 CLINICAL INDICATORS FOR TERMINAL CARE[22]

Q1 Could this patient be in the last days of life?
Clinical indicators of dying may include:

- Confined to bed or chair and unable to self care
- Having difficulty taking oral fluids or not tolerating artificial feeding or hydration
- No longer able to take oral drugs
- Increasingly drowsy

Q2 Was this patient's condition expected to deteriorate in this way? Q3 Is further life prolonging treatment inappropriate?

- Further treatment is likely to be ineffective or too burdensome
- Patient has refused further treatment
- Patient has made a valid advance decision to refuse treatment
- A healthcare proxy has refused further treatment on the patient's behalf

Q4 Have potentially reversible causes of deterioration been excluded?
These may include:

- Infection (for example, urinary, chest)
- Acute renal impairment or dehydration
- Biochemical disorder (calcium, blood sugar)
- Drug toxicity (for example, opioids, sedatives, alcohol)
- Intracranial event or head injury
- Bleeding or severe anaemia
- Hypoxia or respiratory failure
- Delirium
- Depression

If the diagnosis of dying is in doubt, give treatment and review within 24 hours

If the answer to all four questions is "Yes," plan care for a dying patient

---

as long acting analgesia or antiepileptics), a syringe driver should be used to deliver a continuous infusion over 24 hours. It may be useful to have a provisional prescription for a syringe driver in case the need arises out of hours. If a syringe driver is not immediately available, four hourly subcutaneous injections can have the equivalent effect. Box 3 outlines symptom control drugs commonly prescribed in the terminal phase. For prescribing advice, contact your local palliative care team or consult Palliative Care Adult Network guidelines.

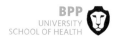

Setting may affect the symptom burden. A trial of hospital at home services for patients with dementia found that significantly fewer patients in the hospital at home group had problems with sleep, agitation, aggression, and feeding compared with those receiving inpatient hospital care.[42] The hypothesis is that a familiar environment helps reduce symptom burden, but evidence for this effect is insufficient in diagnoses other than dementia.

Hydration and nutrition

It is good practice to speak with the patient and family about hydration and nutrition towards the end of life, before specific concerns are raised.[43] It is useful to explain that oral intake gradually decreases in the terminal phase as the body becomes frailer, the coordination of an effective swallow becomes impaired, and the risk of aspiration increases. Simple modifications to diet, such as thickener, can be useful. Good mouth care helps maintain physical comfort.

Administration of parenteral fluids in the terminal phase can increase respiratory secretions and oedema, and in most cases it is unlikely to prolong life or improve quality of life. In certain situations, however, such as identifiable distress associated with thirst, parenteral fluids should be considered. Other such situations include a prolonged period of reduced level of consciousness or of dysphagia, or gastrointestinal obstruction, which make oral intake impossible. In such cases, administration of subcutaneous fluids (such as 1 L normal saline subcutaneously over 12-16 hours) may be useful. In the community setting, these can be prescribed by the GP and administered by district nurses or nursing home staff.

DNACPR

Patients should have a DNACPR (do not attempt cardiopulmonary resuscitation) order in their home or care home, with a copy shared electronically by EPaCC. The DNACPR decision is the responsibility of the doctor in charge of the patient's care (usually the GP). It should be discussed in advance with family and carers and also with the patient, if appropriate, unless it is likely to cause "undue distress."[44] It may be useful to explain that when a patient is deteriorating from incurable disease with no reversible cause and is expected to die within days or weeks, cardiopulmonary resuscitation is futile.[41] Framing the DNACPR order within the context of the patient's and family's goals for end of life care can be helpful. Explanation that a DNACPR order helps support a dignified death in the patient's place of choice and does not affect care up until the point that the heart and lungs have stopped (natural death has occurred) can also help. Families may seek reassurance that medical and nursing care will continue to be provided, including close attention to symptom control needs plus assessment for other medical interventions (such as antibiotics, bisphosphonate treatment of hypercalcaemia) as appropriate.

What should be done after death?

Care of the body after death should be guided by cultural and religious beliefs. Family and carers may need practical advice regarding verification of death, death certification, and registration of death. These procedures vary by country. In England, death can be verified by medical staff (for example, the patient's GP or out of hours GP) or appropriately trained nursing staff (for example, the district nurse). The death certificate should then be completed by a doctor who has seen the patient within the preceding two weeks (usually the patient's GP), otherwise discussion with the coroner is needed. If the coroner (or in Scotland, the procurator fiscal) will definitely need to be consulted (such as in cases of mesothelioma or death from an unknown diagnosis), it may be best to speak to the family about this process in advance because it may delay funeral arrangements. If the coroner does not need to be involved, after verification of death, the family can contact the undertaker of their choice directly to collect the body from the house.

What is the doctor's role in bereavement support?

Bereavement is one of the most stressful of all life events and is associated with subsequent worse mental and physical health.[45] Most people choose informal bereavement support from friends and family. The need for formal bereavement support is associated with poor social support and the nature of the death.

The effectiveness of risk assessment tools in predicting who will benefit most from formal bereavement support is unclear. Risk factors for complicated grief include multiple recent losses, low acceptance of impending death, and death in hospital.[45] Those who are bereaved may be best

---

BOX 3 SYMPTOM CONTROL DRUGS COMMONLY PRESCRIBED IN THE TERMINAL PHASE (BASED ON ROUTINE PRACTICE FROM AUTHORS EXTENSIVE EXPERIENCE IN THE UK AND AUSTRALIA)

Opioid analgesics (for pain and shortness of breath)
For example, morphine sulfate 10 mg/24 h subcutaneously through a syringe driver plus 2.5 mg subcutaneously as needed, or oxycodone 5 mg/24 h subcutaneously through a syringe driver plus 1 mg subcutaneously as needed

Anxiolytics (for anxiety or agitation and seizure prophylaxis)
For example, midazolam 10 mg/24 h subcutaneously through a syringe driver plus 2.5 mg subcutaneously as needed

Antiemetics (for nausea and agitation)
For example, levomepromazine 6.25 mg/24 h subcutaneously through a syringe driver plus 3.125 mg subcutaneously as needed, or haloperidol 1 mg/24 h subcutaneously through a syringe driver plus 0.5 mg subcutaneously as needed

Antimuscarinic drugs (for secretions)
For example, glycopyrronium 1.2 mg/24 h subcutaneously through a syringe driver plus 0.4 mg subcutaneously as needed, or hyoscine butylbromide 120 mg/24 h subcutaneously through a syringe driver plus 20 mg subcutaneously as needed
Tailor the prescription to the individual, taking account of the medical history. Doses given are examples of starting doses in a patient who is not taking opioid analgesia or on a complex symptom management regimen

---

BOX 4 NATIONAL INSTITUTE FOR HEALTH AND CARE EXCELLENCE'S THREE COMPONENT MODEL OF BEREAVEMENT SUPPORT[46]

Component 1
Grief is normal after bereavement and most people manage without professional intervention. Many people, however, lack understanding of grief immediately after bereavement. Health and social care professionals should offer bereaved people information about the experience of bereavement and how to access other forms of support. Family and friends will provide much of this support.

Component 2
Some people need a more formal opportunity to review and reflect on their loss experience, but this does not necessarily have to involve professionals. Volunteer bereavement support workers and befrienders, self help groups, faith groups, and community groups will provide much of the support at this level. These people must establish a process to ensure that people with more complex needs are referred to appropriate health and social care professionals who can deliver component 3 interventions.

Component 3
A minority of people will require specialist interventions. This will involve mental health services, psychological support services, specialist palliative care services, and general bereavement services. Such services will include provision for meeting the specialist need of bereaved children and young people.

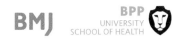

placed to judge their need for formal support.[45] GPs play a key role in ensuring links between hospital and voluntary sector bereavement support (box 4).[46]

Studies of effectiveness of bereavement support are scarce, particularly in care homes. The strongest evidence is from small non-randomised studies of complex grief reactions. In one systematic review,[47] relatives considered bereavement support to be an important aspect of the GP's role and expected contact from the GP immediately after bereavement.

QUESTIONS AND AREAS FOR FUTURE RESEARCH

- Research in end of life care in the community poses complex logistical, methodological, and ethical challenges. Respecting patient choice poses challenges to randomisation, so prospective audits are the favoured study design
- Key research outcomes should include:
- -Meeting patient preferences for end of life care, including good communication, continuity of care, home nursing, 24 hour access to care, preferred place of care
- -Control of pain and other symptoms
- -Avoidance of unwanted hospital admissions
- -Cost effectiveness and impact on healthcare resources
- -Burden on care givers
- -Impact of end of life care pathways on quality of care

TIPS FOR NON-SPECIALISTS

- Patient cues or a change in care setting provide a good trigger for anticipatory care planning discussions—for example, after discharge from hospital
- Always assess the patient and family's current level of understanding before embarking on complex communications
- Frame the do not attempt resuscitation discussion around the patient's goals of care
- Ensure that dying patients who are at home or in a care home are reviewed regularly and are prescribed drugs for symptom control in anticipation
- If in doubt call the local palliative care team for advice and support

---

ADDITIONAL EDUCATIONAL RESOURCES

Resources for healthcare professionals

- Supportive and palliative care indicators tool. Evidence based single page guide to identifying people at risk of dying within the next 12 months. www.palliativecareguidelines.scot.nhs.uk/documents/SPICT_Sept2012.pdf
- Gold Standards Framework (www.goldstandardsframework.org.uk/)—Evidence based framework to optimise delivery of end of life care at home and in care homes
- Palliative Care Adult Network guidelines[plus]. Detailed electronic symptom control guidelines including opioid dose calculator and syringe driver drug compatibility resource. iPhone app available: http://book.pallcare.info/
- e-Learning for Healthcare (www.e-lfh.org.uk/projects/end-of-life-care/)—More than 50 modules on end of life care including advance care planning, assessment, communication skills, and symptom management
- Death and dying: religious practices. A two page guide to the general principles. www.cumbria.gov.uk/elibrary/Content/Internet/536/656/3838485955.pdf

Resources for patients and carers

- Information about the dying process. www.palliativecareguidelines.scot.nhs.uk/documents/DyingwhatHappens[1].pdf
- Dying Matters (www.dyingmatters.org/overview/need-support)—Support with all aspects of dying, death, and bereavement
- Marie Curie Cancer Care (www.mariecurie.org.uk/en-GB/patients-carers/)—Help with being cared for in your place of choice
- Macmillan Cancer Support (www.macmillan.org.uk/Cancerinformation/Livingwithandaftercancer/Financialissues/Financialissues.aspx)—Provides help with financial problems
- Macmillan Cancer Support (www.macmillan.org.uk/Cancerinformation/Endoflife/Afterdeath.aspx)—Practical support with what to do after a death
- UK Government (www.gov.uk/after-a-death)—Practical support with what to do after a death

---

What changes are needed?

Communication and coordination

Improved collaboration between health and social care plus acute and community services could improve the quality of care, reduce emergency admissions, and allow more people to die in the place of their choosing.[4 48] The National Institute for Health and Care Excellence recommends that this collaboration extends to the third (voluntary) sector, with specialists and generalists working together to deliver an integrated model of end of life care.[46]

Retrospective studies of relatives' experience of end of life care show that poor communication is the main reason for an unsatisfactory experience.[30 47 49] The most valued aspects of home care are individualised care and quality of communication.[50] Strategies to improve communication include anticipatory care planning and coordination of care supported by increasingly sophisticated information technology systems (EPaCCS).

Education

In the past, undergraduate and postgraduate medical curriculums have failed to incorporate the complex communication skills and palliative care training that are central to providing good end of life care. There are signs that this is improving. Palliative medicine has this year been awarded specialty status in the US. Improved multidisciplinary education in end of life care is a recognised requirement, particularly in care homes.[51] One recommended tool is more widespread implementation of the gold standards framework. Collaborative working between specialists and generalists helps support workplace based learning in end of life care.

Improved community resources

The need for 24 hour community services, including access to GP home visits and urgent care, is highlighted across studies.[16 50 51 52] Recommendations include coordination of care by a multidisciplinary team with access to a doctor,[52] support for carers, and provision of night services.[53] In the UK, existing end of life care services have been mapped so that gaps can be identified.[54] A more extensive end of life home care service has been recommended in Norway to reduce hospital admissions.[55]

The challenge is to provide end of life care for increasing numbers of patients with dementia, long term conditions, and multimorbidities across all community settings, from home to care homes.[6 7 51] The number of patients needing palliative care is increasing, so increased provision of such services is recommended.[56] It has been suggested that resources should be reallocated to the community to make the proposed savings from the acute sector.[51] A recent Cochrane review found evidence to support the effectiveness of home palliative care services but insufficient evidence to support its cost effectiveness.[17] The palliative care funding review should help answer this question.[57]

Patient centred approach

Learning from carers' experiences of end of life care is crucial to improving patient care.[49] Patient centred outcomes need to be defined and monitored. At all times the patient should remain the focus around which the proposed integrated care structure for end of life care revolves. Patient choice and carer support are key. Meticulous planning for end of life care with the best intentions will fail unless we place the patient and family at the centre.

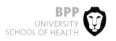

Thanks to Katherine E Sleeman, clinical lecturer in palliative medicine, Cicely Saunders Institute, King's College London, who helped review early drafts of the article and suggested insightful changes to structure and content. Thanks also to Cherry Armstrong, GP (Roundwood Park Medical Centre) and clinical lead for end of life care, Brent Clinical Commissioning Group , London, UK, who contributed to the initial design of article and gave valuable input to the article's content from a GP's perspective.

Contributors: EC had a leading role in the conception and design of the article. She contributed to the literature review, drafting and revision of the article, and approval of the final version. RA-Q contributed to the literature review; drafting, design, and revision of the article; and approval of the final version.

Competing interests: We have read and understood the BMJ Group policy on declaration of interests and declare the following interests: None.

Provenance and peer review: Commissioned; externally peer reviewed.

1 Department of Health. End of life care strategy—promoting high quality care for all adults at the end of life. 2008. https://www.gov.uk/government/uploads/system/uploads/attachment_data/file/136431/End_of_life_strategy.pdf.

2 Gomes B, Higginson I, Calanzani N, Cohen J, Deliens L, Daveson B, et al; on behalf of PRISMA. Preferences for place of death if faced with advanced cancer: a population survey in England, Flanders, Germany, Italy, the Netherlands, Portugal and Spain. Ann Oncol 2012;23:2006-15.

3 Grunier A, Mor V, Weitzen S, Truchil R, Teno J, Roy J. Where people die: a multilevel approach to understanding influences on site of death in America. Med Care Res Rev 2007;64:351-78.

4 National Audit Office. End of life care. 2008. www.nao.org.uk/wp-content/uploads/2008/11/07081043.pdf.

5 Gomes B, Calanzani N, Higginson I. Reversal of the British trends in place of death [poster]. BMJ Support Palliat Care 2012;2:6.

6 Hasselaar J, Engels Y, Menten J, Jaspers B, Vissers K. The burden of non-acute dying on society: dying of cancer and chronic disease in the European Union. BMJ Support Palliat Care 2012;2:4.

7 Houttekier D, Cohen J, Bilsen J, Addington-Hall J, Onwuteaka-Philipsen B, Deliens L. Place of death of older persons with dementia. A study in five European countries. J Am Geriatr Soc 2010;58:751-6.

8 Pritchard RS, Fisher ES, Teno JM, Sharp SM, Reding DJ, Knaus WA, et al. Influence of patient preferences and local health system characteristics on the place of death. SUPPORT Investigators, study to understand prognoses and preferences for risks and outcomes of treatment. J Am Geriatr Soc 1998;46:1242-50.

9 Gomes B, Calanzani N, Higginson IJ. Local preferences and place of death in regions within England 2010. Cicely Saunders International, 2011. www.csi.kcl.ac.uk/files/Local%20preferences%20and%20place%20of%20death%20in%20regions%20within%20England.pdf.

10 Gomes B, Calanzani N, Gysels M, Hall S, Higginson I. Heterogeneity and changes in preferences for dying at home: a systematic review. BMC Palliat Care 2013;12:7.

11 Gomes B, Higginson I. Where people die (1974 to 2030): past trends, future projections and implications for care. Palliat Med 2008;22:33-41.

12 National Center for Health Statistics. Health, United States, 2010. With special feature on death and dying. 2011. www.cdc.gov/nchs/data/hus/hus10.pdf.

13 Gao W, Ho Y, Verne J, Glickman M, Higginson I. Changing patterns in place of cancer death in England: a population-based study. PLoS Med 2013;10:e1001410.

14 Murtagh F, Bausewein C, Petkova H, Sleeman K, Dodd R, Gysels M, et al. Understanding place of death for patients with non malignant conditions: a systematic literature review. Final report. NIHR Service Delivery and Organisational Programme; 2012. www.netscc.ac.uk/hsdr/files/project/SDO_FR_08-1813-257_V01.pdf.

15 Gomes B, Higginson I. Factors influencing death at home in terminally ill patients with cancer: systematic review. BMJ 2006;332:515-21.

16 Shepperd S, Wee B, Straus SE. Hospital at home: home-based end of life care. Cochrane Database Syst Rev 2011;7:CD009231.

17 Gomes B, Calanzani N, Curiale V, McCrone, Higginson I. Effectiveness and cost-effectiveness of home palliative care services for adults with advanced illness and their caregivers. Cochrane Database Syst Rev 2013;6:CD007760.

18 Gott M, Seymour J, Bellamy G, Clark D, Ahmedzai S. Older people's views about home as a place of care at the end of life. Palliat Med 2004;18:460-7.

19 Dying Matters. Find your 1%: supporting GPs in delivering quality end of life care. www.dyingmatters.org/gp?utm_source=Find+Your+1%25+campaign&utm_campaign=e85bab1600-Find+Your+1%25&utm_medium=email&utm_source=Find+Your+1%25+campaign&utm_campaign=7a5e97d498-Find+Your+1%25&utm_medium=email.

20 Brumley R, Enguidanos S, Cherin D. Effectiveness of a home-based palliative care program for end-of-life. J Palliat Med 2003;6:715-24.

21 Supportive and Palliative Care Indicators Tool (SPICT). www.palliativecareguidelines.scot.nhs.uk/documents/SPICT_Sept2012.pdf.

22 Boyd K, Murray SA. Recognising and managing key transitions in end of life care. BMJ 2010;341:c4863.

23 Thoonsen B, Engels Y, van Rijswijk E, Verhagen S, van Weel C, Groot M, et al. Early identification of palliative care patients in general practice: development of RADboud indicators for PAlliative Care Needs (RADPAC). Br J Gen Pract 2012;62:e625-31.

24 Grbich C, Maddocks I, Parker D, Brown M, Willis E, Piller N, et al. Identification of patients with non-cancer diseases for palliative care services. Palliat Support Care 2005;3:5-14.

25 Gómez-Batiste X, Martínez-Muñoz M, Blay C, Amblàs J, Vila L, Costa X, et al. Identifying patients with chronic conditions in need of palliative care in the general population: development of the NECPAL tool and preliminary prevalence rates in Catalonia. BMJ Support Palliat Care 2012; published online 14 December.

26 Harrison N, Cavers D, Campbell C, Murray SA. Are UK primary care teams formally identifying patients for palliative care before they die? Br J Gen Pract 2012;62:e344-52.

27 Candy B, Jones L, Varagunam M, Speck P, Tookman A, King M. Spiritual and religious interventions for well-being of adults in the terminal phase of disease. Cochrane Database Syst Rev 2012;5:CD007544.

28 Grant L, Murray SA, Sheikh A. Spiritual dimensions of dying in pluralist societies. BMJ 2010;341:c4859.

29 Abel J, Pring A, Rich A, Malik T, and Verne J The impact of advance care planning of place of death, a hospice retrospective cohort study. BMJ Support Palliat Care 2013;3:168-73.

30 Travis S, Bernard M, Dixon S, McAuley W, Loving G, McClanahan L. Obstacles to palliation and end-of-life care in a long-term care facility. Gerontologist 2002;42:342-9.

31 Boyd K, Mason B, Kendall M, Barclay S, Chinn D, Thomas K, et al. Advance care planning for cancer patients in primary care: a feasibility study. Br J Gen Pract 2010;60:e449-58.

32 Harding R, Simms V, Calanzani N, Higginson I, Hall S, Gysels M, et al; on behalf of PRISMA. If you had less than a year to live, would you want to know? A seven-country European population survey of public preferences for disclosure of poor prognosis Psychooncology 2013; published online 18 March.

33 Lyons P, Verne V. National policy in England on advance care planning; patterns of hospital admission in the final year of life. BMJ Support Palliat Care 2011;1:81-2.

34 Gold Standards Framework (GSF) http://www.goldstandardsframework.org.uk/.

35 Hughes P, Bath P, Ahmed N, Noble B. What progress has been made towards implementing national guidance on end of life care? A national survey of UK general practices. Palliat Med 2010;24:68-78.

36 Thomas K, Noble B. Improving the delivery of palliative care in general practice: an evaluation of the first phase of the Gold Standards Framework. Palliat Med 2007;21:49-53.

37 Dale J, Petrova M, Munday D, Koistinen-Harris J, Lall R, Thomas K. A national facilitation project to improve primary palliative care: impact of the Gold Standards Framework on process and self-ratings of quality. Qual Safe Health Care 2009;18:174-80.

38 Bomba P. How ePOLST will improve the standard, informed medical decision-making: applying the eMOLST experience in New York. ACPEL abstracts. Oral abstracts—concurrent session 3. Use of IT. BMJ Support Palliat Care 2012;2:184.

39 Millington-Sanders C. EPaCCS: the national context 2013. www.healthcareconferencesuk.co.uk/presentations/downloads/WEB_-_Dr_C_Millington-Sanders.pdf.

40 Department of Health. Independent review of Liverpool Care Pathway to be chaired by Baroness Neuberger. Press Release. January 2013. https://www.gov.uk/government/news/independent-review-of-liverpool-care-pathway-to-be-chaired-by-baroness-neuberger.

41 Sleeman K, Collis E. Caring for a dying patient in hospital. BMJ 2013;346:f2174.

42 Tibaldi V, Aimonino N, Ponzetto M, Stasi MF, Amati D, Raspo S, et al. A randomized controlled trial of a home hospital intervention for frail elderly demented patients: behavioral disturbances and caregiver's stress. Arch Gerontol Geriatr Suppl 2004;9:431-6.

43 Royal College of Physicians and British Society of Gastroenterology. Oral feeding difficulties and dilemmas: a guide to practical care, particularly towards the end of life. 2010.

44 General Medical Council. Treatment and care towards end of life: good practice in medical decision making. 2010. www.gmc-uk.org/static/documents/content/End_of_life_9_May_2013.pdf.

45 Arthur A, Wilson E, James M, Stanton W, Seymour J. Bereavement care services: a synthesis of the literature. Final Report of review commissioned by DH to support implementation of the end of life care strategy. 2011. https://www.gov.uk/government/uploads/system/uploads/attachment_data/file/147509/dh_123810.pdf.pdf.

46 National Institute for Clinical Excellence. Improving supportive and palliative care for adults with cancer. 2004. www.nice.org.uk/nicemedia/live/10893/28816/28816.pdf.

47 Mitchell GK. How well do general practitioners deliver palliative care? A systematic review. Palliat Med 2002;16:457-64.

48 Department of Health. Overview of health and care structures. The Health and Social Care Act 2012. 2013. https://www.gov.uk/government/uploads/system/uploads/attachment_data/file/138258/A3.-Factsheet-Overview-of-health-and-care-structures-240412.pdf.

49 Department of Health. First national VOICES survey of bereaved people key findings report. 2012. https://www.gov.uk/government/uploads/system/uploads/attachment_data/file/156113/First-national-VOICES-survey-of-bereaved-people-key-findings-report-final.pdf.pdf.

50 Jones J, Wilson A, Parker H, Wynn A, Jagger C, Spiers N, et al. Economic evaluation of hospital at home versus hospital care: cost minimisation analysis of data from randomised controlled trial. BMJ 1999;319:1547-50.

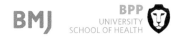

51 Royal College of General Practitioners. RCGP commissioning guidance in end of life care. 2013. www.rcgp.org.uk/revalidation-and-cpd/~/media/Files/CIRC/EOLC/RCGP-EOLC-Guidelines-Apr-2013.ashx.

52 Shepperd S, Doll H, Angus R, Clarke M, Iliffe S, Kalra L, et al. Hospital at home admission avoidance. *Cochrane Database Syst Rev* 2008;4:CD007491.

53 Grande G, Farquhar MC, Barclay SIG. Caregiver bereavement outcome: relationship with hospital at home, satisfaction with care and home death. *J Palliat Care* 2004;20:69-77.

54 Marie Curie. End of life care atlas. www.mariecurie.org.uk/en-GB/Commissioners-and-referrers/Resources/Marie-Curie-Atlas/.

55 Jordhøy MS, Fayers P, Saltnes T, Ahlner-Elmqvist M, Jannert M, Kaasa S. A palliative care intervention and death at home: a cluster randomized trial. *Lancet* 2000;356:888-93.

56 Calanzani N, Higginson I, Gomes B. Current and future needs for hospice care: an evidence- based report. Cecily Saunders International, 2013.

57 Hughes-Hallett T, Craft A, Davies C, Mackay I, Nielsson T. Funding the right care and support for everyone. Creating a fair and transparent funding system; the final report of the palliative care funding review. 2011. http://palliativecarefunding.org.uk/PCFRFinal%20Report.pdf.

Related links

bmj.com
- Get CME credits for this article

bmj.com/archive
Previous articles in this series
- Multiple myeloma (2013;346:f3863)
- Diagnosis and management of first trimester miscarriage (2013;346:f3676)
- Glaucoma (2013;346:f3518)
- Managing unscheduled bleeding in non-pregnant premenopausal women (2013;346:f3251)
- Diagnosis and management of recurrent urinary tract infections in non-pregnant women (2013;346:f3140)

More titles in The BMJ Clinical Review Series

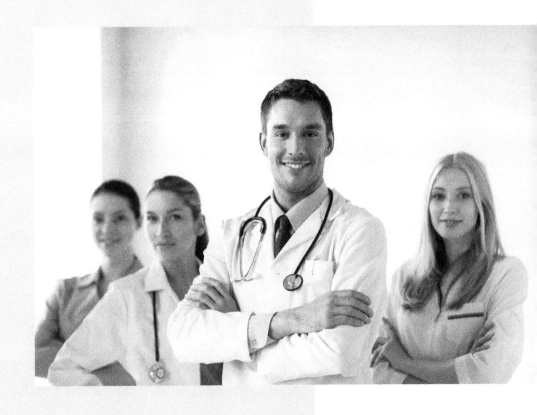

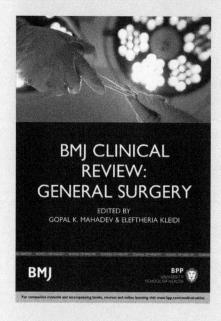
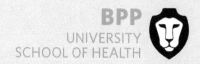

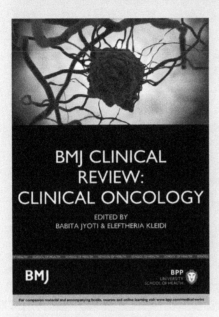
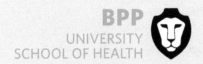

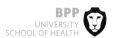
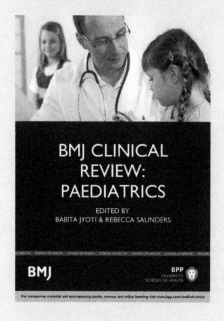
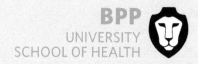

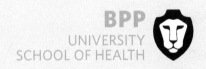
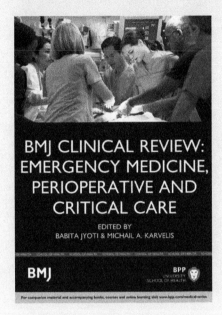

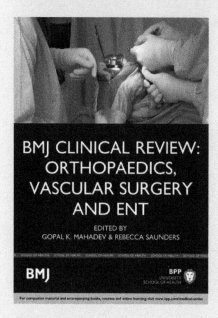
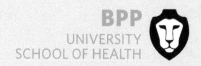

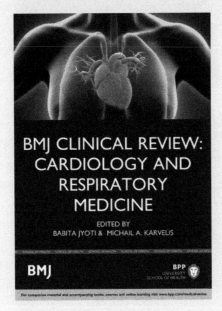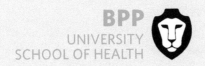

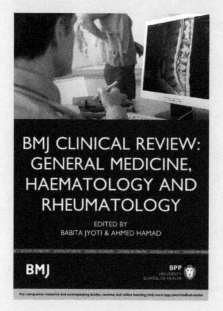
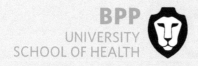

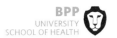

More titles in The Progressing your Medical Career Series

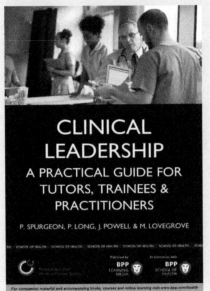

CLINICAL
LEADERSHIP
A PRACTICAL GUIDE FOR
TUTORS, TRAINEES &
PRACTITIONERS

P. SPURGEON, P. LONG, J. POWELL & M. LOVEGROVE

£24.99

June 2015

Paperback

978-1-472727-83-1

Are you a healthcare professional or student who wishes to acquire and develop your leadership and management skills? Do you recognise the role and influence of strong leadership and management in modern healthcare?

Clinical leadership is something in which all healthcare professionals can participate in, in terms of driving forward high quality care for their patients. In this up-to-date guide, the authors take you through the latest leadership and management thinking, and how this links in with the Clinical Leadership Competency Framework. As well as influencing undergraduate curricula this framework forms the basis of the leadership component of the curricula for all healthcare specialties, so a practical knowledge of it is essential for all healthcare professionals in training.

Using case studies and practical exercises to provide a strong work-based emphasis, this practical guide will enable you to build on your existing experiences to develop your leadership and management skills, and to develop strategies and approaches to improving care for your patients.

This book addresses:

- Why strong leadership and management are crucial to delivering high quality care;
- The theory and evidence behind the Clinical Leadership Competency Framework;
- The practical aspects of leadership learning in a wide range of clinical environments
- How clinical professionals and trainers can best facilitate leadership learning for their trainees and students within the clinical work-place.

Whether you are a student just starting out on your career, or an established healthcare professional wishing to develop yourself as a clinical leader, this practical, easy-to-use guide will give you the techniques and knowledge you require to excel.

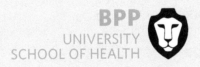

BPP
UNIVERSITY
SCHOOL OF HEALTH

www.bpp.com/medical-series

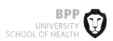

More titles in The Progressing your Medical Career Series

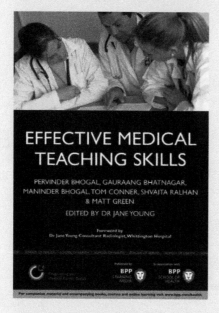

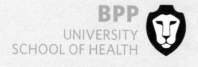

£19.99

September 2011

Paperback

978-1-445379-56-2

BPP
UNIVERSITY
SCHOOL OF HEALTH

We can all remember a teacher that inspired us, encouraged us and helped us to excel. But what is it that makes a good teacher and are these skills that can be learned and improved?

As doctors and healthcare professionals we are all expected to teach, to a greater or lesser degree, and this carries a great deal of responsibility. We are helping to develop the next generation and it is essential to pass on the knowledge that we have gained during our experience to date.

This book aims to cover the fundamentals of medical education. It has been designed to be a guide for the budding teacher with practical advice, hints, tips and essential points of reflection designed to encourage the reader to think about what they are doing at each step.

By taking the time to read through this book and completing the exercises contained within it you should:

- Understand the needs of the learner
- Understand the skills required to be an effective teacher
- Understanding the various different teaching scenarios, from lectures to problem based teaching, and how to use them effectively
- Understand the importance and sources of feedback
- Be aware of assessment techniques, appraisal and revalidation

This book aims to provide you with a foundation in medical education upon which you can build the skills and attributes to become a competent and skilled teacher.

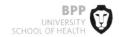

More titles in The Progressing your Medical Career Series

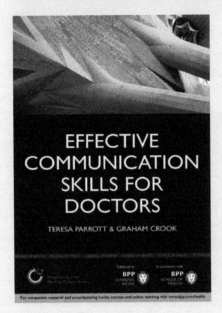

EFFECTIVE COMMUNICATION SKILLS FOR DOCTORS

TERESA PARROTT & GRAHAM CROOK

£19.99
September 2011
Paperback
978-1-445379-56-2

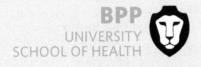

BPP
UNIVERSITY
SCHOOL OF HEALTH

Would you like to know how to improve your communication skills? Are you looking for a clearly written book which explores all aspects of effective medical communication?

There is an urgent need to improve doctors' communication skills. Research has shown that poor communication can contribute to patient dissatisfaction, lack of compliance and increased medico-legal problems. Improved communication skills will impact positively on all of these areas.

The last fifteen years have seen unprecedented changes in medicine and the role of doctors. Effective communication skills are vital to these new roles. But communication is not just related to personality. Skills can be learned which can make your communication more effective, and help you to improve your relationships with patients, their families and fellow doctors.

This book shows how to learn those skills and outlines why we all need to communicate more effectively. Healthcare is increasingly a partnership. Change is happening at all levels, from government directives to patient expectations. Communication is a bridge between the wisdom of the past and the vision of the future.

Readers of this book can also gain free access to an online module which upon successful completion can download a certificate for their portfolio of learning/ Revalidation/CPD records.

This easy-to-read guide will help medical students and doctors at all stages of their careers improve their communication within a hospital environment.

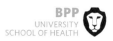

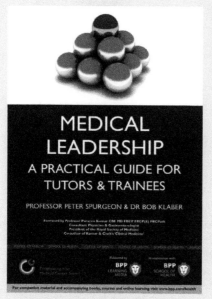
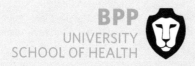

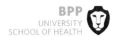
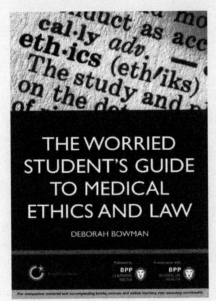
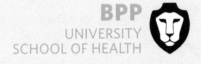

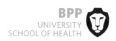
More Titles in The Progressing Your Medical Career Series

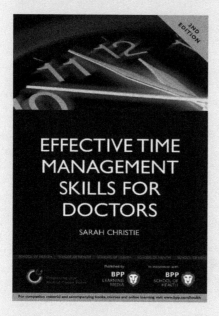

EFFECTIVE TIME MANAGEMENT SKILLS FOR DOCTORS

SARAH CHRISTIE

£19.99

October 2011

Paperback

978-1-906839-08-6

Do you find it difficult to achieve a work-life balance? Would you like to know how you can become more effective with the time you have?

With the introduction of the European Working Time Directive, which will severely limit the hours in the working week, it is more important than ever that doctors improve their personal effectiveness and time management skills. This interactive book will enable you to focus on what activities are needlessly taking up your time and what steps you can take to manage your time better.

By taking the time to read through, complete the exercises and follow the advice contained within this book you will begin to:

- Understand where your time is being needlessly wasted

- Discover how to be more assertive and learn how to say 'No'

- Set yourself priorities and stick to them

- Learn how to complete tasks more efficiently

- Plan better so you can spend more time doing the things you enjoy

In recent years, with the introduction of the NHS Plan and Lord Darzi's commitment to improve the quality of healthcare provision, there is a need for doctors to become more effective within their working environment. This book will offer you the chance to regain some clarity on how you actually spend your time and give you the impetus to ensure you achieve the tasks and goals which are important to you.

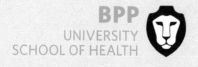

BPP
UNIVERSITY
SCHOOL OF HEALTH

www.bpp.com/medical-series

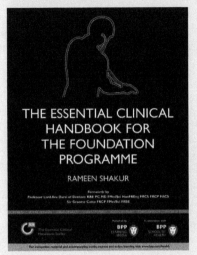
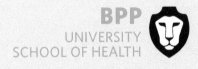

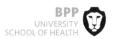
More titles in The Essential Clinical Handbook Series

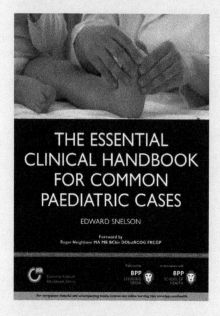

THE ESSENTIAL CLINICAL HANDBOOK FOR COMMON PAEDIATRIC CASES

EDWARD SNELSON

Foreword by
Roger Neighbour MA MB BChir DObstRCOG FRCGP

September 2011

Paperback

978-1-445379-60-9

Not sure what to do when faced with a crying baby and demanding parent on the ward? Would you like a definitive guide on how to manage commonly encountered paediatric cases?

This clear and concise clinical handbook has been written to help healthcare professionals approach the initial assessment and management of paediatric cases commonly encountered by Junior Doctors, GPs, GP Specialty Trainee's and allied healthcare professionals. The children who make paediatrics so fun, can also make it more than a little daunting for even the most confident person. This insightful guide has been written based on the author's extensive experience within both a General Practice and hospital setting.

Intended as a practical guide to common paediatric problems it will increase confidence and satisfaction in managing these conditions. Each chapter provides a clear structure for investigating potential paediatric illnesses including clinical and non-clinical advice covering: background, how to assess, pitfalls to avoid, FAQs and what to tell parents. This helpful guide provides :

- A problem/symptom based approach to common paediatric conditions

- As essential guide for any doctor assessing children on the front line

- Provides easy-to-follow and step-by-step guidance on how to approach different paediatric conditions

- Useful both as a textbook and a quick reference guide when needed on the ward

This engaging and easy to use guide will provide you with the knowledge, skills and confidence required to effectively diagnose and manage commonly encountered paediatric cases both within a primary and secondary care setting.

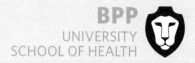

BPP
UNIVERSITY
SCHOOL OF HEALTH

www.bpp.com/medical-series